Guide to Evidence-Based Physical Therapy Practice

Dianne V. Jewell, PT, PhD, CCS, FAACVPR
Assistant Professor
Department of Physical Therapy
Virginia Commonwealth University
Richmond, Virginia

JONES AND BARTLETT PUBLISHERS
Sudbury, Massachusetts
BOSTON TORONTO LONDON SINGAPORE

World Headquarters
Jones and Bartlett Publishers
40 Tall Pine Drive
Sudbury, MA 01776
978-443-5000
info@jbpub.com
www.jbpub.com

Jones and Bartlett Publishers Canada
6339 Ormindale Way
Mississauga, Ontario L5V 1J2
Canada

Jones and Bartlett Publishers International
Barb House, Barb Mews
London W6 7PA
United Kingdom

Jones and Bartlett's books and products are available through most bookstores and online booksellers. To contact Jones and Bartlett Publishers directly, call 800-832-0034, fax 978-443-8000, or visit our website www.jbpub.com.

The authors, editor, and publisher have made every effort to provide accurate information. However, they are not responsible for errors, omissions, or for any outcomes related to the use of the contents of this book and take no responsibility for the use of the products and procedures described. Treatments and side effects described in this book may not be applicable to all people; likewise, some people may require a dose or experience a side effect that is not described herein. Drugs and medical devices are discussed that may have limited availability controlled by the Food and Drug Administration (FDA) for use only in a research study or clinical trial. Research, clinical practice, and government regulations often change the accepted standard in this field. When consideration is being given to use of any drug in the clinical setting, the health care provider or reader is responsible for determining FDA status of the drug, reading the package insert, and reviewing prescribing information for the most up-to-date recommendations on dose, precautions, and contraindications, and determining the appropriate usage for the product. This is especially important in the case of drugs that are new or seldom used.

Library of Congress Cataloging-in-Publication Data
Jewell, Dianne V.
Guide to evidence-based physical therapy practice / Dianne V. Jewell.
p. ; cm.
Includes bibliographical references and index.
ISBN-13: 978-0-7637-3443-5
ISBN-10: 0-7637-3443-8
1. Physical therapy. 2. Evidence-based medicine. I. Title.
[DNLM: 1. Physical Therapy Modalities. 2. Evidence-Based Medicine. WB 460 J59g 2008]
RM700.J49 2007
615.8′2—dc22
2007005811

6048

Production Credits
Executive Editor: David Cella
Production Director: Amy Rose
Production Editor: Renée Sekerak
Editorial Assistant: Lisa Gordon
Associate Marketing Manager: Jennifer Bengtson
Manufacturing Buyer: Amy Bacus
Composition: Auburn Associates, Inc.
Cover Design: Kristin E. Ohlin

Printed in the United States of America
11 10 09 08 10 9 8 7 6 5 4 3

Dedication

To my teachers and colleagues, who inspire me to aim high and keep climbing;

To my students, who challenge me to become a world-class teacher;

To my family and friends, who love and encourage me even when they have taken a back seat to my computer.

Contents

Preface

This book was created to address a challenge I face each time I teach evidence-based physical therapy practice to professional and post-professional students—that is, the need to order two texts to cover the information in my course. What I really wanted was one resource that provided sufficient information regarding research methods to allow the nonresearcher to understand and appraise studies, but that also was sized and structured for routine application of evidence to actual patients in clinical settings. This book attempts to marry the best elements of multiple texts into a single accessible guide to evidence-based physical therapy practice for students and clinicians alike.

The content is organized in four parts. Part I, Principles of Evidence-Based Physical Therapy Practice (EBPT), is comprised of three chapters that set the stage for the use of evidence in patient/client management. Chapter 1 addresses the history behind the evidence-based practice movement in health care, the various labels and definitions used to describe this approach to patient care, and the barriers to its application in real-time clinical practice. The material is placed in the context of the disablement model, as articulated in the American Physical Therapy Association's *Guide to Physical Therapist Practice, 2nd ed.* Chapter 2 examines the nature of evidence and its different forms, including the uses and limitations of hierarchies structured according to the quality of different study designs. A key point is that different research designs are suited to answering different types of clinical questions therapists may have about their patients/clients. Chapter 3 guides readers in the development of clinical questions regarding diagnosis, prognosis, interventions, and outcomes, and describes tools and strategies available to help locate studies of interest.

Part II, Elements of Evidence, reviews the different components of a research article (Chapters 4–7) with an emphasis on features that enhance or diminish a study's quality. The goal is not to teach readers how to become researchers; rather it is to increase their understanding of and confidence in interpreting what they are reading. Chapter 8 is devoted to a discussion of research validity—a key consideration in the evidence appraisal process. Chapter 9 is an attempt to demystify the most intimidating feature of research for many readers by illustrating the parallels between statistical tools and the instruments used in clinical practice.

Part III, Appraising the Evidence, provides the information needed to evaluate evidence about diagnostic tests and measures (Chapter 10), prognostic factors (Chapter 11), interventions (Chapter 12), and outcomes (Chapter 13). To my knowledge, the chapter on outcomes is unique to this textbook. Chapter 14 focuses on the appraisal of summaries of evidence in the form of systematic reviews and practice guidelines. An underlying principle of all of these chapters is that EBPT requires students and clinicians to work with the best available evidence that oftentimes is weakly designed. Physical therapy research still has a long way to go to address (with sophisticated methods) all of the questions we have about the wide variety of patients/clients with whom we work. Until such studies are completed, readers must determine for themselves whether the evidence they locate is useful *despite* its limitations.

Part IV, Evidence in Practice, discusses applications of evidence in practice from the patient/client's point of view and presents illustrations using hypothetical patient/client scenarios. Chapter 15 considers the challenge of integrating evidence with patient/client values and preferences in the context of ethical decision making and patient-centered care. The influence of subjects' values and preferences on study outcomes, and efforts to conduct trials that address these challenges, also are discussed. Chapter 16 ties all of the material together in demonstrations designed to help readers "see how it is done."

Finally, the appendices provide additional information and resources to assist with critical appraisal of the evidence.

My intent throughout is to make this material user-friendly for students and clinicians who are new to the material, as well as for those who already have adopted an evidence-based approach to patient/client management. Terms are defined at the beginning of each chapter to help readers learn and remember the vocabulary of research and its applications. The exercises at the conclusion of each chapter are designed to reinforce the learning objectives stated at the beginning. The examples used to illustrate key concepts and points are specific to physical therapy and, where possible, are drawn directly from the published literature. Readers should recognize that inclusion of these works does not imply superior quality over other articles I may have selected. Similarly, these papers are not intended to reflect standards of practice to which readers should adhere. Readers must decide for themselves whether these studies are useful and relevant based on their own merits.

As readers will discover, I am but one of many authors who have tackled this subject over the years. In reality, this book was possible because of the fine work created by those who pioneered efforts to promote and communicate evidence-based medicine (practice) methods well before I ever heard those terms. David Sackett, MD, Gordon Guyatt, MD, Drummond Rennie, MD, and colleagues have written books and articles that are justifiably classics on this topic and that are cited frequently throughout this text. I have read and re-read their material and each time I do, I come away with a deeper understanding of the content and of my obligations in teaching it. My hope is that I have been able to reorient the information to reflect contemporary physical therapy practice while remaining faithful to the fundamental elements and concepts of evidence-based medicine (practice) that transcend professional disciplines.

In closing, I must remind readers of the principle of specificity of training. Just like any other skill we acquire, EBPT takes practice in order to increase one's efficiency and effectiveness with the process. My students have taught me that practice is easiest when they are working in a culture that encourages and guides their efforts. Not surprisingly, a didactic course on the topic is a natural setting in which to receive this level of support. Once in clinical practice, however, one's momentum may slow in the absence of colleagues and administrators who also are committed to this approach to patient/client management. The challenge is to avoid losing heart as we work to evolve our EBPT skills.

I am a firm believer in the value of small steps. We tell our patients/clients every day to appreciate little victories in their quest to recover or improve their abilities. We must allow ourselves that same opportunity where EBPT is concerned. My hope is that individuals will find this book to be an accessible resource with which to propel their efforts, even when they are "an n-of-1" in their clinical setting.

Dianne V. Jewell, PT, PhD, CCS, FAACVPR

Acknowledgments

Writing a textbook about material I teach every day was a more difficult task than I ever imagined. This book would not be possible without the assistance of Jack Bruggeman, David Cella, and Lisa Gordon at Jones & Bartlett. Their editorial support is only surpassed by their immeasurable patience and persistence! I also have an entirely new appreciation for "details" now that I have seen the work of the J&B production editors Daniel Stone and Renée Sekerak. Thanks to them for helping me avoid the "I know what I mean" syndrome in my manuscript. Finally, I would also like to thank Karen J. Sparrow, PT, PhD, for her contributions to Chapter 16. She truly understands how to apply evidence-based physical therapy principles to clinincal practice.

Part I

Principles of Evidence-Based Physical Therapy Practice

Chapter 1

Evidence-Based Physical Therapy Practice

Nothing could be more humanistic than using evidence to find the best possible approaches to care.

—Jules Rothstein, PT, PhD[1]

Objectives

Upon completion of this chapter the student/practitioner will be able to:

1. Discuss the circumstances that have resulted in an increased emphasis on the use of evidence in practice.
2. Distinguish among definitions of evidence-based medicine, evidence-based practice and evidence-based physical therapy.
3. Discuss the use of evidence in physical therapy decision-making in the context of the *Guide to Physical Therapist Practice*.[2]
4. Describe evidence-based physical therapy focus areas.
5. Describe the general steps involved in evidence-based physical therapy practice.
6. Discuss the barriers to evidence-based physical therapy and possible strategies for reducing them in clinical practice.

Terms in This Chapter

Clinical Expertise: Proficiency of clinical skills and abilities, informed by continually expanding knowledge, that individual clinicians develop through experience, learning, and reflection about their practice.[3,4]

Diagnosis: "A process that integrates and evaluates data" obtained during a patient/client examination, often resulting in a classification that guides prognosis, the plan of care, and subsequent interventions.[2(p. 45),4]

Disability: "The inability or restricted ability to perform actions, tasks, and activities related to required self-care, home management, work (job/school/play), community, and leisure roles in the individual's sociocultural context and physical environment."[2(p. 31)]

Evaluation: "A dynamic process in which the physical therapist makes clinical judgments based on data gathered during the examination."[2(p. 43)]

Evidence: "Any empirical observation about the apparent relation between events constitutes potential evidence."[5(p. 6)]

Examination: "A comprehensive screening and specific testing process leading to diagnostic classification or, as appropriate, referral to another practitioner."[2(p. 42)]

Functional Limitations: "Occur when impairments result in a restriction of the ability to perform a physical action, task or activity in an efficient, typically expected, or competent manner."[2(p. 30)]

Impairment: "Alterations in the anatomical, physiological or psychological structures or functions that both (1) results from underlying changes in the normal state and (2) contributes to illness."[2(p. 30)]

Intervention: The purposeful use of various physical therapy procedures and techniques, in collaboration with the patient/client and, when appropriate, other care providers, in order to effect a change in the patient/client's condition.[2]

Outcome: "The end result of patient/client management, which include the impact of physical therapy interventions;" may be measured by the physical therapist or determined by self-report from the patient/client.[2(p. 43)]

Pathology: A disease, disorder, or condition that is "primarily identified at the cellular level" and is "(1) characterized by a particular cluster of signs and symptoms and (2) recognized by either the patient/client or the practitioner as 'abnormal.'"[2(p. 29)]

Patient-Centered Care: Health care that "customizes treatment recommendations and decision making in response to patients' preferences and beliefs. . . . This partnership also is characterized by informed, shared decision making, development of patient knowledge, skills needed for self-management of illness, and preventive behaviors."[6(p. 3)]

Prevention: Activities that attempt to (1) prevent a "target condition in susceptible or potentially susceptible populations" (primary prevention); (2) decrease the "duration of illness, severity of disease, and sequelae through early diagnosis and intervention" (secondary prevention), and (3) limit "the degree of disability and promote rehabilitation and restoration of function in patients with chronic and irreversible diseases" (tertiary prevention).[2(p. 41)]

Prognosis: Prediction of the natural course of a condition, or its development based upon previously-identified risk factors; also, "the predicted optimal level of improvement through intervention and the amount of time required to achieve that level."[2(p. 46)]

INTRODUCTION

Use of *evidence* in clinical decision-making is promoted extensively across health care professions and practice settings. Gordon Guyatt, MD, David L. Sackett, MD, and their respective colleagues have published the definitive works that instruct physicians in the use of evidence in medical practice.[5,7] In addition, federal agencies including the Agency for Healthcare Research and Quality and the Centers for Medicare and Medicaid Services evaluate the strength of published evidence during the development of health care policies and clinical guidelines.[8,9] Professional associations such as the American Medical Association, the American Heart Association, and the American Occupational Therapy Association have developed resources to help their members and consumers access evidence regarding a wide variety of diseases, treatments, and outcomes.[10,11,12]

The physical therapy profession also has expressed a commitment to the development and use of evidence. The American Physical Therapy Association envisions that by the year 2020 physical therapists will be autonomous practitioners that, among other things, use evidence in practice.[13] Numerous articles regarding the methods for, benefits of, and barriers to evidence-based practice have been published in the journal *Physical Therapy*.[14,15,16,17] For several years the journal also included a recurring feature "Evidence in Practice" in which a patient case was described and the subsequent search for, evaluation and application of evidence was illustrated.[18] Finally, the American Physical Therapy Association has created "Hooked on Evidence," a database of research articles regarding physical therapy interventions, for use by its members in clinical practice.[19]

The ground swell of interest in the use of evidence in health care has resulted from the convergence of multiple issues, including: a) extensive documentation of apparently unexplained practice variation in the management of a variety of conditions; b) the continued increase in health care costs disproportionate to inflation; c) publicity surrounding medical errors; d) identification of potential or actual harm resulting from previously approved medications; and e) trends in technology assessment and outcomes research.[20,21,22,23] In addition, the rapid evolution of Internet technology has increased both the dissemination of and access to health care research. Related issues have stimulated the drive for evidence-based physical therapy practice, the most important of which is the use of evidence by commercial and government payers as a basis for their coverage decisions. For example, the American Physical Therapy Association was able to convince the Centers for Medicare and Medicaid Services to approve Medicare benefit coverage for electrical stimulation to treat chronic wounds based on the evidence submitted demonstrating the effectiveness of this technique.[24] In light of these important developments, physical therapists should have an understanding of what evidence-based practice is, how it works, and how it may improve their clinical practice.

EVIDENCE-BASED WHAT?

The use of evidence in health care is referred to by a variety of labels with essentially similar meanings. "Evidence-based medicine," a term relevant to physicians, is defined as: "the conscientious, explicit, and judicious use of current best evidence in making decisions about the care of individual patients. The practice of evidence-based medicine means integrating individual clinical expertise with the best available clinical evidence from systematic research."[3(p. 71)]

"Evidence-based practice" and "evidence-based healthcare" are labels that have been created to link the behavior described by evidence-based medicine to other health care professionals. Hicks provides this expanded definition: "care that 'takes place when decisions that affect the care of patients are taken with due weight accorded to all valid, relevant information.' "[25(p. 8)] In both definitions, evidence does not replace *clinical expertise*; rather, evidence is used to inform more fully a decision-making process in which expertise provides one perspective to the clinical problem.

Regardless of the label used, the implicit message in all cases is that the use of evidence in clinical decision making is a movement away from unquestioning reliance upon knowledge gained from authority or tradition. Authority may be attributed to established experts in the field, as well as to revered teachers in professional training programs. Tradition may be thought of as practice habits expressed by the phrase "this is what I have always done." Habits may be instilled by eminent authority figures, but also they may be based upon local or regional practice norms that are reinforced by their use in payment formulas ("usual and customary") and in legal proceedings ("local standard of care"). Knowledge derived from these sources often reflects an initial understanding of clinical phenomena from which diagnostic and treatment approaches are developed based on biological plausibility ("this is how the body works") and anecdotal experience. As such, this form of knowledge will continue to have a role as new clinical problems are encountered that require new solutions. The fundamental weakness in a clinician's dependence on this type of knowledge, however, is the potential for selection of ineffective, or even harmful, treatments as a result of the lack of inquiry into their "true" effects.

Straus *et al.* offer as an example the use of hormone replacement therapy in women without a uterus or those who are post-menopausal.[26] Women in these situations were observed to have an increased risk of heart disease that, from a biological perspective, appeared connected to the loss of estrogen and progestin. Replacing the lost hormones in an effort to reduce the risk of heart disease in these women made sense. The success of this treatment was confirmed further by observational studies and small randomized controlled trials.[27] However, the early termination in 2002 of a large National Institutes of Health-sponsored hormone replacement therapy trial challenged the concept of protective effects from this intervention. The study's initial results indicated, among other things, that estrogen replacement *did not* protect post-menopausal women against cardiovascular disease as had been hypothesized. Moreover, long-term estrogen plus progestin therapy increased a woman's risk for the development of heart attacks, strokes, blood clots, and breast cancer.[22] In effect, years of clinical behavior based upon a biologically plausible theory supported by lower quality evidence were invalidated by a well-designed piece of evidence. This example is extreme, but it makes the point that health care providers should willingly and knowingly re-evaluate the assumptions that underlie practice that is based on authority and tradition supported by limited evidence.

EVIDENCE-BASED PHYSICAL THERAPY PRACTICE

With that background in mind, this text has adopted the term "Evidence-Based Physical Therapy Practice" (EBPT) in order to narrow the professional and clinical frame of reference. The definition of EBPT should be consistent with previously established concepts regarding the use of evidence, but also should reflect the specific nature of physical therapy practice.

The *Guide to Physical Therapist Practice, 2nd edition* establishes physical therapy as a profession that is grounded in an expanded disablement model originally articulated by Nagi,[2] illustrated here in Figure 1–1. This model reflects the clinical aspects of a patient/client's situation, as well as the social context that shapes perceptions of illness and disability for each individual. Within this framework physical therapists examine, evaluate, diagnose, prognosticate, and intervene with individuals with identified *pathology*, *impairments*, *functional limitations* and *disabilities*, as well as with persons with health, *prevention*, and wellness needs. These professional behaviors are summarized in the term "patient/client management." Finally, the management process incorporates the individual patient or client as a participant whose knowledge, understanding, goals, preferences, and appraisal of their situa-

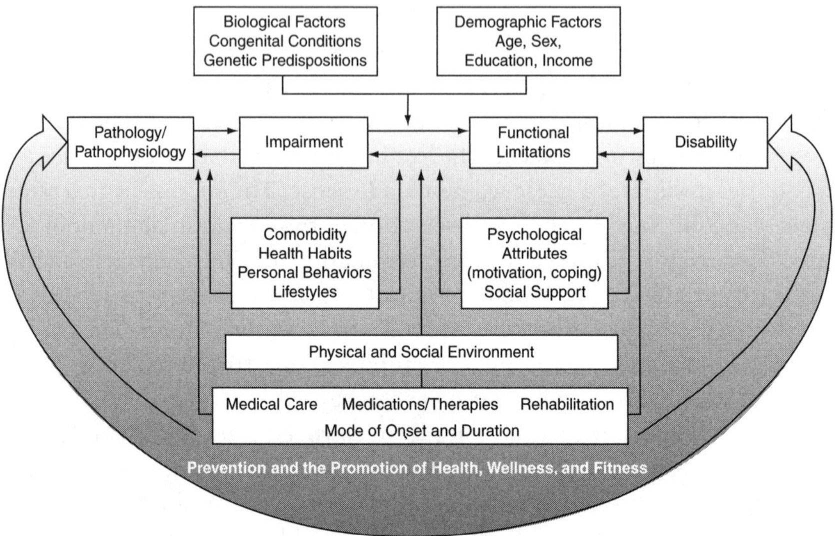

[a] *Adapted with permission of the American Physical Association from Guccione AA. Arthritis and the process of disablement.* Phys Ther. *1994; 74:410.*

Figure 1–1 An expanded disablement model, showing interactions among individual and environmental factors, prevention, and the promotion of health, wellness, and fitness.[a]

Source: Reprinted from Guide to Physical Therapist Practice. 2nd ed. *Phys Ther.* 2001; 81(1):9–746 with permission of the American Physical Therapy Association. This material is copyrighted, and any further reproduction or distribution is prohibited.

tion are integral to the development and implementation of a physical therapy plan of care.

A definition of EBPT that reflects the intent of evidence-based medicine as well as the nature of physical therapy practice is offered here:[2,28]

> Evidence-based physical therapy practice is "open and thoughtful clinical decision-making" about the physical therapy management of a patient/client that integrates the "best available evidence with clinical judgement" and the patient/client's preferences and values, and that further considers the larger social context in which physical therapy services are provided, to optimize patient/client outcomes and quality of life.

The term "open" implies a process in which the physical therapist is able to articulate in understandable terms the details of his or her recommendations including the: 1) steps taken to arrive at this conclusion; 2) underlying rationale; and, 3) potential impact of taking, and of refusing action. "Thoughtful clinical decision-making" refers to the physical therapist's appraisal of the risks and benefits of various options within a professional context that includes ethics, standards of care, and legal or regulatory considerations.[29] "Best available evidence" will be operationally defined in Chapter 2. "Preferences and values" are the patient/client's "unique preferences, concerns and expectations"[7] against which each option should be weighed and which ultimately must be reflected in a collaborative decision-making process between the therapist and the patient/client. This point is consistent with the emphasis on *patient-centered care* as articulated by the Institute of Medicine.[6] Finally, "larger social context" refers to the social, cultural, economic, and political influences that shape health policy including rules governing the delivery of and payment for health care services.[30] Figure 1-2 provides an illustration of EBPT.

Evidence-Based Physical Therapy Practice Focus Areas

A clinician interested in evidence-based physical therapy practice rightly might ask "evidence for what?". The patient/client management model

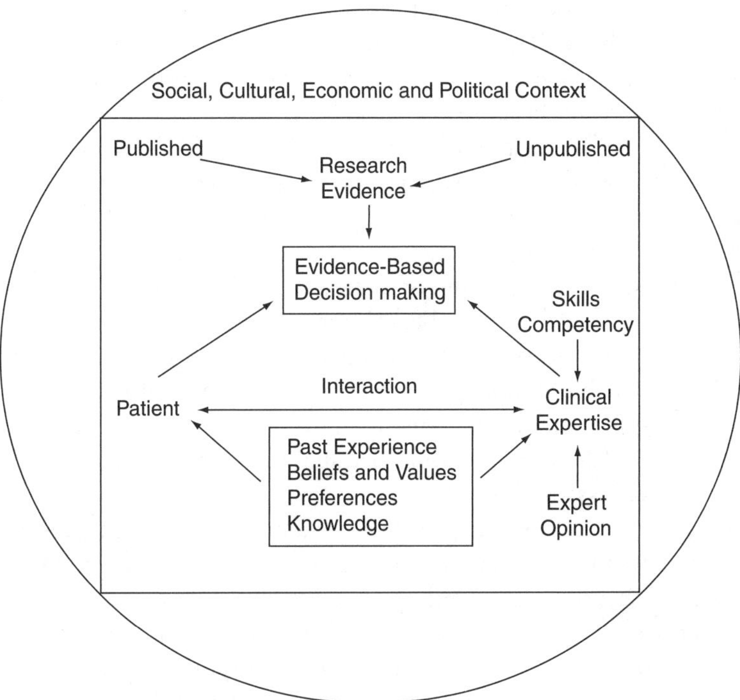

Figure 1-2 Evidence-based physical therapy practice in a societal context.
Source: Reprinted from *Evidence-Based Healthcare: A Practical Guide for Therapists,* Tracy Bury & Judy Mead. Page 10. Copyright (1999), with permission from Elsevier.

provides the answer to this question when one considers its individual elements.[2] In order to conduct an *examination* and *evaluation*, physical therapists must choose, apply, and interpret findings from a wide variety of tests and measures, such as ligament stress techniques and quantifications of strength and range of motion. Similarly, accurate *diagnosis* of conditions resulting in pain depends upon a properly constructed and tested classification scheme. Evidence may assist the physical therapist in selecting the best techniques to correctly identify, quantify, and classify the patient/client's problem, a result that will enhance the efficiency and effectiveness of service delivery.

Prognosis refers to a prediction of the future status of the patient/client that may reflect the natural course of a condition or result following physical therapy treatments or prevention activities. Predictive ability depends upon the physical therapist's understanding of the phenomenon in question (i.e., accurate diagnosis), as well as the identification of indicators or risk factors that signal a particular direction. In all cases the therapist must determine which of the numerous characteristics about the patient/client's physical, psychological, behavioral, and environmental situation will be most predictive of the outcome of interest. Evidence may identify the most salient factors that will produce the most accurate prediction.

The choice of *interventions* is the step in the patient care process that carries particular weight because of the dual responsibilities of the provider to "do good" (beneficence) and to "do no harm" (non-maleficence). The stakes in this balancing act increase when the intervention in question has with it a risk of serious consequences, such as permanent disability or mortality. Most physical therapy treatment options are not "high risk" in this sense; however, the application of low risk interventions that produce no positive effect does not meet the test of beneficence. A common clinical scenario is one in which a patient presents with a painful condition and the therapist must decide which physical agents, exercise, or some combination of both, will be most effective for this individual. Evidence may assist the therapist and the patient/client in a risk-benefit analysis by providing information about effectiveness and harm.

The end product of the patient/client management process is referred to as the *outcome*. Outcomes should be distinguished from treatment effects.[30] The former focus on results from the patient/client's point of view that occurred at the conclusion of the episode of care. For example, return-to-work represents a commonly-used outcome following outpatient orthopedic physical therapy management. On the other hand, treatment effects represent the change, if any, in the underlying problems that prevented the individual from working. Outcomes usually are stated in functional terms such as "The patient will work six hours without pain." Such statements reflect the patient/client's goals for the physical therapy episode of care. Use of standardized outcome measures, however, permits an analysis of progress over the course of an episode for a single individual, as well as a comparison across patients/clients with similar issues. As with the selection of tests and measures, a physical therapist must decide which standardized outcome instrument will provide the most discriminating information with respect to changes in impairment, function, or health-related quality of life. A review of available evidence may assist the therapist in determining what outcomes are possible and which measurement tool is able to detect change in a consistent and meaningful fashion.

The Process of Evidence-Based Physical Therapy Practice

Evidence-based physical therapy practice as a process starts with a question in response to a patient/client's problem or concern. A search for relevant evidence to answer the question is then followed by a critical appraisal of its merits and conclusions, as well as a determination of its applicability to the patient/client. At the conclusion of the appraisal, the therapist will consider the evidence in the context of his or her clinical expertise and the patient/client's values and preferences during an explicit discussion with that patient/client.[5] Finally, the therapist and the patient/client will collaborate to identify and implement the next steps in the management process.

The process of EBPT depends upon a variety of factors. First, physical therapists require sufficient knowledge about their patient/client's condition in order to recognize what is unknown. In other words, physical therapists must be willing to suspend the assumption that they have complete information about a patient/client's situation. In addition, physical therapists must have, or have access to, knowledge of the evidence appraisal process—that is, which features characterize stronger versus weaker evidence. Second, therapists need access to the evidence, a situation that has improved considerably with the advent of online databases and electronic publication of journals. Availability of these resources, however, does not ensure their efficient use, particularly when it comes to developing effective search strategies. Third, physical therapists need the time to search for, appraise, and integrate the evidence into their practice. In busy clinical settings, time is a limited commodity that usually is dedicated to administrative tasks, such as documentation of services and discussions with referral sources and payers. Unless the entire clinic or department adopts the EBPT philosophy, it may be difficult for a single physical therapist to incorporate the behavior into his or her patient/client management routine.

Results from a survey conducted by Jette *et al.* suggest that some of the requirements of EBPT are obstacles to its implementation.[16] Although the majority of respondents (n=488) believed evidence was necessary for practice and improved quality of care, 67 percent of the subjects listed lack of time as one of the top three barriers to implementation of EBPT. Nearly all respondents (96%) indicated they had access to evidence; however, 65 percent reported performing searches for evidence less than twice in a typical month. In addition, notable proportions of the sample indicated lower confidence levels in their abilities to execute effective search strategies (34%), appraise the evidence (44%), and interpret results for terms such as "odds ratio" (47%) and "confidence interval" (37%). Finally, older therapists with more years since licensure were less likely to have the necessary training, familiarity with, and confidence in the skills necessary for effective EBPT.

So, what can be done to reduce the barriers to effective EBPT? Clearly a philosophical shift is required to develop consistent behavior during a busy day of patient/client care. Management support in terms of the technology (e.g., Internet access), as well as time allotted in a therapist's schedule, would reflect the type of commitment needed. The time issue also may be helped by the use of services that locate, summarize, and appraise the evidence for easy review by practitioners. Some of these services will be discussed at the end of Chapter 3; however, it should be noted that physical therapists must determine whether or not the methodology used by these services is sufficiently stringent to provide an appropriate assessment of evidence quality. Databases dedicated to physical therapy evidence also may enhance the efficiency of the search process.

Ultimately, the ability to engage in EBPT in a consistent fashion requires practice just like any other skill. The process starts with the individual patient/client and the questions generated from the initial encounter, such as:

- Which tests will provide accurate classification of this person's problem?
- What functional limitations can I anticipate if this problem is not addressed?
- What is the most effective intervention I can offer for documented impairments?
- How will we know if we have been successful?
- What does the patient/client want to get out of this episode of care?

A physical therapist's willingness to consider *consciously* these questions is the first step of EBPT. The word "consciously" is emphasized because it takes practice to develop the habit of openly challenging one's assumptions and current state of knowledge. Until this behavior becomes a routine part of one's practice, EBPT will be difficult to implement in a consistent and time efficient manner.

SUMMARY

The use of evidence in clinical decision making is promoted among many health professions in response to documented practice variation and increasing health care costs, as well as in response to a desire for improved quality of care. Evidence-based practice in any profession promotes less dependence on knowledge derived from authority or tradition through the use of evidence to evaluate previously unquestioned information. Evidence-based physical therapy practice is open, thoughtful decision making about the physical therapy management of a patient/client that integrates the best available evidence, as well as the patient/client's preferences and values, within the larger social context of the patient/client and the therapist. Evidence may be used to assist decision making regarding measurement, diagnosis, prognosis, interventions, and outcomes. Requirements for EBPT include: a willingness to challenge one's assumptions, the ability to develop relevant clinical questions about a patient/client, access to evidence, knowledge regarding evidence appraisal, the time to make it all happen, as well as a willingness to acquire and practice the necessary skills described in this book.

Exercises

1. Describe two factors that have prompted the emphasis on evidence-based practice in health care. How might evidence address these issues or concerns?
2. Discuss the strengths and weaknesses of clinical knowledge derived from:
   a. Authority
   b. Evidence
   c. Tradition

   Describe a specific example of each type of knowledge in current physical therapy practice.
3. Discuss the potential contribution of evidence to each step of the patient/client management process.
4. Discuss the role of the patient/client in EBPT.
5. Complete the survey in Figure 1-3 modified from Jette *et al.*[16] What do your answers tell you about your willingness and readiness to participate in EBPT?

Appendix.
Evidence-Based Practice (EBP) Questionnaire

This section of the questionnaire inquires about personal attitudes toward, use of, and perceived benefits and limitations of EBP.

For the following items, place a mark ☒ in the appropriate box that indicates your response.

1. Application of EBP is necessary in the practice of physical therapy.
   ☐ Strongly disagree ☐ Disagree ☐ Neutral ☐ Agree ☐ Strongly Agree
2. Literature and research findings are useful in my day-to-day practice.
   ☐ Strongly disagree ☐ Disagree ☐ Neutral ☐ Agree ☐ Strongly Agree
3. I need to increase the use of evidence in my daily practice.
   ☐ Strongly Disagree ☐ Disagree ☐ Neutral ☐ Agree ☐ Strongly Agree
4. The adoption of EBP places an unreasonable demand on physical therapists.
   ☐ Strongly Disagree ☐ Disagree ☐ Neutral ☐ Agree ☐ Strongly Agree
5. I am interested in learning or improving the skills necessary to incorporate EBP into my practice.
   ☐ Strongly Disagree ☐ Disagree ☐ Neutral ☐ Agree ☐ Strongly Agree
6. EBP improves the quality of patient care.
   ☐ Strongly Disagree ☐ Disagree ☐ Neutral ☐ Agree ☐ Strongly Agree
7. EBP does not take into account the limitations of my clinical practice setting.
   ☐ Strongly Disagree ☐ Disagree ☐ Neutral ☐ Agree ☐ Strongly Agree
8. My reimbursement rate will increase if I incorporate EBP into my practice.
   ☐ Strongly Disagree ☐ Disagree ☐ Neutral ☐ Agree ☐ Strongly Agree
9. Strong evidence is lacking to support most of the interventions I use with my patients.
   ☐ Strongly Disagree ☐ Disagree ☐ Neutral ☐ Agree ☐ Strongly Agree
10. EBP helps me make decisions about patient care.
    ☐ Strongly Disagree ☐ Disagree ☐ Neutral ☐ Agree ☐ Strongly Agree
11. EBP does not take into account patient preferences.
    ☐ Strongly Disagree ☐ Disagree ☐ Neutral ☐ Agree ☐ Strongly Agree

For the following items, place a mark ☒ in the appropriate box that indicates your response for a typical month.

12. Read/review research/literature related to my clinical practice.
    ☐ ≤1 article ☐ 2–5 articles ☐ 6–10 articles ☐ 11–15 articles ☐ 16+ articles
13. Use professional literature and research findings in the process of clinical decision making.
    ☐ ≤1 time ☐ 2–5 times ☐ 6–10 times ☐ 11–15 times ☐ 16+ times
14. Use MEDLINE or other databases to search for practice-relevant literature/research.
    ☐ ≤1 time ☐ 2–5 times ☐ 6–10 times ☐ 11–15 times ☐ 16+ times

The following section inquires about personal use and understanding of clinical practice guidelines. Practice guidelines provide a description of standard specifications for care of patients with specific diseases and are developed through a formal, consensus-building process that incorporates the best scientific evidence of effectiveness and expert opinion available.

For the following items, place a mark ☒ in the appropriate box that indicates your response.

15. Practice guidelines are available for topics related to my practice.
☐ Yes ☐ No ☐ Do Not Know

16. I actively seek practice guidelines pertaining to areas of my practice.
☐ Strongly Disagree ☐ Disagree ☐ Neutral ☐ Agree ☐ Strongly Agree

17. I use practice guidelines in my practice.
☐ Strongly Disagree ☐ Disagree ☐ Neutral ☐ Agree ☐ Strongly Agree

18. I am aware that practice guidelines are available online.
☐ Yes ☐ No

19. I am able to access practice guidelines online.
☐ Yes ☐ No

20. I am able to incorporate patient preferences with practice guidelines.
☐ Strongly Disagree ☐ Disagree ☐ Neutral ☐ Agree ☐ Strongly Agree

The following section inquires about availability of resources to access information and personal skills in using those resources.

For the following items, place a mark ☒ in the appropriate box that indicates your response. In items referring to your "facility," consider the practice setting in which you do the majority of your clinical care.

21. I have access to current research through professional journals in their paper form.
☐ Yes ☐ No

22. I have the ability to access relevant databases and the Internet at my facility.
☐ Yes ☐ No ☐ Do Not Know

23. I have the ability to access relevant databases and the Internet at home or locations other than my facility.
☐ Yes ☐ No ☐ Do Not Know

24. My facility supports the use of current research in practice.
☐ Strongly Disagree ☐ Disagree ☐ Neutral ☐ Agree ☐ Strongly Agree

continues

Figure 1–3 Survey of beliefs and attitudes regarding evidence-based physical therapy practice.

Source: Reprinted from Jette DU, Bacon K, Batty C, Carlson M, Ferland A, *et al.* Evidence-based practice: beliefs, attitudes, knowledge, and behaviors of physical therapists. *Phys Ther.* 2003; 83(9):786–805 with permission of the American Physical Therapy Association.

25. I learned the foundations for EBP as part of my academic preparation.
    ☐ Strongly Disagree ☐ Disagree ☐ Neutral ☐ Agree ☐ Strongly Agree
26. I have received formal training in search strategies for finding research relevant to my practice.
    ☐ Strongly Disagree ☐ Disagree ☐ Neutral ☐ Agree ☐ Strongly Agree
27. I am familiar with the medical search engines (e.g., MEDLINE, CINAHL).
    ☐ Strongly Disagree ☐ Disagree ☐ Neutral ☐ Agree ☐ Strongly Agree
28. I received formal training in critical appraisal of research literature as part of my academic preparation.
    ☐ Strongly Disagree ☐ Disagree ☐ Neutral ☐ Agree ☐ Strongly Agree
29. I am confident in my ability to critically review professional literature.
    ☐ Strongly Disagree ☐ Disagree ☐ Neutral ☐ Agree ☐ Strongly Agree
30. I am confident in my ability to find relevant research to answer my clinical questions.
    ☐ Strongly Disagree ☐ Disagree ☐ Neutral ☐ Agree ☐ Strongly Agree

For the following item, place a mark ☒ in one box in the row for each term.

31. My understanding of the following terms is:

Term	**Understand Completely**	**Understand Somewhat**	**Do Not Understand**
a) Relative risk	☐	☐	☐
b) Absolute risk	☐	☐	☐
c) Systematic review	☐	☐	☐
d) Odds ratio	☐	☐	☐
e) Meta-analysis	☐	☐	☐
f) Confidence interval	☐	☐	☐
g) Heterogeneity	☐	☐	☐
h) Publication bias	☐	☐	☐

For the following items, rank your top 3 choices by placing numbers in the appropriate boxes (1 = most important).

32. Rank your 3 greatest barriers to the use of EBP in your clinical practice.
    ☐ Insufficient time
    ☐ Lack of information resources
    ☐ Lack of research skills
    ☐ Poor ability to critically appraise the literature
    ☐ Lack of generalizability of the literature findings to my patient population
    ☐ Inability to apply research findings to individual patients with unique characteristics
    ☐ Lack of understanding of statistical analysis
    ☐ Lack of collective support among my colleagues in my facility
    ☐ Lack of interest

Figure 1–3 Survey of beliefs and attitudes regarding evidence-based physical therapy practice. (*continued*).

6. Based upon your results from the previous question, identify two changes that you would need to make to enhance your ability to participate in EBPT. For each change, identify one strategy that you could implement to move you in the right direction.

References

1. Rothstein JM. Thirty-Second Mary McMillan Lecture: Journeys beyond the horizon. *Phys Ther.* 2001; 81(11):1817–1829.
2. American Physical Therapy Association, Guide to Physical Therapist Practice. 2d ed. *Phys Ther.* 2001; 81(1):9–746.
3. Sackett DL, Rosenberg WMC, Gray JAM, Haynes RB, Richardson WS. Evidence-based medicine: What it is and what it isn't." *BMJ.* 1996; 312(7023):71–72.
4. Higgs J, Jones M. *Clinical Reasoning in the Health Professions.* 2d ed. Oxford, England: Butterworth Heinemann; 2000.
5. Guyatt G, Rennie D. *Users' Guides to the Medical Literature: A Manual for Evidence-Based Clinical Practice.* Chicago, IL: AMA Press; 2002.
6. Knebel E. *Educating Health Professionals to be Patient-Centered.* Institute of Medicine Web site. Available at: http://www.iom.edu/Object.File/Master/10/460/Patient.pdf. Accessed February 15, 2006.
7. Sackett DL, Straus SE, Richardson WS, Rosenberg W, Haynes RB. *Evidence-based Medicine: How to Practice and Teach EBM.* 2d ed. Edinburgh, Scotland: Churchill Livingstone; 2000.
8. Evidence in Practice: Agency for Healthcare Research and Quality Web site. Available at: http://www.ahrq.gov/clinic/epcix.htm. Accessed February 15, 2006.
9. Medicare Announces Draft Guidance for National Coverage Determinations with Evidence Development: Centers for Medicare and Medicaid Services Web site. Available at: http://new.cms.hhs.gov/apps/media/press/release.asp?Counter=1423. Accessed February 15, 2006.
10. Users' Guides. American Medical Association Web site. Available at: http://www.usersguides.org/. Accessed February 15, 2006.
11. American Heart Association Web site. Available at: http://www.americanheart.org/presenter.jhtml?identifier=1200409. Accessed February 15, 2006.
12. American Occupational Therapy Association Web site. Available at: http://www.aota.org/. Accessed February 15, 2006.
13. Vision 2020. American Physical Therapy Association Web site. Available at: http://www.apta.org/AM/Template.cfm?Section=About_APTA&Template=/TaggedPage/TaggedPageDisplay.cfm&TPLID=41&ContentID=23725. Accessed February 15, 2006.
14. Fritz JM, Wainner RS. Examining diagnostic tests: an evidence-based perspective. *Phys Ther.* 2001; 81(9):1546–1564.
15. Scalzitti DA. Evidence-based guidelines: Application to clinical practice. *Phys Ther.* 2001; 81(10):1622–1628.

16. Jette DU, Bacon K, Batty C, Carlson M, Ferland A *et al.* Evidence-based practice: beliefs, attitudes, knowledge, and behaviors of physical therapists. *Phys Ther.* 2003; 83(9):786–805.
17. Maher CG, Sherrington C, Elkins M, Herbert RD, Moseley AM. Challenges for evidence-based physical therapy: Accessing and interpreting high-quality evidence on therapy. *Phys Ther.* 2004; 84(7):644–654.
18. Evidence in Practice. American Physical Therapy Association Web site. Available at: http://www.ptjournal.org/info/eipList.cfm. Accessed February 15, 2006.
19. Hooked on Evidence. American Physical Therapy Association Web site. Available at: http://www.hookedonevidence.com/. Accessed February 15, 2006.
20. Eddy DM. Evidence-based medicine: a unified approach. *Health Affairs.* 2005; 24(1):9–17.
21. Steinberg EP, Luce BR. Evidence based? Caveat emptor! *Health Affairs.* 2005; 24(1):80–92.
22. Women's Health Initiative Participant Information. National Institutes of Health Web site. Available at: http://www.whi.org/. Accessed February 15, 2006.
23. Institute of Medicine Web site. Available at: http://www.iom.edu/. Accessed February 15, 2006.
24. E-Stim Coverage for Wound Care Celebrated at Board Meeting. American Physical Therapy Association Web site. Available at: http://www.apta.org/AM/Template.cfm?Section=Coding&TEMPLATE=/CM/HTMLDisplay.cfm&CONTENTID=8664. Accessed February 15, 2006.
25. Hicks N. Evidence-Based Healthcare. *Bandolier.* 1997; 4(39):8.
26. Straus SE, Richardson WS, Glaziou P, Haynes RB. *Evidence-Based Medicine: How to Practice and Teach EBM.* 3d ed. Edinburgh, Scotland: Elsevier Churchill Livingstone; 2005.
27. Mobasseri S, Liebson PR, Klein LW. Hormone therapy and selective receptor modulators for prevention of coronary heart disease in postmenopausal women: Estrogen replacement from the cardiologist's perspective. *Cardiol Rev.* 2004; 12(6):287–298.
28. Normative Model of Physical Therapist Education: Version 2004. Alexandria, VA: American Physical Therapy Association; 2004.
29. Guyatt GH, Haynes RB, Jaeschke RZ, Cook DJ, Green L *et al.* Users' guides to the medical literature XXV. Evidence-based medicine: principles for applying the users' guides to patient care. *JAMA.* 2000; 284(10):1290–1296.
30. Herbert R, Jamtvedt G, Mead J, Hagen KB. *Practical Evidence-Based Physiotherapy.* Edinburgh, Scotland: Elsevier Butterworth Heinemann; 2005.

Chapter 2

What Is Evidence?

The most savage controversies are those about matters as to which there is no good evidence either way.

—Bertrand Russell

Objectives

Upon completion of this chapter the student/practitioner will be able to:

1. Discuss the concept of "best available clinical evidence."
2. Describe the general content and procedural characteristics of desirable evidence and their implications for the selection of studies to evaluate.
3. Describe different forms of evidence and their uses for answering clinical questions in physical therapy practice.
4. Discuss and apply the principles and purposes of evidence hierarchies for each type of clinical question.
5. Discuss the limitations of evidence hierarchies and their implications for the use of evidence in practice.

Terms in this Chapter

Bias: Results or inferences that systematically deviate from the truth "or the processes leading to such deviation."[1(p. 251)]

Case Report: A detailed description of the management of a patient/client that may serve as a basis for future research.[2]

Cross-Sectional Study: A study that collects data about a phenomenon during a single point in time or once within a defined time interval.[3]

Effectiveness: The extent to which an intervention or service produces a desired outcome under typical clinical conditions.[1]

Efficacy: The extent to which an intervention or service produces a desired outcome under ideal conditions.[1]

Evidence: "Any empirical observation about the apparent relation between events constitutes potential evidence."[4(p. 6)]

Experimental Design: A research design in which the behavior of randomly-assigned groups of subjects is measured following the purposeful manipulation of an independent variable(s) in at least one of the groups; used to examine cause-and-effect relationships between an independent variable(s) and an outcome(s).[5,6]

Longitudinal Study: A study that looks at a phenomenon occurring over time.[1]

Narrative Review (also referred to as a Summary or Literature Review): A description of prior research without a systematic search and selection strategy or critical appraisal of the studies' merits.[7]

Observational Study (also referred to as a Non-Experimental Design): A study in which controlled manipulation of the subjects is lacking;[5] in addition, if groups are present, assignment is predetermined based upon naturally occurring subject characteristics or activities.[3]

Peer Review: A process by which research is appraised by one or more content experts; commonly utilized when articles are submitted to journals for publication and when grant proposals are submitted for funding.[1]

Physiologic Study: A study that focuses on the cellular- or physiologic-systems level of the subjects; often performed in a laboratory.[3]

Prospective Design: A research design that follows subjects forward over a specified period of time.

Quasi-Experimental Design: A research design in which there is only one subject group or in which randomization to more than one subject group is lacking; controlled manipulation of the subjects is preserved.[8]

Randomized Clinical Trial (also referred to as a Randomized Controlled Trial and a Randomized Controlled Clinical Trial)[RCT]: A clinical study that uses a randomization process to assign subjects to either an experimental group(s) or a control (or comparison) group. Subjects in the experimental group receive the intervention or preventive measure of interest and then are compared to the subjects in the control (or comparison) group who did not receive the experimental manipulation.[5]

Retrospective Design: A research design that uses historical (past) data from sources such as medical records, insurance claims, or outcomes databases.

Single-System Design: A quasi-experimental research design in which one subject receives in an alternating fashion both the experimental and control (or comparison) condition.[5]

Systematic Review: A method by which a collection of research is gathered and critically appraised in an effort to reach an unbiased conclusion about the cumulative weight of the evidence on a particular topic.[3]

INTRODUCTION

Chapter 1 made the case that physical therapists should use *evidence* to inform their decision making during the patient/client management process. This claim raises the question "what qualifies as evidence"? Guyatt and Rennie's statement "any empirical observation about the apparent relation between events constitutes potential evidence"[4(p. 6)] suggests that a variety of types of evidence exist that may be integrated with clinical decisions. Options may include, but are not limited to, published research articles, clinical guidelines, patient/client records, and recall of prior patient/client cases. Sackett's use of the modifier "best available clinical evidence," however, indicates that a method of prioritizing the evidence according to its merits is required to guide the clinician's selection of relevant information.[9] This chapter will discuss the forms and general characteristics of evidence available, as well as the hierarchies that have been developed to rank them.

GENERAL CHARACTERISTICS OF DESIRABLE EVIDENCE

In light of the variety of evidence potentially available to physical therapists, it is helpful to have some general characteristics to consider during the initial search. Desirable attributes relate both to content, as well as to procedural considerations that serve as preliminary indicators of quality.

The first content criterion pertains to the type of question a physical therapist wants to answer. The patient/client management elements of examination, diagnosis, prognosis, intervention (including preventive measures), and outcomes provide potential focus areas for evidence development and application. Ideally, the evidence located will address specifically the test, classification system, risk factor, treatment technique, or outcome that the physical therapist is considering relative to an individual patient/client.

The second content criterion pertains to the subjects studied. Desirable evidence includes subjects whose characteristics are similar to the patient/client in order to increase the therapist's ability to apply the research findings to this individual person. Common attributes of interest may include, but are not limited to, the subjects' diagnosis, stage of illness, duration of the problem(s), functional status, level of disability, age, gender, race, and clinical setting in which the patient/client management is occurring.

There are two basic procedural characteristics that have relevance in the evidence selection process as well. Whether or not a research article is peer-reviewed is an important consideration. *Peer review* is the process by which research articles are evaluated by identified content experts to determine their merit for publication. Evaluation criteria usually include the credibility of the research in terms of its design and execution, relevance of the findings for the field and/or the specific journal, contribution to the body of knowledge about the topic, and, to a lesser degree, writing style.[1] The scrutiny of peer review provides an initial screening process which allows lower quality research efforts to be weeded out.

The time of publication may be another procedural feature of interest given that articles often appear in journals a year or more after the completion of the research project.[5] Direct Internet publication undoubtedly has reduced this time line in many cases. Nevertheless, the rapid evolution of medical technology and pharmaceuticals continues to alter health care dramatically. As a result, older research may not reflect current patient management. A hypothetical example might be a 15-year-old study evaluating the effectiveness of an aerobic training program in patients with multiple sclerosis that has limited relevance now that multiple disease-modifying drugs are available.[10] On the other hand, studies should not be rejected outright because of their age if the techniques in question, and the context in which they were evaluated, have remained relatively unchanged since the research was conducted.

Table 2–1 summarizes the four general characteristics of evidence that are preferable. It is important to note that these attributes are labeled "desirable," not "mandatory." This word choice is purposeful because there is much work to be done to expand the depth and breadth of physical therapy research. Many of the clinical questions physical therapists have about their patients/clients have not been explored or have been addressed in a limited fashion. A search for the "best available clinical evidence" may result in the identification of studies that are not peer-reviewed or that do not include subjects that look like a therapist's individual patient/client. Similarly, stud-

Table 2–1 Four desirable characteristics of research identified during a search for evidence.

1) The study addresses the specific clinical question the physical therapist is trying to answer.
2) The subjects in the study have characteristics that are similar to the patient/client about whom the physical therapist has a clinical question.
3) The study was published in a peer-reviewed medium (paper, electronic).
4) The context of the study and/or the technique of interest are consistent with contemporary health care.

ies may not exist that include a test or technique of interest in the clinical setting. The evidence-based physical therapy practice challenge is to decide how best to use evidence that is limited in these ways when it is the only evidence available.

FORMS OF EVIDENCE

As noted previously, forms of evidence may include anything from published research to patient records and clinical recall. Evidence-based practice in health care emphasizes the use of research to inform clinical decisions because of its potential to provide objective, unbiased results. A variety of research design options exist, many of the details of which are discussed in Chapter 5. A key point is that different research designs are suited to answering different types of clinical questions therapists may have about their patients/clients. The usefulness of a diagnostic test must be evaluated with methods that are different than those used to determine whether an intervention works. As a result, therapists should anticipate looking for evidence with different research designs depending upon what they want to know. The remainder of this chapter provides highlights of these different designs and their relative merits.

Research Designs–Overview

Forms of evidence fall along a continuum that is dictated by the presence and strength of a research design. At one end of the continuum is research that attempts to impose maximum control within the design in order to reduce the chance that bias will influence the study's results. *Bias* is a systematic deviation from the truth that occurs as a result of uncontrolled (and unwanted) influences during the study.[1] Various authors refer to research designs with the best features to minimize bias as *randomized clinical trials*, *randomized controlled trials*, or *randomized controlled clinical trials*.[1,3,5] The acronym used for all three is "RCT." These studies also are categorized as *experimental designs*. Irrespective of the label, the researchers' intention is the same: to reduce unwanted influences in the study through randomization of study participants to two or more groups and through controlled manipulation of the experimental intervention. A variant of this approach is the *single-system design* in which only one person is studied who receives, on an alternating basis, both the experimental and control (or comparison) conditions.[5]

An RCT or single-system design is best suited to answer questions about whether an experimental intervention has an effect and whether that effect is beneficial or harmful to the subjects. When conducted under ideal conditions—that is, when a high degree of control is achieved—these studies are focused on treatment *efficacy*. An example might be a study in which individual subjects with traumatic brain injuries are randomized to an experimental balance-training program that is performed in a quiet research laboratory. Such an environment is free of distractions that may interfere with the subjects' ability to pay attention to directions and focus on the required activities. Alternatively, if the same subjects perform the experimental balance-training program during their regular physical therapy appointment in the outpatient rehabilitation center, then the RCT is focused on treatment *effectiveness*.[11] Investigators in this version of the study want to know if the balance program works in a natural clinical environment full of noise and activity.

Randomized controlled clinical trials and single-system designs are approaches used to conduct an original research project focusing on one or more persons. These individual studies themselves may serve as the focus of another type of controlled research design referred to as a systematic review. *Systematic reviews* synthesize original evidence that has been selected and critically appraised according to pre-established criteria.[3] The goal of this research design is to draw conclusions from the cumulative weight of studies that, individually, may not provide enough evidence to provide a definitive answer. The pre-established criteria are used to minimize bias that may be introduced when investigators make decisions about which prior studies to include and when judgments are made about their quality. Systematic reviews may address any type of clinical question; however, most commonly they focus on well-controlled studies of interventions—in other words, on RCTs.

At the other end of the evidence continuum is the unsystematic collection of patient/client data that occurs in daily physical therapy practice. The term "unsystematic" is not meant to imply substandard care; rather, it is an indication that clinical practice is focused on the individual patient/client rather than on groups of subjects upon whom controls are imposed for the purposes of ensuring research integrity. This type of evidence often is labeled "anecdotal"[9] and frequently is put to use when therapists recall from memory prior experiences with patients/clients similar to the person with whom they are currently dealing. In response to regulatory and reimbursement pressures, many clinical settings are creating a degree of consistency in data collection with their implementation of standardized instruments and databases to capture patient/client outcomes. As a result, physical therapists working in these settings may find some evidence that is useful to inform their practice.

In between the two ends of the evidence continuum are study designs that lack one or more of the following characteristics:

a) Randomization techniques to distribute subjects into groups;
b) The use of more than one group in order to make a comparison;
c) Controlled experimental manipulation of the subjects;
d) Measures at the patient/client level (e.g., impairment, function, disability); and/or,
e) A systematic method for collecting and analyzing information.

These designs have fewer features with which to minimize bias and/or shift their focus away from patient/client-centered outcomes. For example, *quasi-experimental designs* maintain the purposeful manipulation of the experimental technique, but may not randomize subjects to groups or may have only one subject group to evaluate.[8] *Observational*, or *non-experimental*, designs have even less control than quasi-experimental studies because they have the same limitations with respect to their group(s) *and* they do not include experimental manipulation of subjects.[5] In spite of their less rigorous designs, both quasi-experimental and observational studies are used to evaluate the effectiveness of interventions, often due to ethical or pragmatic reasons related to the use of patients in research. In addition, observational designs are used to answer questions about diagnostic tests, prognostic indicators, and patient/client outcomes.

Below quasi-experimental and observational designs on the continuum are research efforts that focus only on cellular, anatomical, or physiological systems. These studies often have a high degree of control because they are grounded in the scientific method that is the hallmark of good bench research. They are lower on the continuum not because of their potential for bias, but because they do not focus on person level function. For this reason they are referred to as *physiologic studies*.[4]

Even lower on the continuum are case reports and narrative reviews. These study approaches have different purposes. *Case reports* simply describe what occurred with a patient/client while *narrative reviews* summarize prior research.[2,7] In spite of these differences, these designs have one common element that puts them both at the bottom of the continuum: they lack a systematic approach to the issue or topic of interest. It is important to note, however, that the content of a case report or narrative review may provide a stimulus to conduct a more rigorous research project. Table 2-2 provides a list of citations from physical therapy literature that represent each type of study design described here.

Table 2-2 Citations from physical therapy research illustrating different study designs.[15]

Study Design	Citation
Systematic Review	Milne S, Brosseau L, Robinson V, Noel MJ, Davis J *et al.* Continuous passive motion following total knee arthroplasty. *Cochrane Database Syst Rev.* 2003; (2):CD004260.
Randomized Clinical Trial	Johansson KM, Adolfsson LE, Foldevi MOM. Effects of acupuncture versus ultrasound in patients with impingement syndrome: randomized clinical trial. *Phys Ther.* 2005; 85(6):490–501.
Single-System Design	Carr S, Fairleigh A, Backman C. Use of continuous passive motion to increase hand range of motion in a woman with scleroderma: a single-subject study. *Physiother Can.* 1997; 49(4):292–296.
Quasi-Experimental Study	Kileff J, Ashburn A. A pilot study of the effect of aerobic exercise on people with moderate disability multiple sclerosis. *Clin Rehabil.* 2005; 19(2):165–169.
Observational Study	Kirk-Sanchez NJ. Factors related to activity limitations in a group of Cuban Americans before and after hip fracture. *Phys Ther.* 2004; 84(5):408–418.
Physiologic Study	DeSimone NA, Christiansen C, Dore D. Bactericidal effect of 0.95-mW helium-neon and 5-mW indium-gallium-aluminum-phosphate laser irradiation at exposure times of 30, 60, and 120 seconds on photosensitized *Staphylococcus aureus* and *Pseudomonas aeruginosa* in vitro. *Phys Ther.* 1999; 79(9):839–846.
Case Report	Shrader JA, Siegel KL. Nonoperative management of functional hallux limitus in a patient with rheumatoid arthritis. *Phys Ther.* 2003; 83(9):831–843.
Summary	Ciesla ND. Chest physical therapy for patients in the intensive care unit. *Phys Ther.* 1996; 76(6):609–625.

Research Designs–Timing

Research designs also may be categorized according to the time line used in the study. For example, physical therapy researchers may want to know the relationship between the number of visits to an outpatient orthopedic clinic and the worker's compensation insurance status of patients treated over a three-year period. Such a question may be answered through a historical analysis of three years of patient records from the clinic. This *retrospective* approach has as an opposite form—a *prospective design*—in which the investigators collect data over time from new patients that are admitted to the clinic.

In a similar fashion, researchers may be interested in a single point in time or a limited time interval (e.g., *cross-sectional study*) or they may wish to study a phenomenon over a period of time (e.g., *longitudinal study*). In the cross-sectional approach, investigators may have an interest in the outcome at discharge from the hospital of patients receiving physical therapy following total hip replacement. On the other hand, a longitudinal approach would include follow-up of these patients to assess outcomes at discharge *and* at a specified point or points in time in the future (e.g., 3 months, 6 months, 1 year).

The sequence of events across time in a study is important, particularly when an investigator is trying to determine whether a change in the patient/client's condition was the direct result of the intervention or preventive measure applied. Specifically, the intervention must have occurred *before* the outcome was measured in order to increase one's confidence that it was the technique of interest that made a difference in the subjects.

Research Designs–What Is the Question?

Remember that the clinical question the physical therapist wants to answer will determine which of these forms of evidence to seek. For example, a question about the best test to identify a rotator cuff tear (diagnosis) is likely to be addressed by a cross-sectional observational study of patients that are suspected to have the problem based on clinical exam. On the other hand, a question about risk factors for falls in the elderly may be answered in one of two ways: 1) a longitudinal study in which two groups of elderly subjects are followed to determine who falls and who does not, or 2) a retrospective study that starts with subjects with documented falls and evaluates possible precipitating characteristics (e.g., visual deficits) in comparison to nonfallers. Finally, a question about the effectiveness of joint mobilization in the management of neck pain is best answered by a prospective randomized clinical trial of patients classified with neck pain. Physical therapists should anticipate these differences when planning their search strategies in order to increase the efficiency of the process.

One must also recall that a search for the "best available clinical evidence" may result in the discovery of research that is limited in content and/or quality. In other words, the current state of knowledge in an area may be such that the best (and only) evidence available is from studies in which the chance of bias is higher because of weaknesses in the research designs. Physical therapists will find this scenario to be true for many of the clinical questions they pose in practice. This reality is not a reason to reject evidence-based physical therapy practice; rather, it is a reaffirmation that clinical judgment and experience are required in order to decide how to use evidence that is limited in form.

HIERARCHIES OF EVIDENCE

Previous research has identified a number of barriers to using evidence in physical therapy practice, one of which is the lack of time available to search for, select, and read professional literature.[12] The selection process may be eased somewhat by ranking research designs based on their ability to minimize bias. Proponents of evidence-based medicine have attempted to make the study selection process easier by developing hierarchies, or levels, of evidence.[13] Guyatt and colleagues have focused on a hierarchy for studies about treatment[4] while Sackett *et al.*[14(p.6)] and the Oxford Center for Evidence-Based Medicine in the United Kingdom[15] have developed separate hierarchies for diagnosis, prognosis, treatment, and economic and decision analysis studies. The variety of hierarchies is necessary because of the point made previously: different research designs are required to answer different types of clinical questions. Understanding the nuances of each hierarchy is an important skill to develop in order to use them appropriately.

The remainder of this chapter focuses on the hierarchies adapted from the Oxford Center for Evidence-Based Medicine Web site.[15] Table 2–3 depicts the hierarchy for intervention papers. All of the hierarchies are included in Appendix A.

These ranking schemes are similar to one another in that they place systematic reviews at the top of each list. Systematic reviews are valued because they may produce conclusions based on a critical appraisal of a number of individual studies that have been selected according to pre-established criteria. Ideally, the studies reviewed: have research designs that minimize the chance of bias (e.g., "high quality evidence"), are pertinent to the therapist's question, and provide a more definitive answer to the question. This ideal is akin to the "holy grail" in evidence-based practice; however, systematic reviews also have their limitations as will be discussed in Chapter 14.

At the other end of each hierarchy are several forms of evidence that are least desirable because of their potential for bias or because of their lack of focus on patient/client level information, including:

- Expert opinion without critical appraisal;
- Anecdotal evidence;
- Physiologic studies; and,
- Studies based only on biological plausibility.

Clinicians who locate studies that fall into this level of evidence must identify, and consider the implications and limitations for, each study type when

Table 2–3 Hierarchy of evidence for articles about therapy.[15]

Level	Therapy/Prevention, Etiology/Harm
1a	• Systematic Review of Randomized Clinical Trials that *do not* have statistically significant variation in the direction or degrees of results
1b	• Individual Randomized Clinical Trial with narrow confidence interval
1c	• All-or-none study[a]
2a	• Systematic Review of Cohort Studies [b] that *do not* have statistically significant variation in the direction or degrees of results
2b	• Individual Cohort Study (including low quality Randomized Clinical Trial; e.g., <80% subject follow-up)
2c	• "Outcomes" Research[c]
3a	• Systematic Review of Case-Control Studies[d] that *do not* have statistically significant variation in the direction or degrees of results
3b	• Individual Case-Control Study
4	• Case-Series Study[e]
	• Cohort or Case-Control Study that did not
	– define comparison groups adequately; or,
	– did not measure exposures and outcomes objectively or in a blinded fashion; or,
	– control for confounders; or,
	– have sufficient follow-up (cohort studies only)
5	• Expert Opinion without explicit critical appraisal, or based on physiology, bench research, or "first principles"[f]

a. *All-or-none Study:* A study in which some or all patients died before treatment became available, and then none die after the treatment.

b. *Cohort Study:* In intervention papers, a prospective research design used to evaluate the relationship between a treatment and an outcome; two groups of subjects—one of which receives the intervention and one of which does not—are monitored over time to determine who develops the outcome and who does not. This label also could be applied to quasi-experimental and non-experimental research designs in which two non-randomized groups of subjects are evaluated.

c. *Outcomes Research:* Non-experimental research that evaluates outcomes of care in "real world" clinical conditions.

d. *Case-Control Study:* A retrospective epidemiological research design used to evaluate the relationship between a potential risk factor and a disease or disorder; two groups of subjects—one of which has the disease/disorder (the case) and one which does not (the control)—are compared to determine which group has a greater proportion of individuals with the risk factor.

e. *Case Series:* A description of the management of several patients/clients for the same purposes as a case report; the use of multiple individuals increases the potential importance of the observations as the basis for future research.

f. *First Principles:* Biologically plausible rationales for management of pathophysiology.

Source: Adapted with permission from Oxford Center for Evidence-Based Medicine (www.cebm.net).

deciding whether to use the information with a patient/client. Despite their limitations, however, it is worth noting that these study types are included in the hierarchies because they constitute evidence.

Details for each level between these end points on the hierarchies vary because of the types of questions being addressed; however, some additional common themes can be identified. First, level of rank depends upon the strength of the study design. For example, a randomized clinical trial is highly ranked because it is a more rigorous research design than an observational study for investigation of the therapeutic effects of joint mobilization in patients with neck pain. Second, individual studies with strong designs are ranked more highly than systematic reviews of studies with weaker designs. For example, a single prospective study of fall risk in the elderly that includes a comprehensive list of predisposing factors for falls is more valuable than a systematic review of retrospective studies that failed to include medications, living environment, and mental status as potential contributors to fall risk. Third, systematic reviews of studies with similar directions and degrees of results (e.g., subjects improved in most studies) are ranked higher as a result of this homogeneity than systematic reviews of studies with significant variation in their individual findings (e.g., subjects improved in some studies and not others). Figure 2–1 summarizes the commonalities among evidence hierarchies.

Selection of studies through the use of hierarchies may improve the efficiency of the search process for busy clinicians. These schemas also are used regularly to grade evidence in order to facilitate the decision-making process about which information to use. This strategy is most apparent in published clinical guidelines. National and international government agencies and professional associations produce guidelines in an effort to promote effective and efficient health care. A few examples relevant to physical therapy include the:

- Agency for Healthcare Policy and Research's (AHCPR) clinical practice guideline "Treatment of Pressure Ulcers" (1994);[16]

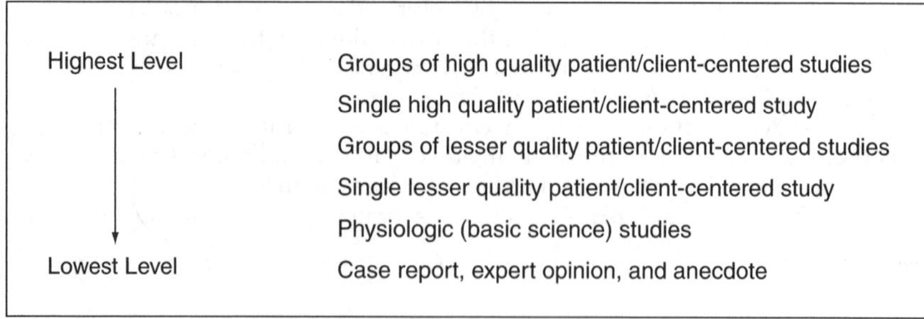

Figure 2–1 General ranking of evidence within hierarchies.

- American College of Chest Physicians & American Association of Cardiovascular & Pulmonary Rehabilitation's "Pulmonary rehabilitation: joint ACCP/AACVPR evidence-based guidelines" (1997);[17]
- The Ottawa Panel Evidence-Based Clinical Practice Guidelines for Therapeutic Exercises in the Management of Rheumatoid Arthritis in Adults (2004).[18]

Each of these documents, as well as numerous other similar publications, contain recommendations based upon a review and ranking of available evidence. Grading schemes are described in the guidelines and are used to qualify the recommendations made. For example, the AHCPR assigned the letter grades A, B, and C based upon the quality and quantity of the evidence. The letter "A" is the highest designation and signifies that a recommendation in the guideline is supported by "two or more randomized controlled clinical trials on pressure ulcers in humans."[16(p. 24)] The letters "B" and "C" indicate that recommendations are supported by fewer studies and/or by studies with weaker designs as compared to randomized trials. In fact, the letter "C" also includes "expert opinion" as an option.

In theory, physical therapists using any of these guidelines could go straight to the recommendations and make decisions about how to change their practice based upon these evidence grades. However, there are several limitations to these levels that should be recognized before a clinician blindly adopts the practice behaviors addressed in the guidelines.

Limitations of Evidence Hierarchies

In 2002, the Agency for Healthcare Research and Quality (formerly known as the Agency for Healthcare Policy and Research) published an evidence report entitled "Systems to Rate the Strength of Scientific Evidence."[13] The authors of this report performed an extensive literature review to identify quality assessment methods used to assess the strength of evidence for systematic reviews and meta-analyses, randomized controlled trials, observational studies, and diagnostic studies, as well as methods for evaluating the strength of an entire body of evidence on a particular topic. In addition, they examined evidence evaluation methods used by agency-sponsored Evidence-based Practice Centers and other organizations focused on evidence-based medicine, such as the Cochrane Collaboration.

Of the 121 systems reviewed, only 26 fully addressed quality criteria established by the authors for each type of study. Many of these lengthy systems required an inconvenient amount of time to complete. Also noted was the greater number of quality assessment methods for randomized controlled trials as compared to other types of research. The other 95 assessment methods the authors reviewed were limited either in the quality domains addressed, by a "one-size-fits-all" approach that did not distinguish among critical features of different study designs, or by lack of validation. Few of the methods had been tested for reliability. The take home message from this report is that the strength of evidence depends, in part, on the scale against which it is being rated. In response to the potential misuse of evidence grading systems, Glasziou *et al.* suggested that quality ratings or scales should address different types of research and would be improved by the addition of qualitative statements, as well as details regarding ratings criteria.[19]

Understanding the details and bases for evidence hierarchies will help physical therapists select evidence to answer clinical questions about patients/clients. However, a hierarchy is only a tool to facilitate the process; it should not be used to make a final judgment about a study's value and relevance. Physical therapists must still read and critically appraise the evidence they find before incorporating any results into their clinical decisions. This point is emphasized by an ongoing debate about the relative merits of RCTs versus quasi-experimental and observational studies. Some evidence indicates that the bias in the latter study designs results in overestimations of treatment effects, whereas other authors have reported that none of the study designs consistently estimate an intervention's impact.[20,21] As noted in Chapter 1, clinical judgment and expertise are essential to evidence-based physical therapy. The variability in research quality requires that physical therapists use their knowledge and skills to determine whether the evidence they find, no matter how high or low on a hierarchy, is useful for an individual patient/client.

SUMMARY

Evidence-based physical therapy practice requires clinicians to select the "best available evidence" from studies whose quality depends upon their relevance to the question asked, their timeliness, and the level of prior scrutiny of their merits, as well as upon their research design and execution. Evidence hierarchies may facilitate study selection because of the ranking structure they create based on important research attributes. Different hierarchies have been designed to address evidence about diagnosis, prognosis, and intervention. Producers of clinical guidelines also have defined various levels of evidence to demonstrate the degree to which their recommendations are supported by research. No matter what form a hierarchy takes, it is only a tool to facilitate the process; it should not be used to make a final judgment about a study's value and relevance. Physical therapists must still read and critically appraise the evidence they find before incorporating any results into their clinical decisions.

Exercises

1. What does the phrase "best available clinical evidence" mean with respect to a physical therapist's selection and use of studies?
2. Discuss the differences between a randomized controlled trial and an observational study. Under which circumstances might each study design be appropriate?
3. Discuss the difference between cross-sectional and longitudinal studies and give an example of each that reflects a study question relevant to physical therapy.
4. Describe the common organizational characteristics of evidence hierarchies.
5. Discuss the rationale behind the creation of different hierarchies for evidence about diagnosis, prognosis, and intervention.
6. Discuss the limitations of evidence hierarchies. Why is a hierarchy only a starting point in evidence-based physical therapy practice?

References

1. Helewa A, Walker JM. *Critical Evaluation of Research in Physical Rehabilitation: Towards Evidence-Based Practice.* Philadelphia, PA: W.B. Saunders Company; 2000.
2. McEwen I. *Writing Case Reports: A How-to Manual for Clinicians.* 2d ed. Alexandria, VA: American Physical Therapy Association; 2001.
3. Straus SE, Richardson WS, Glaziou P, Haynes RB. *Evidence-Based Medicine: How to Practice and Teach EBM.* 3d ed. Edinburgh, Scotland: Elsevier Churchill Livingstone; 2005.
4. Guyatt G, Rennie D. *Users' Guides to the Medical Literature: A Manual for Evidence-Based Clinical Practice.* Chicago, IL: AMA Press; 2002.
5. Domholdt E. *Rehabilitation Research: Principles and Applications.* 3d ed. St Louis, MO: Elsevier Saunders; 2005.
6. Campbell DT, Stanley JC. *Experimental and Quasi-experimental Designs for Research.* Boston, MA: Houghton Mifflin Company; 1963.
7. Herbert R, Jamtvedt G, Mead J, Hagen KB. *Practical Evidence-Based Physical Therapy.* Edinburgh, Scotland: Elsevier Butterworth Heinemann; 2005.
8. Cook TD, Campbell DT. *Quasi-experimentation: Design and Analysis Issues for Field Settings.* Boston, MA: Houghton Mifflin Company; 1979.
9. Sackett DL, Rosenberg WMC, Gray JAM, Haynes RB, Richardson WS. "Evidence-based medicine: What it is and what it isn't." *BMJ.* 1996; 312(7023):71–72.
10. Comparing the Disease-Modifying Drugs. National Multiple Sclerosis Society Web site. Available at: http://www.nationalmssociety.org/Brochures-Comparing.asp. Accessed February 15, 2006.
11. Winstein CJ, Lewthwaite R. *Efficacy and Effectiveness: Issues for Physical Therapy Practice and Research. Examples from PTClinResNet.* Eugene Michels Forum. Combined Sections Meeting. American Physical Therapy Association. 2004.

Available at: http://pt.usc.edu/clinresnet/CSM04/Eugene%20Michels%20pdf%20files/Winstein%20EM%202004.pdf. Accessed February 15, 2006.

12. Jette DU, Bacon K, Batty C, Carlson M, Ferland A *et al.* Evidence-based practice: Beliefs, attitudes, knowledge, and behaviors of physical therapists. *Phys Ther.* 2003; 83(9):786–805.
13. West S, King V, Carey TS, Lohr KN, McKoy N *et al. Systems to Rate the Strength of Scientific Evidence.* Evidence Report/Technology Assessment Number 47 (Prepared by the Research Triangle Institute–University of North Carolina Evidence-Based Practice Center under Contract No. 290-97-0011.). AHRQ Publication No. 02-E016. Rockville, MD: Agency for Health Care Research and Quality; April 2002.
14. Sackett DL, Straus SE, Richardson WS, Rosenberg W, Haynes RB. *Evidence-Based Medicine: How to Practice and Teach EBM.* 2d ed. Edinburgh, Scotland: Churchill Livingstone; 2000.
15. Levels of Evidence. Oxford Center for Evidence-Based Medicine Web site. Available at: www.cebm.net. Accessed July 15, 2005.
16. Guidelines for Treatment of Pressure Ulcers. Agency for Health Care Policy and Research Web site. Available at: http://www.guideline.gov/summary/summary.aspx?ss=15&doc_id=810&nbr=8. Accessed July 15, 2005.
17. Pulmonary Rehabilitation: Joint ACCP/AACVPR Evidence-Based Guidelines. Available at: http://www.chestjournal.org/cgi/reprint/112/5/1363.pdf. Accessed July 15, 2005.
18. Ottawa Panel Evidence-Based Clinical Practice Guidelines for Therapeutic Exercises in the Management of Rheumatoid Arthritis in Adults. *Phys Ther.* 2004; 84(10):934–972.
19. Glasziou P, Vandenbroucke J, Chalmer I. Assessing the quality of research. *BMJ.* 2004; 328(7430):39–41.
20. Britton A, McKee M, Black N, McPherson K, Sanderson C *et al.* Choosing between randomized and non-randomised studies: A systematic review. *Health Technol Assess.* 1998; 2(13):i–iv, 1–124.
21. MacLehose RR, Reeves BC, Harvey IM, Sheldon TA, Russell IT *et al.* A systematic review of comparisons of effect sizes derived from randomised and non-randomised studies. *Health Technol Assess.* 2000; 4(34):1–154.

Chapter 3

The Quest for Evidence: Getting Started

The outcome of any serious research can only be to make two questions grow where only one grew before.

—Thorstein Veblen

Objectives

Upon completion of this chapter the student/practitioner will be able to:

1. Distinguish between, and provide examples of, background and foreground clinical questions.
2. Write questions pertaining to physical therapy:
   a) Diagnostic tests and measures;
   b) Prognoses;
   c) Interventions;
   d) Outcomes.
3. Use electronic databases reviewed in this chapter to search for evidence about a clinical question.
4. Identify research review services that may be helpful in physical therapy practice.

Terms in This Chapter:

Boolean: The words AND, OR, NOT and NEAR; used to combine search terms in electronic evidence databases and other search engines.

Diagnosis: "A process that integrates and evaluates data" obtained during a patient/client examination, often resulting in a classification that guides prognosis, the plan of care, and subsequent interventions.[1,2(p. 45)]

Examination: "A comprehensive screening and specific testing process leading to diagnostic classification or, as appropriate, referral to another practitioner."[1(p. 42)]

"Hits": A term used to indicate the records retrieved by an electronic search engine that meet the criteria entered into the search function.

Intervention: The purposeful use of various physical therapy procedures and techniques, in collaboration with the patient/client and, when appropriate, other care providers, in order to effect a change in the patient/client's condition.[1]

Keyword(s): The word(s) or term(s) that is/are entered into an electronic database search function to locate evidence pertaining to a clinical question.

MeSH: "Medical subject heading;" the term used to describe approved search vocabulary in the U.S. National Library of Medicine electronic database (PubMed); may be used by other electronic evidence databases.

Outcome: "The end result of patient/client management, which include the impact of physical therapy interventions;" may be measured by the physical therapist or determined by self-report from the patient/client.[1(p. 43)]

Prognosis: Prediction of the natural course of a disease or condition, or its development based upon previously-identified risk factors; also, "the predicted optimal level of improvement through intervention and the amount of time required to achieve that level."[1(p. 46)]

Search String: A combination of keywords, phrases, names, or other information that is entered into an electronic database search function to locate evidence pertaining to a clinical question.

INTRODUCTION

Chapter 1 proposed that the first step toward evidence-based physical therapy practice is a professional commitment to make the attempt as best one can given individual work environments and resource constraints. Once that commitment is made the next step is to consider the questions that arise during the daily management of a patient/client's problems or needs. These questions direct the search for evidence that may inform clinical decision making. This chapter focuses on the types of questions physical therapists and their patients/clients might ask and describes several electronic databases and search techniques that are available to support the quest for evidence.

FORMULATING CLINICAL QUESTIONS

Evidence-based physical therapy practice starts and ends with a physical therapist's patient or client. As the therapeutic relationship develops, questions naturally arise regarding the patient/client's problems and concerns and the best course of action with which to address them. Questions may pertain to: 1) the anatomic, physiologic, or pathophysiologic nature of the problem or issue; 2) the medical and surgical management options; 3) the usefulness of diagnostic tests and measures to identify, classify, and/or quantify the problem; 4) which factors will predict the patient/client's future health status; 5) the benefits and risks of potential interventions; and/or 6) the nature of the outcomes themselves and how to measure them. Any of these questions may prompt a search for evidence to help inform the answer.

When formulating a clinical question it is important to consider how that question is phrased. Questions that are designed to increase understanding about a situation (such as #1 & #2 above) are different than questions used to facilitate clinical decision making (#3–#6). These different forms are referred to as "background questions" and "foreground questions," respectively.[3,4]

Background Questions

Background questions reflect a desire to understand the nature of a patient/client's problem or need. Often these questions focus on the medical aspects of the situation rather than on the physical therapy component. Here are some examples:

- "What are the side effects of steroid treatment for asthma?"
- "How long will it take for a total knee arthoplasty incision to heal?"
- "What are the signs and symptoms of an exacerbation of multiple sclerosis?"
- "Will it be possible to play baseball again after elbow surgery?"

Understandably, these are the most common types of questions patients/clients and their families will ask. In addition, these questions are typical of physical therapy students and new graduates who are still learning about the many clinical scenarios they may encounter in practice. Experienced clinicians, on the other hand, will use background questions when a new or unusual situation is encountered, when entering a new practice area, or when returning to practice after a significant absence. Answers to background questions help therapists to understand the clinical context of their patient's situation so that an individual's needs can be anticipated and planned for accordingly. Precautions, contraindications, exercise limits, and other parameters may be determined based on evidence gathered to answer background questions.

Foreground Questions

Foreground questions are the meat of evidence-based physical therapy practice. These questions help clinicians and their patient/clients make decisions about the specific physical therapy management of the problem or issue. Foreground questions contain four key elements:[3,4]

- Patient/client details such as age, gender, diagnosis, acuity, severity, and/or preferences
- A specific test, predictive factor, intervention, or outcome
- [A comparison test, predictive factor, intervention, or outcome]
- The consequence of interest for the test, prediction, intervention, or outcome

The first and second components are included because a good foreground question has sufficient detail to search for answers that are specific to the patient/client about whom the question is asked. The third component, a comparison, is in brackets because there may be times when a simpler question is indicated or when a comparison simply is not available. Clinicians with more expertise in a particular content area may find it easier to ask comparative questions by virtue of their knowledge about a variety of options for tests and measures, predictive factors, interventions, and outcomes. Finally, the fourth component refers to what the therapist or patient/client hopes to achieve during the management step about which the question is raised.

Although questions about diagnosis, prognosis, interventions, and outcomes have this basic structure in common, they also have unique features that are important to recognize. The following sections outline details about each type of question. Table 3–1 provides examples of simple and comparative questions for each content area.

Clinical Questions about Diagnosis

Diagnosis is a process by which physical therapists label and classify a patient/client's problem or need.[1] Tests and measures used during the physical therapy examination provide the objective data for the diagnostic process. Clinical questions about diagnosis usually focus on which tests or measures will provide the most precise and accurate information in a timely manner with the least amount of risk, cost, or both.

Clinical Questions about Prognosis

Prognosis is the process by which therapists make predictions about the future health status of patients/clients.[1] Questions about prognosis arise because therapists and patients/clients want to know which pieces of information—collectively referred to as indicators, predictors, or factors—are most important to consider when predicting the outcomes of preventive

Table 3–1 Clinical questions physical therapists might ask about diagnostic tests and measures, prognosis, interventions, and outcomes.

	Foreground Questions–Simple	Foreground Questions–Comparative
Diagnosis	• Will the "Neer's" test help me detect rotator cuff impingement in a 35-year-old male tennis player with shoulder pain?	• Is the "Neer's" test more accurate than the "Lift Off" test for detecting rotator cuff impingement in a 35-year-old male tennis player with shoulder pain?
Prognosis	• Is muscle strength a predictor of fall risk in a 76-year-old female with diabetes?	• Which is a better predictor of fall risk, muscle strength or proprioception, in a 76-year-old female with diabetes?
Intervention	• Is proprioceptive neuromuscular facilitation (PNF) an effective treatment technique for restoring core trunk stability in a 7-year-old child with right hemiparesis due to stroke?	• Is PNF more effective than the neurodevelopmental technique (NDT) for restoring core trunk stability in a 7-year-old child with right hemiparesis due to stroke?
Outcomes	• Does participation in a cardiac rehabilitation program increase the chance that a 58-year-old man will return to work following a myocardial infarction?	• Does participation in a cardiac rehabilitation program increase the chances of returning to work more than a home walking program in a 58-year-old man following myocardial infarction?
Outcomes	• Will the Minnesota Living with Heart Failure Questionnaire detect change following rehabilitation in a 82-year-old woman with chronic congestive heart failure?	• Is the Minnesota Living with Heart Failure Questionnaire better than the Chronic Heart Failure Questionnaire for detecting change following rehabilitation in an 82-year-old woman with chronic congestive heart failure?

activities, interventions, or inaction. Predictors often take the form of demographic information such as age, gender, race/ethnicity, income, education, and social support; disorder-related information such as stage, severity, time since onset, recurrence, and compliance with a treatment program; and/or, the presence of comorbid conditions.[4]

Clinical Questions about Interventions

Interventions are the techniques and procedures physical therapists use to produce a change in the patient/client.[1] Clinical questions about interventions may focus on the benefits or risks of a treatment technique, or both. The goal is identify which treatment approaches will provide the desired effect in a manner that is consistent with the patient/client's preferences and values. Additional objectives may include a desire to minimize costs and expedite the treatment process.

Clinical Questions about Outcomes

Outcomes are the end results of the patient/client management process.[1] Questions about outcomes may focus on the type of end point(s) possible in response to a particular treatment or on the methods by which the end point can be measured. Outcomes are likely to have the most relevance for a patient/client when they pertain to functional abilities as performed in the context of the individual's daily life. Of particular clinical interest, is the usefulness of self-report instruments that measure outcomes from the patient/client's point of view. These tools usually focus on the impact of a disorder or problem on the individual's health-related quality of life. An ideal instrument captures relevant information, is responsive to change in a patient/client's status, and is logistically reasonable to administer and process.

SEARCHING FOR EVIDENCE

Once a patient/client-centered clinical question is formulated, it is important to plan a general strategy for a search before delving into the various sources of evidence available. The following five steps are recommended as a starting point.

Determine Which Database Will Be Most Useful

There are an enormous variety of sources through which a physical therapist may search for evidence, many of which are available through the Internet. As these electronic databases have proliferated, their focus areas have evolved. Some are broad-based and cover any type of question, while others only focus on interventions. Some databases list citations of original works, while others provide synopses or reviews of research articles. Some only address physical therapy research, while yet others cover medical and allied health topics. Familiarity with the options will help a physical therapist select the database that will provide citations for evidence about the clinical question in an efficient manner.

Readers may be tempted to use more general Internet search engines such as Yahoo or Google because they are familiar to frequent Web users. These services are helpful for numerous reasons, but locating evidence to inform physical therapy practice decisions is not one of them. First, they are not designed to search efficiently through a designated collection of resources devoted to medical or physical therapy practice. Second, they do not have clinically relevant search features, such as the ability to restrict the search according to patient characteristics or type of article or year of publication. These limitations mean that evidence to answer a question may be missed or irrelevant information may be returned. Third, they may or may not provide access to the online journals in which the evidence is published. As a result, evidence-based physical therapists should spend the time necessary to learn the features of the databases described below and save Yahoo and Google for other types of searches.

Identify Search Terms to Enter into the Database

All electronic databases and search engines require input from the user to start the search. The most common form of input is a *keyword* or search term that the database will use to identify relevant information. In evidence-based physical therapy practice the keywords are derived directly from the clinical question of interest. Consider the following example:

> "Does age and prior functional status predict discharge to home following inpatient rehabilitation for a fractured hip in a 92-year-old woman?"

Possible keywords from this question include "age," "predict," "discharge," "home," "inpatient," "rehabilitation," "fracture," "hip," and "woman." Additional terms may be used to reflect concepts in the question such as "function" instead of "functional status" and "elderly" in place of "92-year-old." Finally, some of the words may be combined into phrases—such as "inpatient rehabilitation" and "hip fracture"—to provide a more accurate representation of the question's content.

The challenge is to determine which of these keywords and phrases are the best to use because using all of them would be inefficient. One option is to start simply by using a few words or phrases, such as "predict," "discharge," and "hip fracture." This approach may improve the chances of identifying a wide variety of evidence because of the general nature of the terms. However, the question addresses specific predictive factors, namely age and prior functional status, in an elderly woman. The second option, therefore, is to include more keywords or phrases to narrow the search to evidence directly addressing the question.

In addition to these decisions, therapists also should consider other synonyms that may be useful or necessary to enhance the search. Relevant synonyms in this example include "femur" for "hip" and "female" for "woman." Synonyms will come in handy when a search for evidence returns no citations. Evidence databases usually have specific keyword vocabularies that are used to perform searches. Familiarity with these vocabularies is essential to optimize the efficiency of the search.

Use the Database Features to Streamline the Search

Every electronic database has rules that determine which keywords it will recognize and what letter size (case) and punctuation must be used when entering search terms. Words such as "and," "or," "not," and "near"—collectively referred to as *booleans*—are used universally to create search term combinations. The databases also contain options to limit or to expand the search. "Limiters" or "expanders" often include choice of language, publication date, type of research design, and search basis such as keyword, author, or journal name. There also may be choices available regarding subject characteristics, such as age and gender. Selecting from these options allows the user to keep the number of search terms to a minimum because the search function is "programmed" to work within the specified parameters. Finally, a method for including synonyms or related terms (referred to as "exploding" the search term) usually is available. Some electronic databases will make these rules and choices apparent by the way that they format their search pages. Others require some effort to hunt for the information through the "search help" features. In either case, spending some time on the front end learning these details will save time and frustration during the search.

Be Prepared to Reformulate the Question

A common problem during an evidence search is either excessive numbers of citations (or *"hits"*) or none at all. When this situation happens, the first thing to do is go back to the database features and determine if there are additional options to narrow or expand the search. Keyword and phrase substitutions also may be required. If these approaches are unsuccessful, then it may be time to revise the question. Consider the following example:

> "Which is more effective for symptom relief, land-based or aquatic exercise, in a middle-aged man with joint pain?"

Too many hits using keywords from this question likely indicates that the question is too broad. There are several options for revising the question into a more precise form, including:

1. Using a more specific diagnostic label such as degenerative joint disease or rheumatoid arthritis;
2. Adding more specific details about the patient/client, such as his age; or,
3. Using a more specific outcome, such as pain relief.

A revised question might read:

> "Which is more effective for pain relief, land-based or aquatic exercise, in a 58-year-old man diagnosed with rheumatoid arthritis?"

On the other hand, too few hits may indicate that the question is too specific, or, that there is no evidence yet available to answer it. In that case a broader question may be useful, such as:

> "Is exercise effective for pain relief in a man with arthritis?"

Keep in mind that as questions become more general, there is a greater chance that the evidence located will contain information that is not directly related to the current situation. For example, subjects in a study may be older than the patient or the intervention may be a home walking program rather than a program supervised in the clinic. In these situations physical therapists will be required to use their clinical judgment to determine whether the study is relevant and whether there is enough in common between the patient/client and the subjects studied to extrapolate the results to this specific situation.

In extreme cases there may be difficulty finding any physical therapy-related evidence for a patient/client's disease, disorder or need. Physical therapy management of the sequelae of heart disease is a common example of such a situation. In these instances it may be helpful to search for evidence that includes medical professionals other than physical therapists (e.g., exercise physiologists or nurses). Once again, clinical judgment will be required to determine if it is safe and appropriate to extrapolate and apply any findings from this general evidence to an individual patient/client.

Aim for the Highest Quality Evidence Available

There are two general sources of evidence: primary and secondary. Primary sources provide original research reports via peer-reviewed journals, theses and dissertations, proceedings from professional meetings, and Web sites. Secondary sources such as textbooks, summaries on Web sites, and review papers contain information that is based on primary sources.[5] Understandably, primary sources of evidence are preferred because they provide the original work about which the physical therapist can make an independent critical appraisal. One form of secondary source evidence, the systematic review, also is valued because of the comprehensive and rigorous methodology used to search for, select, and appraise original works about a paritcular topic. As discussed in Chapter 2, evidence hierarchies have been developed to expedite the process of identifying high-quality evidence from primary and secondary sources.

ELECTRONIC DATABASES FOR EVIDENCE-BASED PHYSICAL THERAPY PRACTICE

As mentioned above, a variety of electronic databases are available to search for evidence. This section reviews important features of five that are likely to be most relevant to physical therapists. An entire textbook could be devoted to all of the details required to master searches in each database! Fortunately, there are numerous "help" and tutorial functions to guide a user through the process. Readers of this textbook should plan to spend time on the computer using these functions to learn more about each database and to explore the features highlighted here.

U.S. NATIONAL LIBRARY OF MEDICINE–PUBMED

The U.S. National Library of Medicine has developed a bibliographic database of basic and applied research citations dating back to the late 1800s. The electronic version, PubMed, contains over 15 million citations starting from the 1950s (Figure 3–1).[6]

Advantages of this search engine are that it:

1. is free to the public;
2. is comprehensive;
3. contains links to online journals that provide full text versions of articles;
4. has rigorous standards for determining which journals will be listed (indexed).

Challenges with the database include its size, the complexity of keyword searches, and its exclusion of many physical therapy and other allied health journals due to its indexing standards.

Search Limits

One method available to enhance the efficiency of a search in PubMed is to use the "Limits" function identified as a tab on the main search page (see

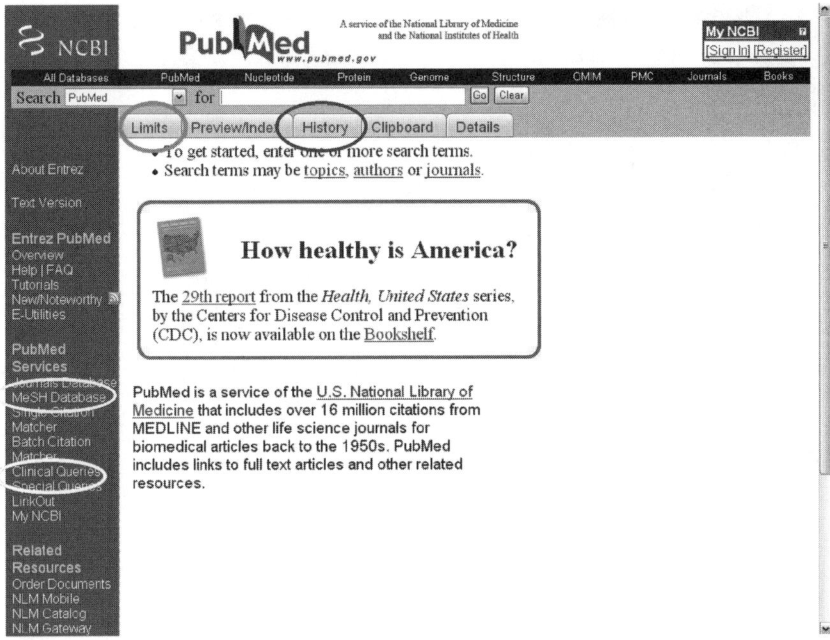

Figure 3–1 PubMed home page.

Source: Screenshot from PubMed (www.pubmed.gov), the U.S. National Library of Medicine, and the National Institutes of Health.

Figure 3–1). This feature provides a variety of drop-down menus to help direct a search (Figure 3–2).

Because EBPT is a patient/client-centered endeavor, it is often practical to select "human" for study subjects. Selection of the language choice "English" is helpful to avoid retrievals of evidence written in a foreign language in which the therapist is not fluent. Users may choose to restrict where the search engine looks for the keywords or phrases by selecting an option such as "title" or "title/abstract" so that only the most relevant hits will be identified; however, this tactic may result in missed citations because abstracts are limited in length and simply may not contain the keywords of interest. A search also may be restricted to author name or journal, among others, through this same limit menu. Other limit options include specifying the age range and gender of the subjects studied, the type of article (e.g., clinical trial, practice guideline, etc.), the date the citation was entered into PubMed, and the publication date of the article. Finally, the entire PubMed database will be searched unless directed otherwise by selecting from the "Subset" drop-down menu. Keep in mind that numerous limits

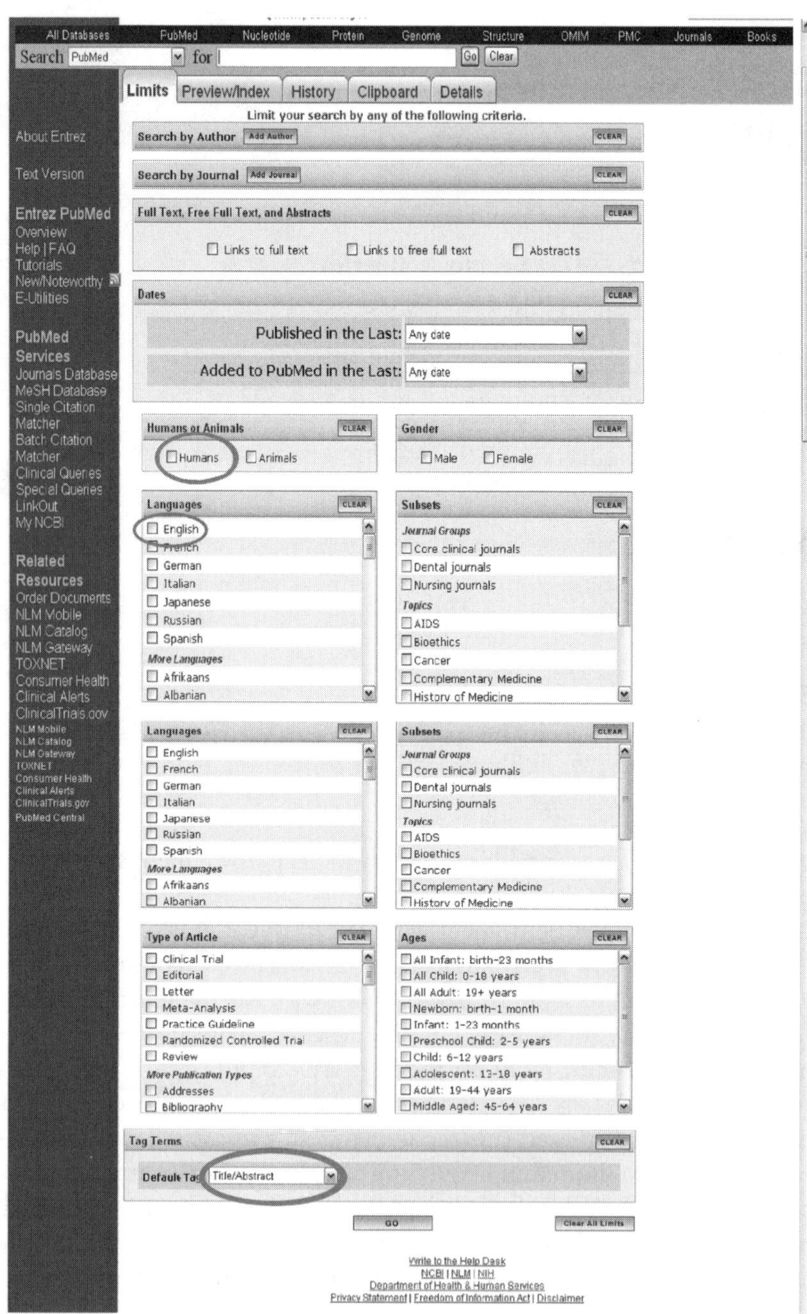

Figure 3–2 PubMed limits page.

Source: Screenshot from PubMed (www.pubmed.gov), the U.S. National Library of Medicine, and the National Institutes of Health.

may result in too few or no citations. If that is the case, then limits should be changed or removed one at a time and the search repeated.

Medical Subject Headings (MeSH)

The complexity of searches in PubMed relates to the database's use of the Medical Subject Heading (*MeSH*) vocabulary to determine which keywords will be recognized in the indexing process. As explained on the PubMed Web site, "MeSH terminology provides a consistent way to retrieve information that may use different terminology for the same concepts."[7] The MeSH database can be accessed through a link on the left hand-side of the PubMed home page (see Figure 3-1). Fortunately, the site provides brief user-friendly animated tutorials to quickly orient individuals to the MeSH function (Figure 3-3). Key features to understand include the ability to select subheadings under a MeSH term, as well as the ability to expand the search to include subcategories of MeSH terms.

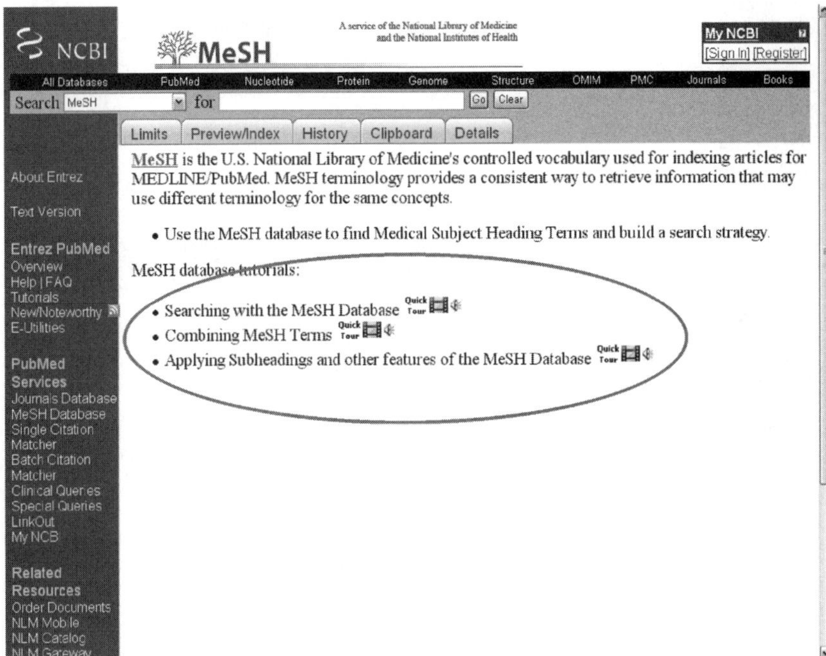

Figure 3-3 PubMed MeSH database page.

Source: Screenshot from PubMed (www.pubmed.gov), the U.S. National Library of Medicine, and the National Institutes of Health.

Recall the hypothetical clinical question: "Which is more effective for pain relief, land-based or aquatic exercise, in a 58-year-old man diagnosed with rheumatoid arthritis?" A search for the words "rheumatoid arthritis" and "exercise" reveals that both are listed in the MeSH vocabulary. The word "aquatic" is not recognized; however a synonym—"water"—is associated with 70 MeSH terms, the first of which is "hydrotherapy." "Hydrotherapy" is defined as the "external application of water for therapeutic purposes"[8] (Figure 3–4). This definition is consistent with the clinical question. Situations like these reinforce the need to think of synonyms for keywords before starting a search so that roadblocks to the process can be addressed efficiently. Figure 3–4 illustrates the search box with the selected MeSH vocabulary terms. Readers should note that when using the MeSH search box booleans are entered automatically and do not need to be typed in by the user.

Once the MeSH terms are selected a search can be executed along with any limits the user chooses. In this example the limits are "English," "humans,"

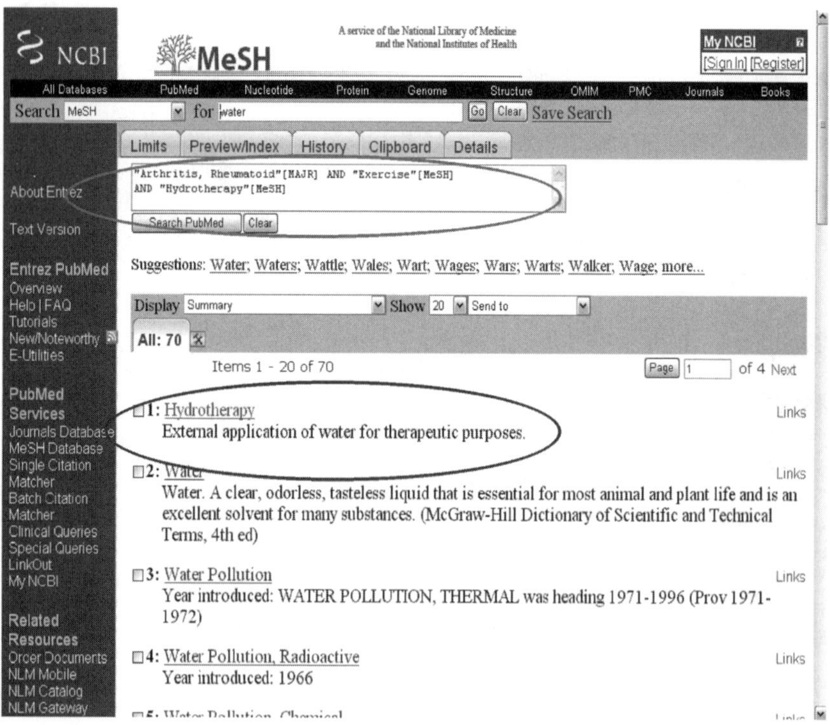

Figure 3–4 PubMed MeSH terms results page.

Source: Screenshot from PubMed (www.pubmed.gov), the U.S. National Library of Medicine, and the National Institutes of Health.

"middle-aged: 45–64," and "male." The first two options are selected for reasons described in the previous section. The age and gender selections are consistent with the patient in the question—a 58-year-old man. This attempt to be specific to the question results in two citations returned, one of which appears specific to the question asked (Figure 3–5). Removing the limit "male" results in four citations returned, two of which were located in the original search. The additional two articles are unrelated to the question or only focused on female subjects. Finally, removing "middle-aged: 45–64" results in eight citations, including the original two; however, these additional studies do not address the question asked.

With so few "hits" a different strategy is to subsitute a new MeSH term into the search box. The most obvious choice for amendment is the term "rheumatoid arthritis," which can be modified to the more general term "arthritis." Making this change results in four citations, two of which are in addition to those obtained in the original search. However, one article is about osteoarthritis and the other is over 30 years old. Alternatively, keeping "rheumatoid arthritis" and switching "hydrotherapy" to the MeSH term

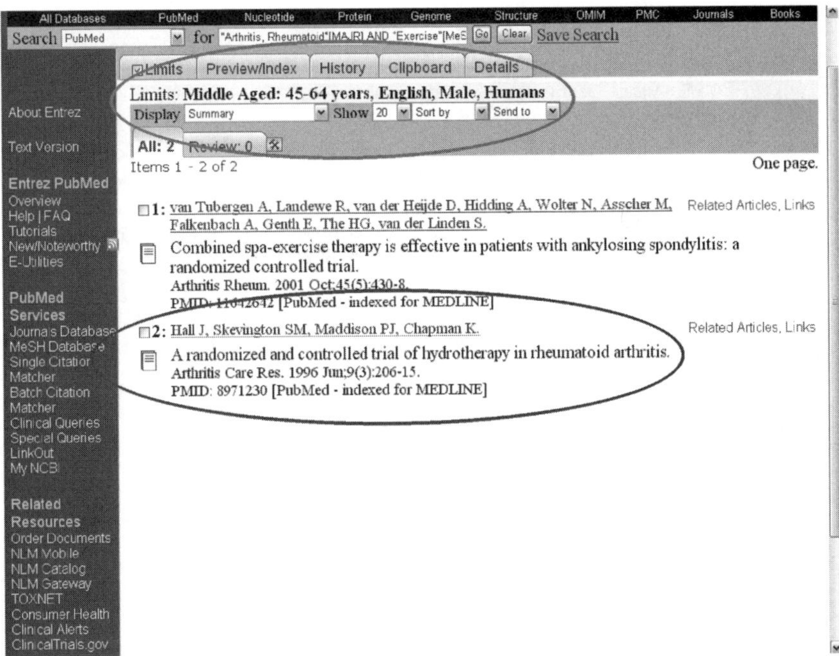

Figure 3–5 PubMed search results using MeSH terms.

Source: Screenshot from PubMed (www.pubmed.gov), the U.S. National Library of Medicine, and the National Institutes of Health.

"water" results in two citations, both of which are unrelated to the question. Finally, making both substitutions produced the same results as the previous search (Figure 3-6). Table 3-2 summarizes the steps taken to expand the search.

General Keyword Search

An alternative to using the MeSH vocabulary is to type keywords or phrases directly into the search box on the PubMed home page. Users may create various combinations of terms with this freestyle approach; however, keyword choice becomes more challenging because the database does not provide definitions of terms it recognizes through this general search feature. Figure 3-7 illustrates an example of what can happen when the wrong keyword combination is selected—in this case, [arthritis AND exercise]. Each of these terms is so broad that 1464 "hits" are returned—too many citations to read through efficiently. Note that the word "AND" must be typed using uppercase or capital letters in order to be recognized as booleans in PubMed.

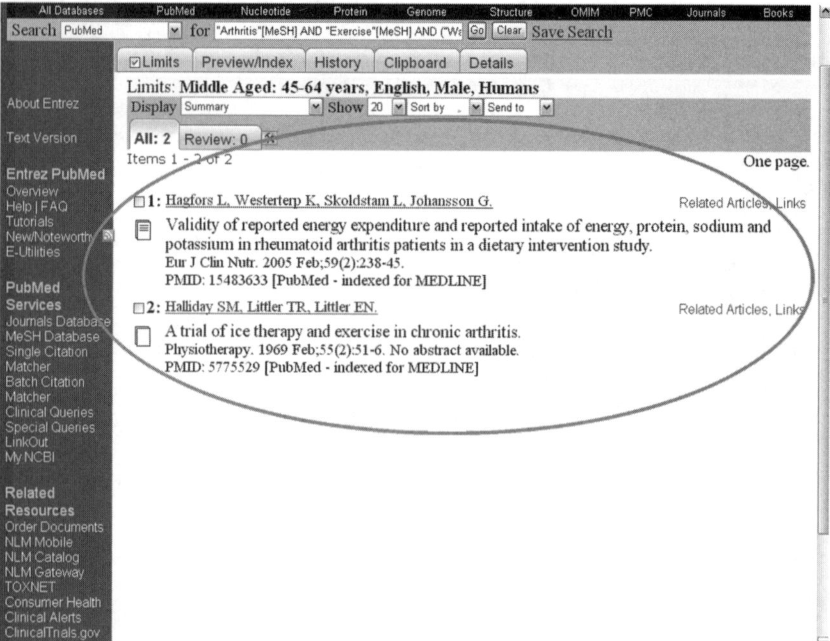

Figure 3-6 PubMed search results using alternative MeSH terms.

Source: Screenshot from PubMed (www.pubmed.gov), the U.S. National Library of Medicine, and the National Institutes of Health.

Table 3–2 Results from search using MeSH terms and limits in PubMed.

Search Method	Number of Hits
MeSH Terms* Plus Limits: • English Language • Human • Middle-Aged: 45–64 • Male	2
MeSH Terms* Plus Limits: • English Language • Human • Middle Aged: 45–64	4
MeSH Terms* Plus Limits: • English Language • Human	8
MeSH Terms† Plus Limits: • English Language • Human • Middle-Aged: 45–64 • Male	4
MeSH Terms‡ Plus Limits: • English Language • Human • Middle-Aged: 45–64 • Male	2
MeSH Terms§ Plus Limits: • English Language • Human • Middle-Aged: 45–64 • Male	2

* MeSH terms: "Arthritis, Rheumatoid," "Exercise," and "Hydrotherapy"

† MeSH terms: "Arthritis," "Exercise," and "Hydrotherapy"

‡ MeSH terms: "Arthritis, Rheumatoid," "Exercise," and "Water"

§ MeSH terms: "Arthritis," "Exercise," and "Water"

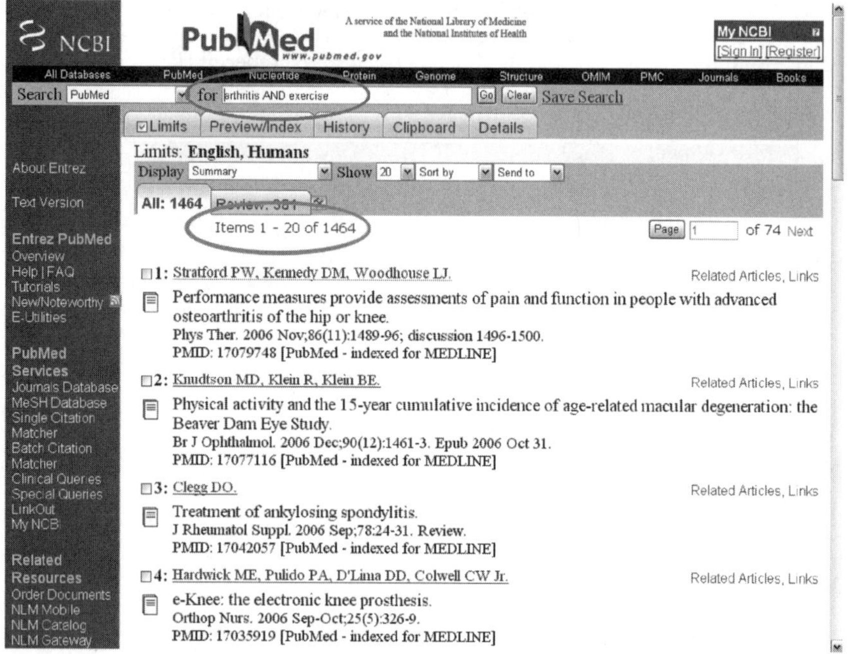

Figure 3–7 PubMed search results using general terms without limits.

Source: Screenshot from PubMed (www.pubmed.gov), the U.S. National Library of Medicine, and the National Institutes of Health.

By comparison, Figure 3–8 illustrates the results obtained using a *search string* that reflects more precisely the content of the clinical question: [rheumatoid arthritis AND aquatic AND exercise] plus the limits "English," "human," "male," and "middle-aged: 45–64." The fact that only two articles are returned suggests that this time the search limits are too restrictive. The results of searches performed with fewer limits are indicated in Table 3–3; the progressive increase in the number of "hits" bears out this assessment of the initial search parameters.

Search History

The "History" function is accessed via a tab on the top of the main PubMed search page (see Figure 3–1). This feature is useful for two reasons: 1) it keeps a record of your search strings; and, 2) it can be used to combine search strings. Keeping track of your different search terms and combinations is important in situations when limits are added or subtracted and when multiple synonyms are exchangd in response to unsuccessful searches.

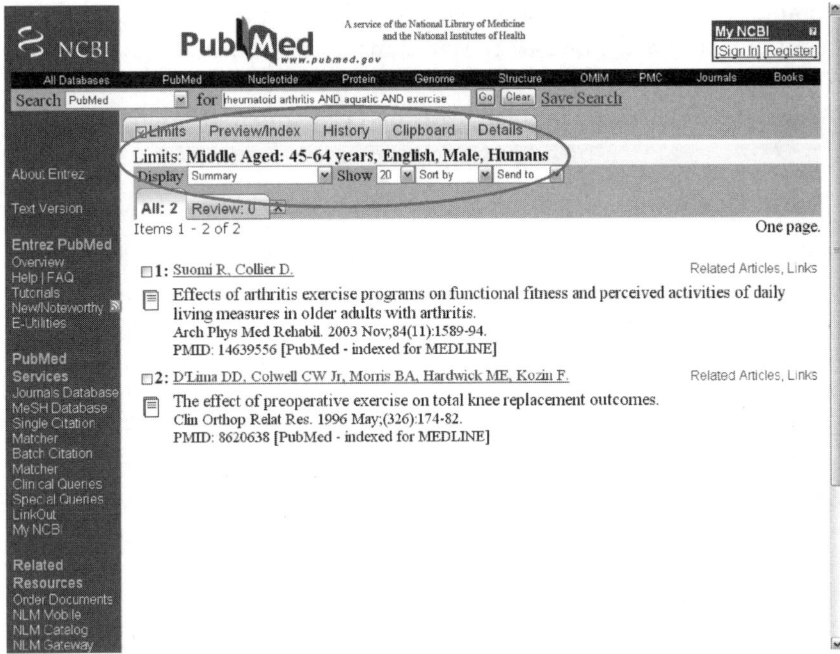

Figure 3–8 PubMed search results using terms specific to question and limits.
Source: Screenshot from PubMed (www.pubmed.gov), the U.S. National Library of Medicine, and the National Institutes of Health.

Table 3–3 Results from a search using keywords other than MeSH terms in PubMed.

Search Method	Number of Hits
Search Terms* Plus Limits: • English Language • Human • Middle-Aged: 45–64 • Male	2
Search Terms* Plus Limits: • English Language • Human • Middle-Aged: 45–64 ~~• Male~~	3
Search Terms* Plus Limits: • English Language • Human ~~• Middle-Aged: 45–64~~ • Male	6

* Search Terms: "Rheumatoid Arthritis," "Aquatic," and "Exercise"

Combining search strings often narrows the search and reduces the number of hits obtained; however, the citations retrieved may be more relevant to the question of interest. Figure 3-9 depicts the history for the search using the string [rheumatoid arthritis AND aquatic AND exercise].

Clinical Queries

"Clinical Queries" is PubMed's version of an evidence-based practice database and is accessible via a link on the left-hand side of the home page (Figure 3-1). This feature allows a more tailored search for studies pertaining to etiology, diagnosis, prognosis, therapy, or clinical prediction rules (Figure 3-10). Depending on which topic area is selected, this feature will automatically add terms that direct the search to the most useful forms of evidence for that practice element. In addition, the user can direct the search engine to narrow or expand the search. Selecting "systematic reviews" may reduce the need to search further if a high-quality, relevant example of this

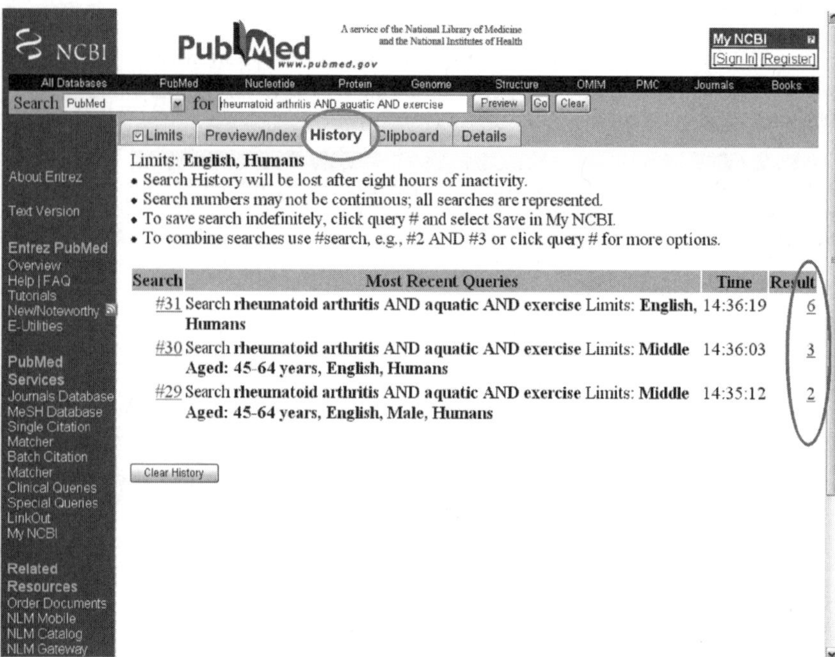

Figure 3-9 PubMed search history page.

Source: Screenshot from PubMed (www.pubmed.gov), the U.S. National Library of Medicine, and the National Institutes of Health.

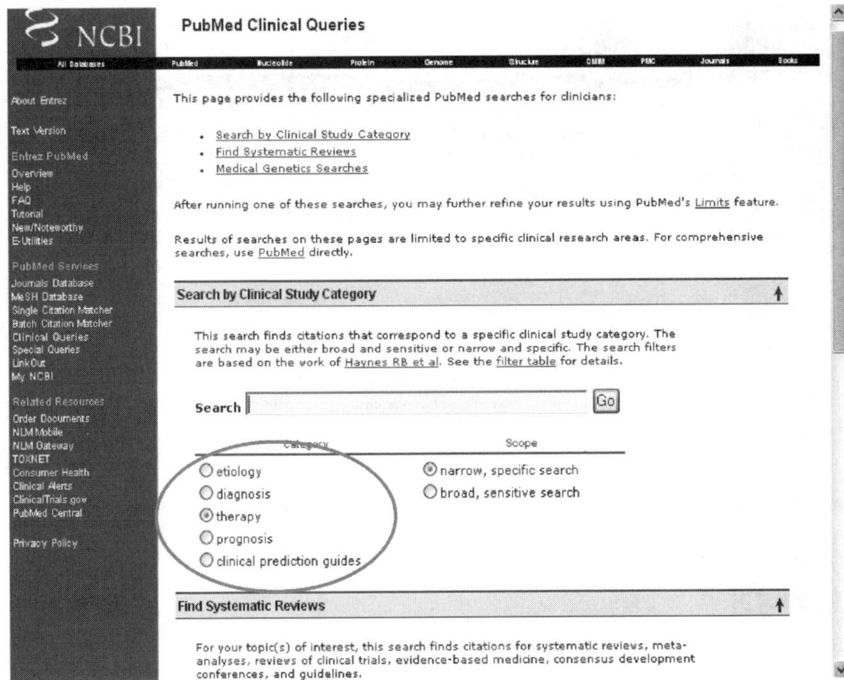

Figure 3–10 PubMed clinical queries page.

Source: Screenshot from PubMed (www.pubmed.gov), the U.S. National Library of Medicine, and the National Institutes of Health.

comprehensive form of evidence is located. Figure 3–11 illustrates the results for the search string [rheumatoid arthritis AND aquatic AND exercise], along with the limits "English," "human," "middle-aged: 45-64," and "male," entered through the "Clinical Queries" function. Note that by selecting "therapy," the search was limited automatically to randomized controlled trials, the highest form of evidence about interventions. This approach yielded the same two citations obtained using the general search feature in the previous example. As noted above, the goal is to find the highest quality evidence available; therefore, using the "Clinical Queries" feature is the more efficient option in this example because of its automatic search for the best research design for intervention studies.

"My NCBI"

"My NCBI" (National Center for Biotechnology Information) allows therapists to individualize a free account on the PubMed Web site that will save search parameters, perform automatic searches for new studies, and e-mail

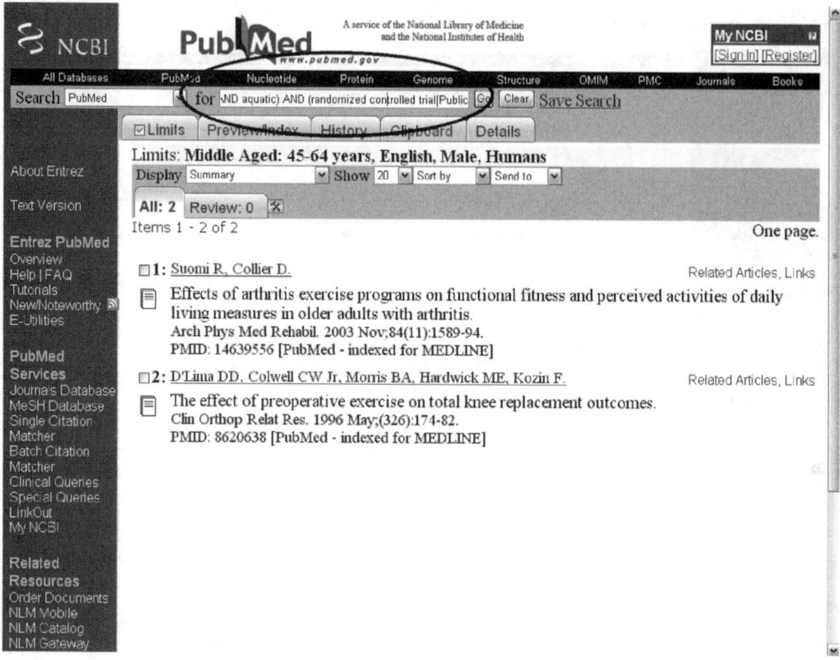

Figure 3-11 PubMed search results using clinical queries.

Source: Screenshot from PubMed (www.pubmed.gov), the U.S. National Library of Medicine, and the National Institutes of Health.

updates about the results of these searches (Figure 3-12). Registration with a password is required. This is a particularly useful feature for therapists who anticipate routine exploration of a particular topic area (e.g., "shoulder pain" or "multiple sclerosis").

CUMULATIVE INDEX OF NURSING AND ALLIED HEALTH LITERATURE (CINAHL)

As its name suggests, CINAHL is a database of citations from journals pertaining to nursing and the allied health professions.[9] Some of these journals are not indexed through the U.S. National Library of Medicine because they do not meet the inclusion criteria. For example, studies published in the *Cardiopulmonary Physical Therapy Journal* are not listed in PubMed because the journal is both a research dissemination vehicle and a format for providing news to Cardiovascular & Pulmonary Section members of the American Physical Therapy Association. However, this journal's articles are

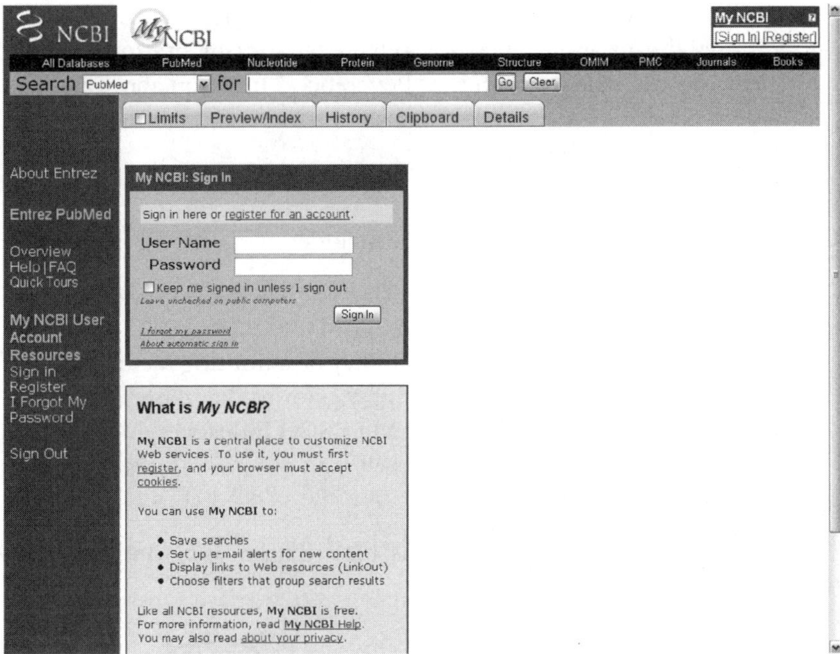

Figure 3–12 PubMed's "My NCBI" page.

Source: Screenshot from PubMed (www.pubmed.gov), the U.S. National Library of Medicine, and the National Institutes of Health.

cited by CINAHL. As a result of this differential in indexing rules, physical therapists may find it useful to start a search with CINAHL rather than with PubMed. Additional advantages of this database include:

- Links to online journals;
- Easy-to-understand search pages;
- Abilities to limit or expand the search by specifying:
  - –Characteristics of the subjects studied (e.g., age, gender, etc.);
  - –Characteristics of the article or publication (e.g., publication date, journal type, etc.);
  - –Treatment setting (e.g., inpatient, outpatient);
  - –Special interest areas (e.g., physical therapy, complementary medicine, etc.);
- Automated suggestions for additional limits returned with search results;

- Ability to view the retrieved "hits" by citation only, citation plus additional details about the study's characteristics, or citation plus the abstract (available through the "Preferences" function above the search page);
- Easy-to-view search history;
- Weekly updates of the database.

Disadvantages of the CINAHL database include:

- A non-MeSH-based search vocabulary, requiring a different set of search terms to learn;
- Citations only back to 1982, which may be a limiting factor if a topic was researched more thoroughly prior to that date; and,
- A subscription fee required through EBSCO Industries, Inc. (EBSCOHost) for individual users who do not have access through an instutional site license.

CINAHL has two search page options: basic (Figure 3–13) and advanced (Figure 3–14).

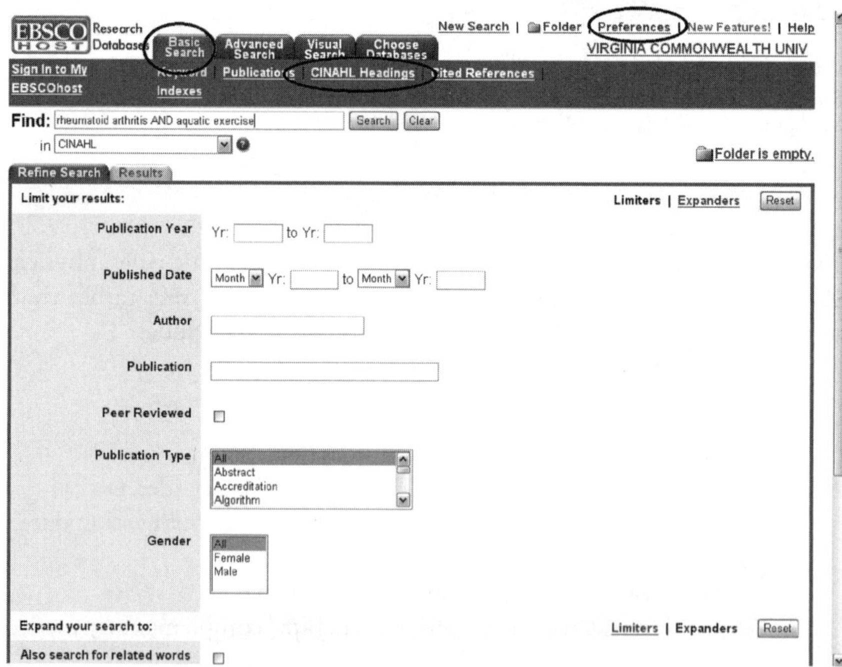

Figure 3–13 CINAHL basic search page.

Source: Screenshot from CINAHL with full text (http://search.ebscohost.com), EBSCOhost, EBSCO Industries, Inc. Accessed February 20, 2006.

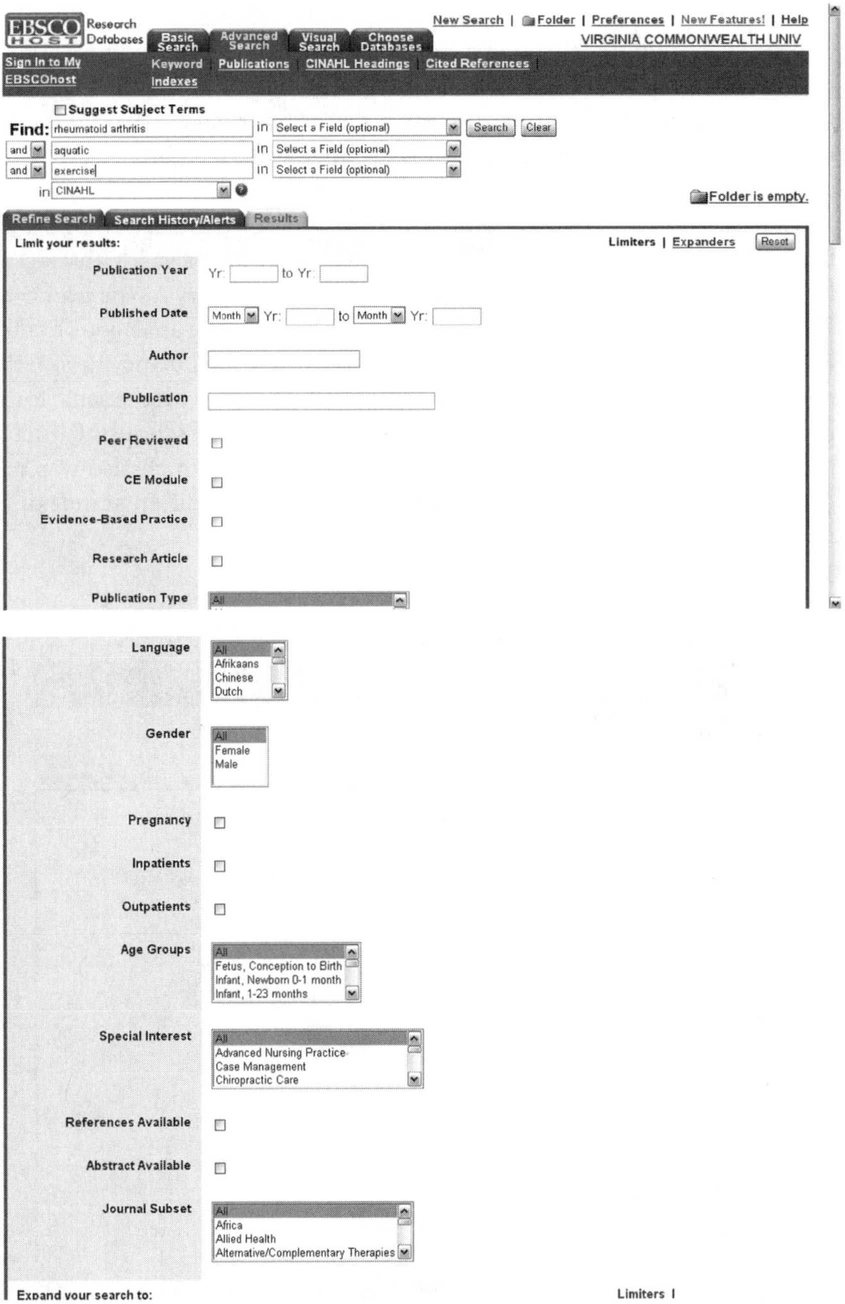

EBSCO HOST Research Databases
Basic Search | Advanced Search | Visual Search | Choose Databases
New Search | Folder | Preferences | New Features! | Help
VIRGINIA COMMONWEALTH UNIV
Sign In to My EBSCOhost
Keyword | Publications | CINAHL Headings | Cited References | Indexes

Suggest Subject Terms
Find: rheumatoid arthritis in Select a Field (optional) Search Clear
and aquatic in Select a Field (optional)
and exercise in Select a Field (optional)
in CINAHL
Folder is empty.

Refine Search | Search History/Alerts | Results

Limit your results: Limiters | Expanders Reset

Publication Year Yr: to Yr:
Published Date Month Yr: to Month Yr:
Author
Publication
Peer Reviewed
CE Module
Evidence-Based Practice
Research Article
Publication Type All
Language All, Afrikaans, Chinese, Dutch
Gender All, Female, Male
Pregnancy
Inpatients
Outpatients
Age Groups All, Fetus, Conception to Birth, Infant, Newborn 0-1 month, Infant, 1-23 months
Special Interest All, Advanced Nursing Practice, Case Management, Chiropractic Care
References Available
Abstract Available
Journal Subset All, Africa, Allied Health, Alternative/Complementary Therapies

Expand your search to: Limiters |

Figure 3–14 CINAHL advanced search page.

Source: Screenshot from CINAHL with full text (http://search.ebscohost.com), EBSCOhost, EBSCO Industries, Inc. Acessed February 20, 2006.

The basic search page contains a search box similar to that used in PubMed that requires the user to type in the search terms along with any booleans. Unlike PubMed, booleans may be entered in lowercase letters in CINAHL. Choices for limiting the search on the basic page are few and primarily pertain to characteristics of the publication or search field. The advanced search page includes more features to limit or expand the search and allows the user to select booleans from a drop-down menu. It is possible to configure the results on both pages so that they appear with abstracts, brief synopses, or simply with citations. CINAHL vocabulary can be searched via the CINAHL Headings function (Figure 3–15), a feature analagous to the PubMed MeSH function. Figure 3–16 illustrates a search using the search string [rheumatoid arthritis AND aquatic AND exercise] with the same four limits used in PubMed. Results were returned in the brief synopsis format. Once again, only two citations were identified, one of which also was retrieved by PubMed. This differential is a reflection of the different indexing methods used by each database.

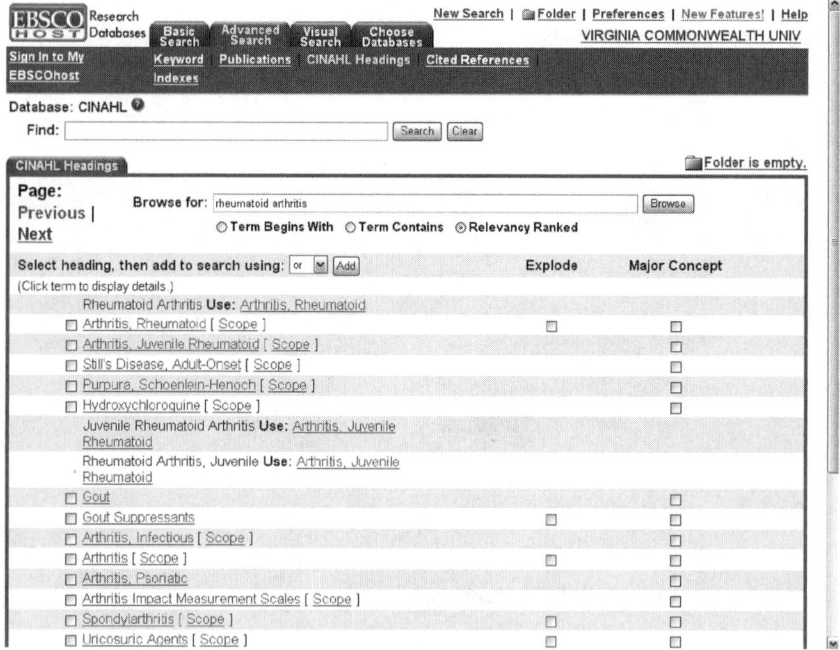

Figure 3–15 CINAHL headings page.

Source: Screenshot from CINAHL with full text (http://search.ebscohost.com), EBSCOhost, EBSCO Industries, Inc. Acessed February 20, 2006.

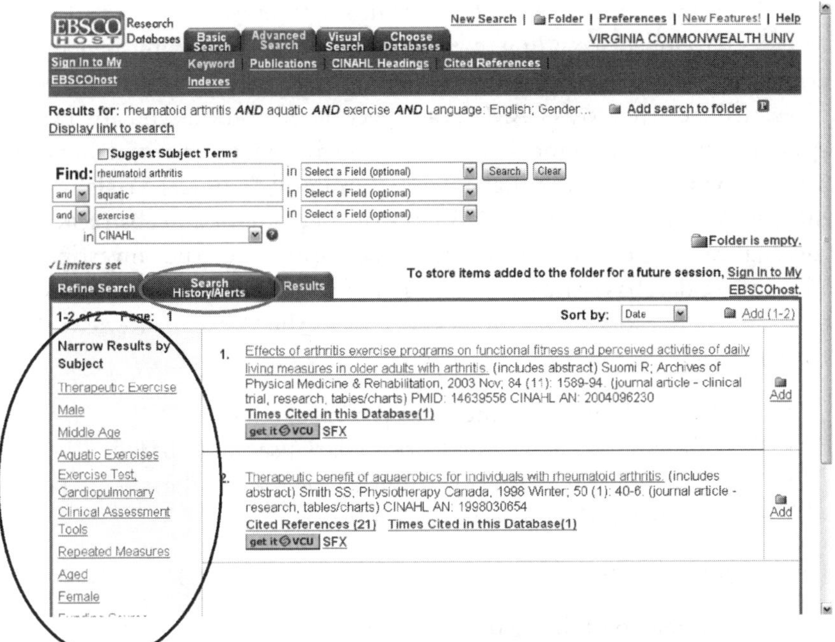

Figure 3–16 CINAHL search results using the brief citation format.

Source: Screenshot from CINAHL with full text (http://search.ebscohost.com), EBSCOhost, EBSCO Industries, Inc. Acessed February 20, 2006.

COCHRANE LIBRARY

The Cochrane Library, developed and maintained by an international organization, the Cochrane Collaboration,[10] offers a potentially more efficient means of searching for evidence about interventions. The Library is actually a collection of five databases and two registries:

- The Cochrane Database of Systematic Reviews (Cochrane Reviews)
- The Database of Abstracts of Reviews of Effects (Other Reviews)
- The Cochrane Central Register of Controlled Trials (Clinical Trials)
- The Cochrane Database of Methodology Reviews (Methods Reviews)
- The Cochrane Methodology Register (Methods Studies)
- Health Technology Assessment Database (Technology Assessments)
- The National Health Service Economic Evaluation Database (Economic Evaluations)

The Cochrane Reviews database contains systematic reviews and meta-analyses developed according to rigorous methodology established and executed by members of the Cochrane Collaboration. "Other Reviews" (previously referred to as DARE) is a collection of citations and abstracts of systematic reviews and meta-analyses performed by other researchers who are not members of the collaboration. Similarly, "Clinical Trials" (previously referred to as CENTRAL) is a database of citations and abstracts of individual randomized controlled trials performed by other investigators. These three databases are the most useful for searching for evidence to answer clinical questions. Advantages specific to the Cochrane Reviews database include:

- Reviews are limited to randomized clinical trials;
- Use of the same MeSH search vocabulary used in PubMed;
- The availability of full-text versions of the reviews that include complete details of the process and results.

Disadvantages include:

- Few reviews pertaining to etiology, diagnosis, and prognosis;
- A limited online overview of the system; however, detailed user guides in Adobe Acrobat "PDF" format are available for downloading and printing;
- A subscription fee is required for individual users who do not have access through an instutional site license.

The remaining databases in the Cochrane Library contain citations pertaining to research methods (Methods Reviews, Methods Studies), health technology appraisals (Technology Assessments) conducted by other investigators or agencies (such as the Agency for Healthcare Research and Quality), and health economics topics (Economic Evaluations). Users may search all of the databases simultaneously or select specific databases.

The Library has both a basic (Figure 3–17) and advanced (Figure 3–18) search page, although neither has nearly the number of options to expand or limit the search as compared to PubMed and CINAHL. Figure 3–19 illustrates the results obtained from the search string [rheumatoid arthritis AND aquatic AND exercise] as entered into the advanced search page. The number of hits found in each of the most relevant databases are circled: four in the Cochrane Reviews, zero in Other Reviews, and six in Clinical Trials. Of the citations in the Cochrane Reviews, two are descriptions of review protocols and two are actual systematic reviews. Unfortunately, the citation title that is relevant to rheumatoid arthritis is the protocol for the review yet to be completed, whereas the reviews are about interventions for

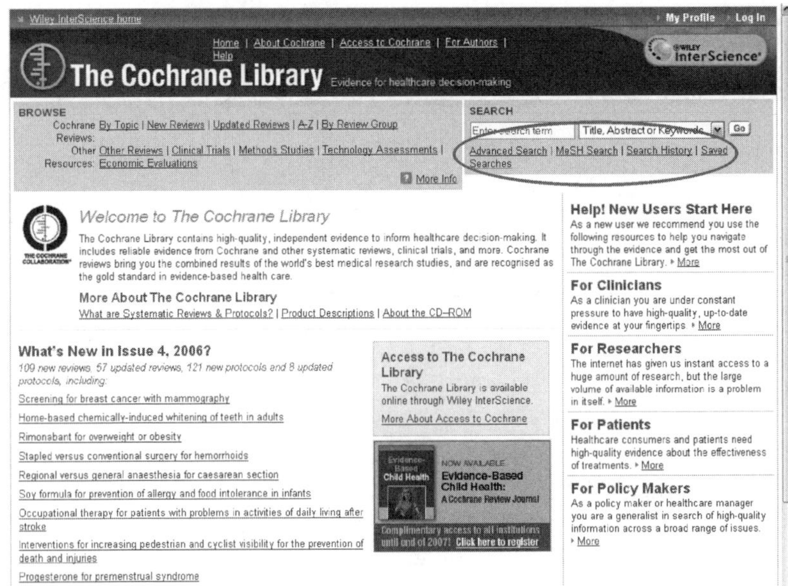

Figure 3–17 The Cochrane Library home page.

Source: Screenshot from John Wiley & Sons, Inc.'s World Wide Web Site. Copyright 1999–2006, John Wiley & Sons, Inc. Reproduced with permission.

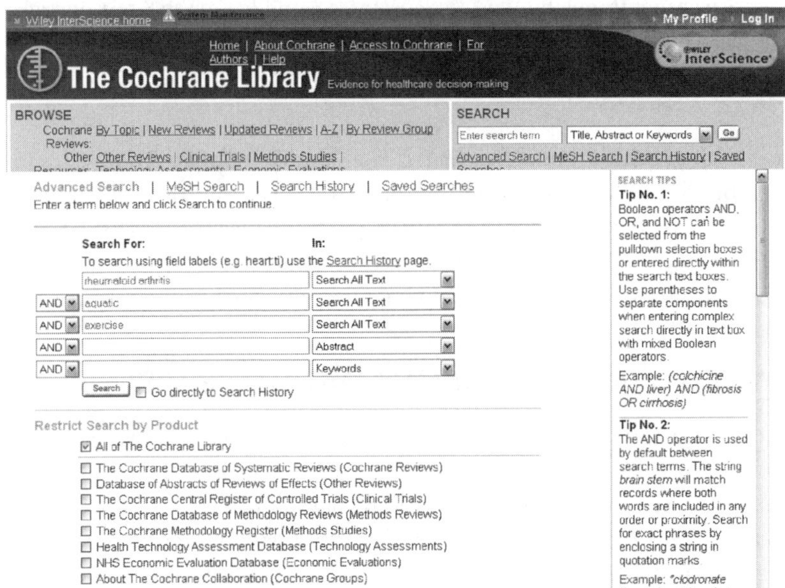

Figure 3–18 The Cochrane Library advanced search page.

Source: Screenshot from John Wiley & Sons, Inc.'s World Wide Web Site. Copyright 1999–2006, John Wiley & Sons, Inc. Reproduced with permission.

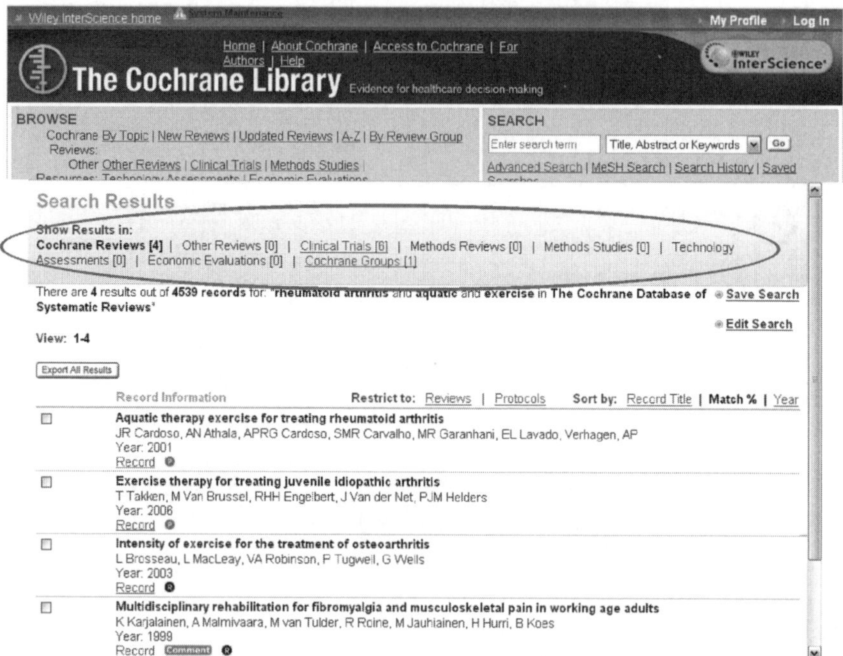

Figure 3–19 The Cochrane Library search results for the Cochrane Reviews database. *Source:* Screenshot from John Wiley & Sons, Inc.'s World Wide Web Site. Copyright 1999–2006, John Wiley & Sons, Inc. Reproduced with permission.

patients with other forms of arthritis. The Library is updated quarterly so the timetable for review production is likely to exceed the time available with the hypothetical patient about whom the clinical question was asked. On the other hand, the six citations in the Clinical Trials database provide leads on individual randomized controlled trials that may be helpful (Figure 3–20).

PHYSIOTHERAPY EVIDENCE DATABASE (PEDro)

PEDro is an initiative of the Centre for Evidence-Based Physiotherapy in Sydney, Australia that provides "bibliographic details and abstracts of randomized controlled trials, systematic reviews, and evidence-based clinical practice guidelines in physiotherapy."[11] Individual trials are rated on a 0–10 scale based on their internal validity and statistical interpretability. The reliability of the total rating score was determined to be "fair" to "good" based on a study by Maher *et al.*[12] The validity of the scoring system has not been published. The rating scores appear next to citations in the search results

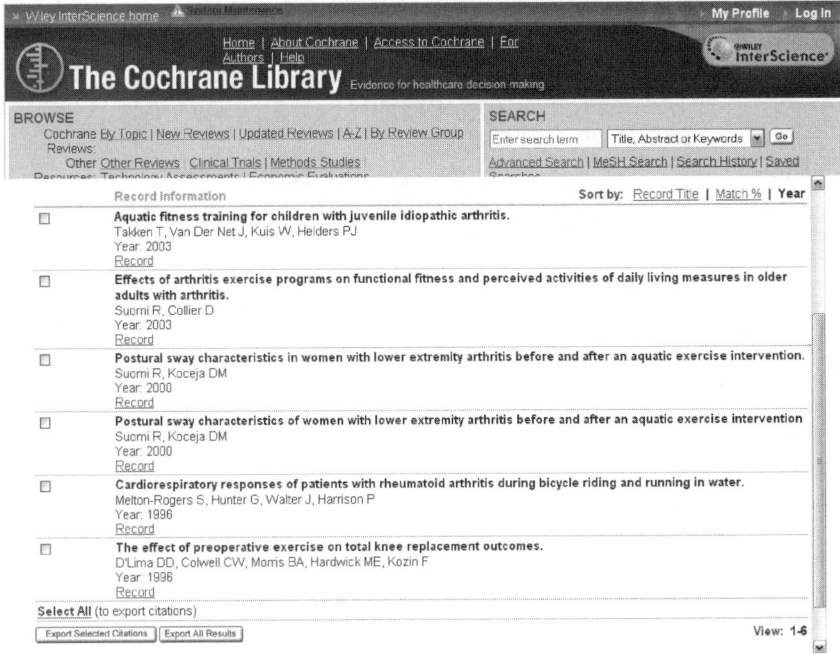

Figure 3–20 The Cochrane Library search results for the Clinical Trials database.
Source: Screenshot from John Wiley & Sons, Inc.'s World Wide Web Site. Copyright 1999–2006, John Wiley & Sons, Inc. Reproduced with permission.

to help the user prioritize which studies to review first. Reviews and practice guidelines are not rated.

The primary reason to use PEDro is its focus on physical therapy research. Like CINAHL and the Cochrane Library this database has a simple (Figure 3–21) and advanced (Figure 3–22) search page.

Other advantages include:

- An ability to search by:
  - –Therapeutic approach
  - –Clinical problem
  - –Body part
  - –Physical therapy subspecialty;
- An ability to write booleans in upper or lowercase;
- A tutorial regarding determination of the internal validity of a clinical trial;
- An opportunity for readers to submit feedback when they disagree with a rating score.

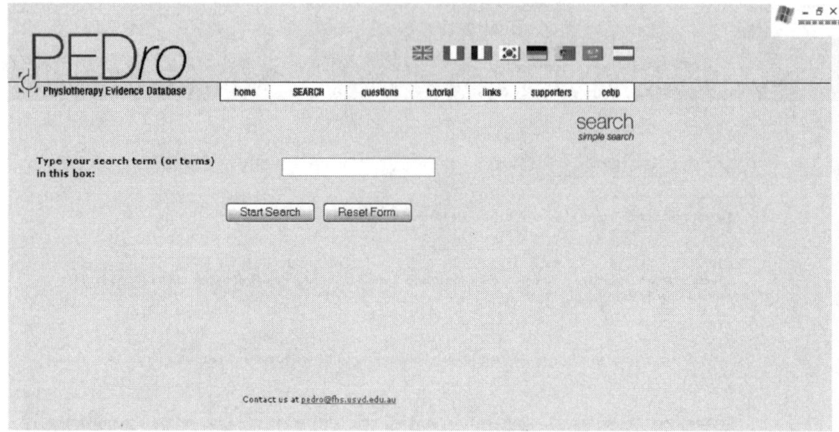

Figure 3–21 PEDro simple search page.

Source: Screenshot from PEDro (http://www.pedro.fhs.usyd.edu.au/index.html), the Center for Evidence-Based Physiotherapy, the School of Physiotherapy at the University of Sydney, Australia.

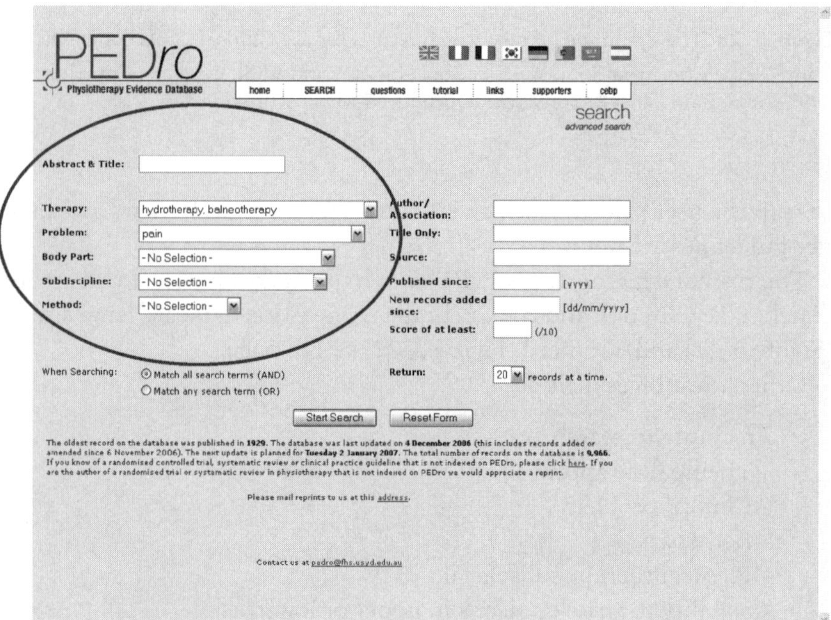

Figure 3–22 PEDro advanced search page.

Source: Screenshot from PEDro (http://www.pedro.fhs.usyd.edu.au/index.html), the Center for Evidence-Based Physiotherapy, the School of Physiotherapy at the University of Sydney, Australia.

Like Cochrane, the primary limitation of PEDro is the lack of citations pertaining to physical therapy diagnosis, prognosis, and outcomes. In addition, the options available to tailor the search are limited to characteristics of the study; more specific details about the subjects are unavailable. Unlike Cochrane, PEDro is free and is updated approximately every two weeks. In addition, the database does not have a specific search vocabulary to learn.

Figure 3–23 illustrates the results returned from a search using the search string [rheumatoid arthritis AND aquatic AND exercise]. Only clinical trials are cited, indicating that there may not be any systematic reviews or clinical practice guidelines pertaining to this search. Note that one of the citations returned is in Danish due to the inability to restrict the search to English language articles. The quality ratings for each citation are circled and are in descending order from highest to lowest quality. One option is to select only those articles that meet a minimum threshold score, such as "greater than or equal to 5/10." There is no evidence to support the selection

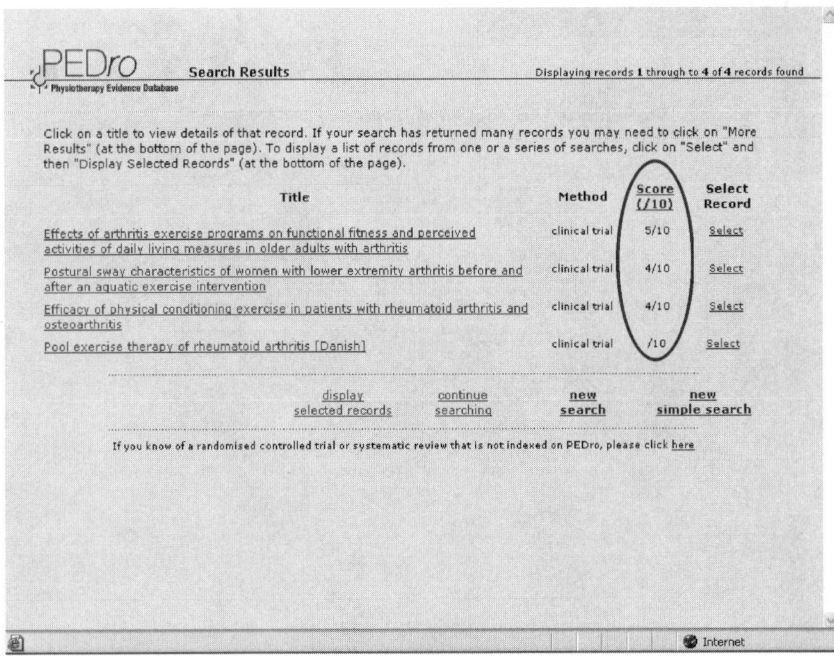

Figure 3–23 PEDro search results page.

Source: Screenshot from PEDro (http://www.pedro.fhs.usyd.edu.au/index.html), the Center for Evidence-Based Physiotherapy, the School of Physiotherapy at the University of Sydney, Australia.

of a threshold, however, so the target value is arbitrary and should be acknowledged as such. Readers are encouraged to pull the most relevant citations and review them on their own merits rather than rely solely on scoring criteria to make a decision.

AMERICAN PHYSICAL THERAPY ASSOCIATION'S *HOOKED ON EVIDENCE*

In response to the emphasis on evidence-based physical therapy practice, the American Physical Therapy Association (APTA) has created "Hooked on Evidence" (Figure 3-24).[13] "Hooked" is a database of citations concerning the effectiveness of physical therapy interventions. Studies of etiology, diagnosis, prognosis, or outcomes are not included. Four criteria must be met in order for studies to be entered in the database:

1. The study is about human subjects;
2. The study investigates at least one physical therapy intervention;

APTA
Hooked on EVIDENCE
Subscribe
FAQs
Contact Us
Welcome to the Hooked on Evidence Website!
Member ID:
Last Name:
Login
The APTA Hooked on Evidence Website represents a "grassroots" effort to develop a database containing current research evidence on the effectiveness of physical therapy interventions. The Hooked on Evidence project was motivated by a concern that clinicians lacked access to the knowledge available from current research, thus hindering evidence-based practice. The website has the following objectives:
• Allow members to search a database of article extractions relevant to the field of physical therapy to build support for evidence-based practice
• Allow members to contribute extractions of the peer-reviewed literature to the database
• List useful web resources and other information consistent with evidence-based practice
• Disseminate clinical practice guidelines based on systematic reviews of the literature
Earn CEUs!
The contents of the site provide learning tools to foster evidence based practice in physical therapy, tutorial information on the Guide to Physical Therapist Practice, and an online input form to allow APTA members to input article extractions on various topics in physical therapy. The website was planned and built by APTA members and the contributions of many are gratefully acknowledged.
Earn Continuing Education Units for Contributing to Hooked on Evidence!
All contents © 2006 American Physical Therapy Association. All Rights Reserved. Disclaimer

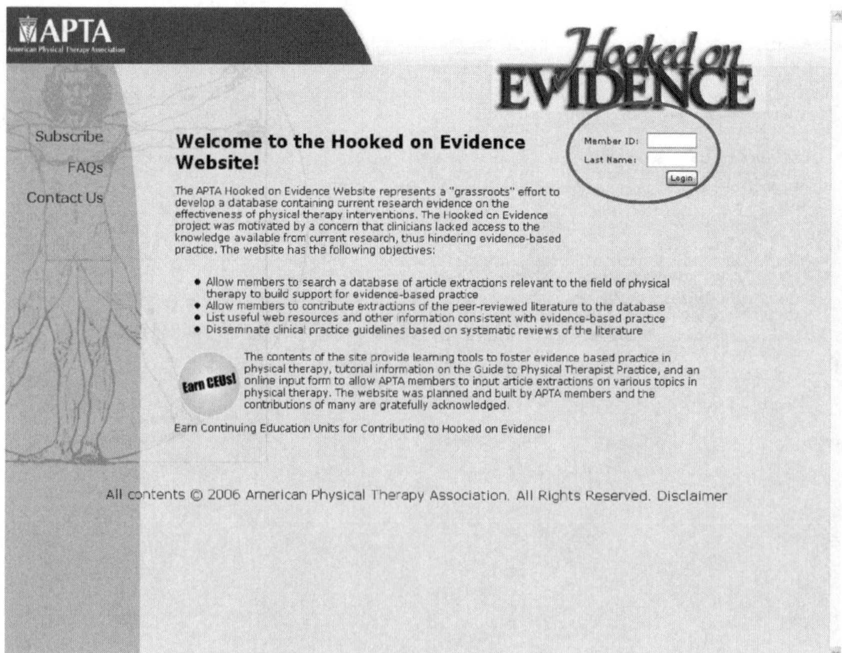

Figure 3-24 APTA's "Hooked on Evidence" log in page.

Source: Reprinted from the American Physical Therapy Association Web site http://www.hookedonevidence.com (2006) with permission of the American Physical Therapy Association. This material is copyrighted, and any further reproduction or distribution is prohibited.

3. The study includes at least one outcome measure of the intervention(s); and,
4. The study was published in an indexed, English-language, peer-reviewed journal.

Unlike PEDro, all study designs are eligible and no rating score is applied. Similar to PEDro, there is no new search vocabulary to learn and booleans may be entered in lower or uppercase.

The primary reason to use "Hooked" is its focus on physical therapy research. Figure 3–25 illustrates the advanced search page with a limited number of options with which to tailor the search (age group, research design, journal). It is also possible to search by diagnostic (ICD-9) code.[14] Using this search function with the phrase [rheumatoid arthritis] reveals no "hits" regardless of which word and limit combinations are used. As with the search using the MeSH vocabulary, using a more general keyword–such as "arthritis"–is an appropriate strategy at this point. Figure 3–26 indicates

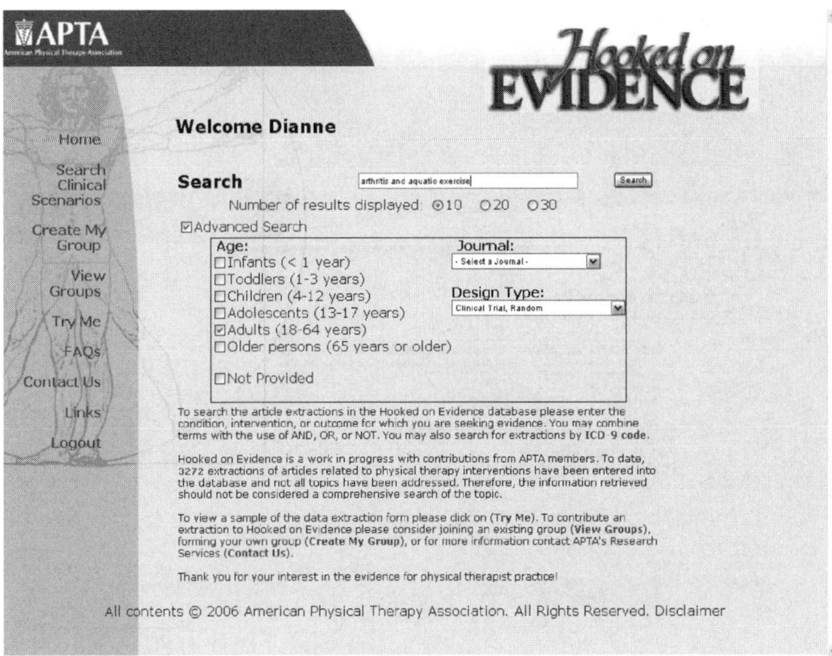

Figure 3–25 APTA's "Hooked on Evidence" advanced search page.

Source: Reprinted from the American Physical Therapy Association Web site http://www.hookedonevidence.com (2006) with permission of the American Physical Therapy Association. This material is copyrighted, and any further reproduction or distribution is prohibited.

that two citations are retrieved when the search string [arthritis AND aquatic AND exercise] are entered along with the limits "Adults 18–64" and "Clinical trial—Random." Removing the "Clinical Trial—Random" results in the same two articles. A third study is obtained when the age limit is deleted; however, its focus is on aquatic exercise effects for children with juvenile rheumatoid arthritis.

A unique benefit of "Hooked" is the type and amount of detail provided in each article extraction. Figure 3–27 illustrates the abbreviated information obtained from the study by Suomi and Koceja that includes the ICD-9 code, *Guide to Physical Therapist Practice*[1] practice pattern, and one measure of treatment effectiveness.[15] Basic details about the study population, interventions, and outcomes of interest also are provided. The "Enhanced Results" page provides additional information about the research design, treatment protocols, and measures of effectives for all eight of the outcomes. This format reminds users of the key elements upon which to focus when appraising evidence about interventions. Figure 3–28 provides a limited view of this information due to the length of the complete extraction.

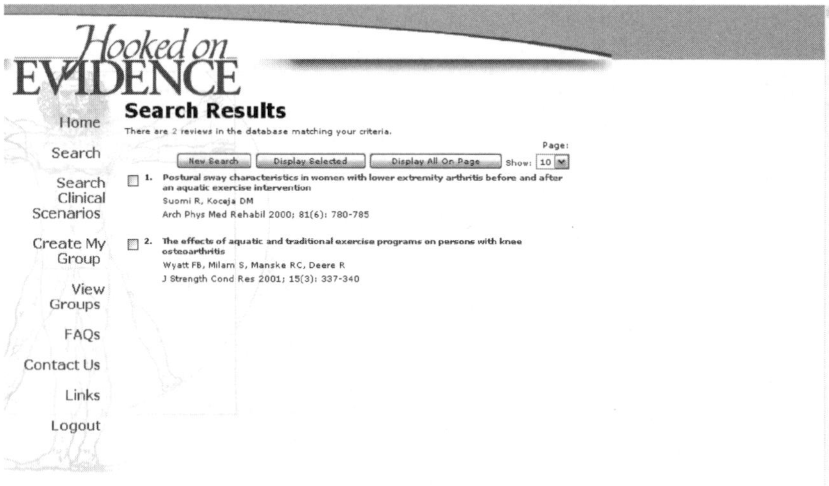

Figure 3–26 APTA's "Hooked on Evidence" search results page.

Source: Reprinted from the American Physical Therapy Association Web site http://www.hookedonevidence.com (2006) with permission of the American Physical Therapy Association. This material is copyrighted, and any further reproduction or distribution is prohibited.

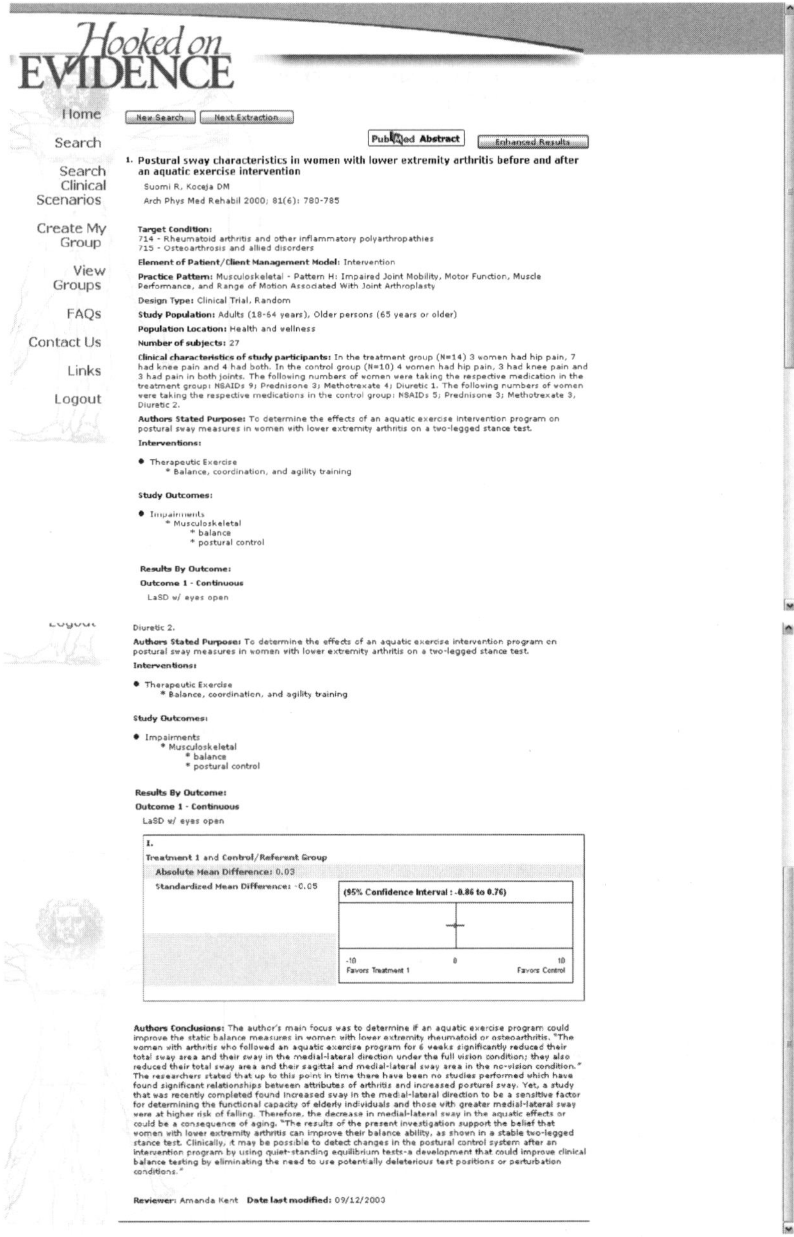

Figure 3–27 APTA's "Hooked on Evidence" citation information.

Source: Reprinted from the American Physical Therapy Association Web site http://www.hooked on evidence.com (2006) with permission of the American Physical Therapy Association. This material is copyrighted, and any further reproduction or distribution is prohibited.

Hooked On Evidence Initiative

Postural sway characteristics in women with lower extremity arthritis before and after an aquatic exercise intervention

Suomi R, Koceja DM

Arch Phys Med Rehabil 2000; 81(6): 780-785

Target Condition:
714 - Rheumatoid arthritis and other inflammatory polyarthropathies
715 - Osteoarthrosis and allied disorders

Element of Patient/Client Management Model: Intervention

Practice Pattern: Musculoskeletal - Pattern H: Impaired Joint Mobility, Motor Function, Muscle Performance, and Range of Motion Associated With Joint Arthroplasty

Design Type: Clinical Trial, Random

Study Population: Adults (18-64 years), Older persons (65 years or older)

Population Location: Health and wellness

Inclusion Criteria: The subjects had to be female and between the ages of 45 and 70 years old. They had to have been diagnosed as having osteoarthritis (OA) or rheumatoid arthritis (RA) of the lower extremities along with a score of 15 or less on the knee/hip Arthritis Impact Measurement scale. The women were to have no medical condition that would restrict them from increased physical activity and have had no involvement in an organized exercise program 3 months prior to the study. The subjects must have also been under a stable medication regimen for the previous 3 months.

Exclusion Criteria: Individuals not included were those who had knee or hip joint replacements or had only upper extremity or spine symptoms of arthritis. Those persons who failed to obtain a physician's permission to participate in the Arthritis Foundation Aquatic Program (AFAP) classes were also excluded.

How were subjects selected: Non-Probability Sample

How many subjects were contacted initially: 58

How many subjects were eligible to participate: 27

How many subjects agreed to participate: 27

Non-clinical characteristics of study participants: All subjects were female. The mean age of the females in the treatment group was 60.7 years old. The average height was 164.4 cm and weight was 73.1 kg for treatment subjects. The mean age of the control group was 54.4 years old, the average height was 163.3 cm and weight was 72.5 kg.

Clinical characteristics of study participants: In the treatment group (N=14) 3 women had hip pain, 7 had knee pain and 4 had both. In the control group (N=10) 4 women had hip pain, 3 had knee pain and 3 had pain in both joints. The following numbers of women were taking the respective medication in the treatment group: NSAIDs 9; Prednisone 3; Methotrexate 4; Diuretic 1. The following numbers of women were taking the respective medications in the control group: NSAIDs 5; Prednisone 3; Methotrexate 3, Diuretic 2.

Blinded Clinicians: No

Blinded Subjects: No

Same person providing treatment and testing measures: No

Blinded assessor: Not Provided

Intention to treat analysis: No

Treatment Group 1 : The treatment group participated in aquatics classes created by the Arthritis Foundation Aquatics Program (AFAP). The AFAP classes consisted of 68 aquatic exercises designed for individuals with arthritis with an emphasis to enhance strength, range of motion, and mobility. The classes were conducted at an area YMCA in a therapeutic pool with controlled temperature and water depth. The participants attended 45-minute training sessions weekly for 6 weeks. The classes were offered three times per week and the women were required to attend a minimum of two classes each week. The subjects completed balance tests under two conditions one week prior to the treatment and one week following the completion of the treatment.

Control/Referent Group: The control subjects were instructed to refrain from participating in any organized physical activity or from beginning any new physical activity for the 6-week duration of the study. Similar to the treatment group, the control group completed balance testing one week prior to and one week following the study.

Figure 3–28 APTA's "Hooked on Evidence" enhanced results page.

Source: Reprinted from the American Physical Therapy Association Web site http://www.hookedonevidence.com (2006) with permission of the American Physical Therapy Association.

Authors Stated Purpose: To determine the effects of an aquatic exercise intervention program on postural sway measures in women with lower extremity arthritis on a two-legged stance test.

Interventions:

- Therapeutic Exercise
    * Balance, coordination, and agility training

Study Outcomes:

- Impairments
    * Musculoskeletal
        * balance
        * postural control

Results By Outcome:

Outcome 1 - Continuous

LaSD w/ eyes open

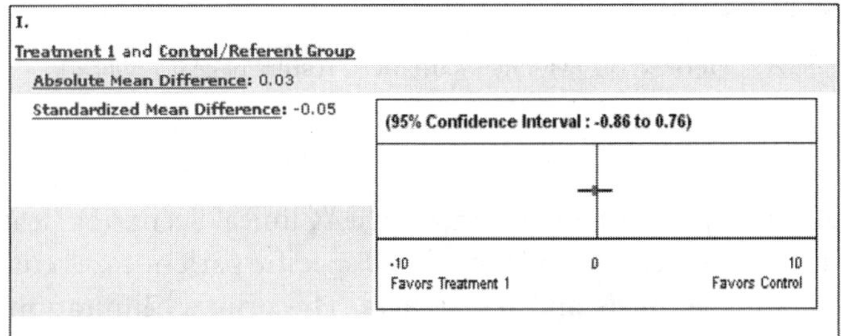

LaSD w/ eyes open

II.

Treatment 1

Number of Subjects: 14

End Mean: 1.88

End Standard Deviation: 0.60

Baseline Mean: 2.56

Baseline Standard Deviation: 0.93

Treatment R

Number of Subjects: 10

End Mean: 1.91

End Standard Deviation: 0.73

Baseline Mean: 1.96

Baseline Standard Deviation: 0.82

Outcome 2 - Continuous

LaSD w/ eyes closed

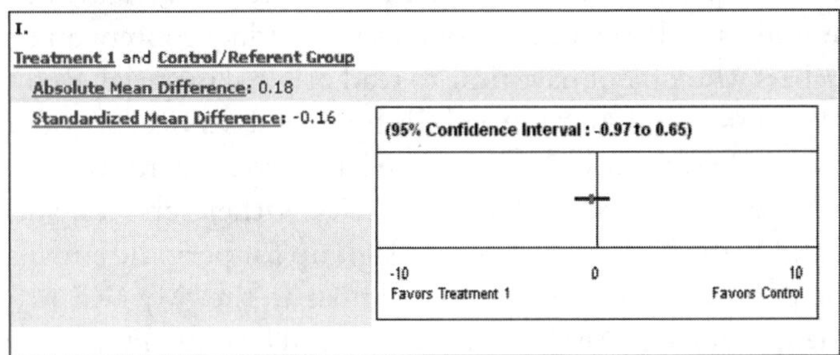

continues

LaSD w/ eyes closed

II.
Treatment 1
Number of Subjects: 14
End Mean: 2.42
End Standard Deviation: 0.97
Baseline Mean: 3.48
Baseline Standard Deviation: 1.43
Treatment R
Number of Subjects: 10
End Mean: 2.60
End Standard Deviation: 1.34
Baseline Mean: 2.64
Baseline Standard Deviation: 1.10

Figure 3–28 APTA's "Hooked on Evidence" enhanced results page (*continued*).

A new addition to Hooked on Evidence is the "Clinical Scenarios" feature that allows users to search for evidence about specific patient cases created by expert physical therapists and researchers. The primary limitations of "Hooked" are the lack of citations pertaining to other elements of the patient/client management process, as well as the dependency upon APTA member submissions of article extractions. Details about the submission and extraction review process, along with other information about the database, is located on the Research page of the APTA Web site.[16] Finally, "Hooked" is viewed as a member benefit; therefore, a therapist must be an APTA member or a paid subscriber to access this database.

OTHER DATABASES AND SERVICES

The search engines discussed above do not comprise an exhaustive list of options. Additional databases such as Bandolier,[17] Netting the Evidence,[18] TRIP,[19] and Evidence in Motion[20] may be useful depending on the type and content of the questions asked. In addition, there are services available that evaluate studies and provide brief synopses regarding content and quality for subscribers who do not have time to read original material. Examples include EBM Online[21] and ACP Journal Club.[22] These services are oriented primarily toward physicians, but are excellent resources regarding the principles and methods of evidence-based practice. Other services, such as Medscape[23] and WebMD,[24] allow users to sign up for periodic e-mails announcing the publication of new studies, similar to the "My NCBI" function in PubMed. Users of these alert services will still have to obtain and read the articles to determine their usefulness.

SUMMARY

Evidence-based physical therapy practice starts with the formulation of a clinical question about a patient/client. Background questions seek information to increase understanding about the patient/client's clinical context. Foreground questions seek information to facilitate clinical decision making with respect to diagnosis, prognosis, interventions, and outcomes. Once the question is formulated, therapists should plan their search strategy and include identification of search terms and databases that will be used. The five electronic databases that are commonly accessed by physical therapists are: PubMed, CINAHL, the Cochrane Library, PEDro and APTA's "Hooked on Evidence." Each database has specific search features with which users should be familiar to enhance the efficiency of the process. Research synthesis and alert services also are available to facilitate identification of relevant evidence; however, therapists will want to review the evidence for themselves to judge its quality and relevance for a specific patient/client.

Exercises

1. Think about a patient/client scenario in which you have an interest and consider what you would like to know about it. Practice writing "background" questions to increase your understanding of the scenario. Write one "foreground" question each pertaining to diagnosis, prognosis, intervention, and outcomes for this scenario.
2. Review all three MeSH database online tutorials on the PubMed Web site.
3. Upon completion of the tutorials, choose one of your "foreground" questions and identify the search terms you might use. Look for these terms in the MeSH database.
4. Perform a PubMed search for evidence about your clinical question using the MeSH terms you identified and any other "Limits" you prefer.
5. Record the following information about your PubMed search:
   - Your initial search term choices
   - Were your keywords in the MeSH database?
     - If not, what keywords did you choose from the MeSH vocabulary instead?
   - What limits did you select? Why?
   - What were your search results?
     - Number of hits?
     - Number of articles that looked promising based on their titles?

- Change your search in some way.
  - What did you change? Why?
  - What was the outcome (more hits, fewer hits)?

6. Try your search with one other database that you think would best help you answer the question.
   - Which electronic database did you choose? Why?
   - Which keywords did you use in this database? Why?
   - Which limits did you use in this database? Why?
   - What were your results?
     - Number of hits?
     - Number of articles that look promising based on their titles?
   - How would you compare this database with PubMed in helping you to answer this question?

References

1. American Physical Therapy Association, Guide to Physical Therapist Practice. 2d ed. *Phys Ther.* 2001; 81(1):9–746.
2. Higgs J, Jones M. *Clinical Reasoning in the Health Professions*. 2d ed. Oxford, England: Butterworth Heinemann; 2000.
3. Sackett DL, Straus SE, Richardson WS, Rosenberg W, Haynes RB. *Evidence-based Medicine. How to Practice and Teach EBM.* 2d ed. Edinburgh, Scotland: Churchill Livingstone; 2000.
4. Guyatt G, Rennie D. *Users' Guides to the Medical Literature: A Manual for Evidence-Based Clinical Practice*. Chicago, IL: AMA Press; 2002.
5. Helewa A, Walker JM. *Critical Evaluation of Research in Physical Rehabilitation: Towards Evidence-Based Practice.* Philadelphia, PA: W.B. Saunders Company; 2000.
6. PubMed. U.S. National Library of Medicine Web site. Available at: http://www.ncbi.nlm.nih.gov/entrez/query.fcgi?DB=pubmed. Accessed February 20, 2006.
7. MeSH. PubMed. U.S. National Library of Medicine Web site. Available at: http://www.ncbi.nlm.nih.gov/entrez/query.fcgi?db=mesh. Accessed February 20, 2006.
8. MeSH Search Results. PubMed. U.S. National Library of Medicine Web site. Available at: http://www.ncbi.nlm.nih.gov./entrez/query.fcgi?CMD=search&DB=mesh. Accessed February 20, 2006.
9. Cumulative Index of Nursing and Allied Health Literature. Available via Ovid's Web site at: http://www.ovid.com/site/catalog/DataBase/40.jsp?top=2&mid=3&bottom=7&subsection=10. Accessed February 20, 2006.
10. The Cochrane Library. The Cochrane Collaboration Web site. Available via Wiley Interscience at: http://www.cochrane.org/. Accessed February 20, 2006.
11. Physiotherapy Evidence Database. Center for Evidence-Based Physiotherapy Web site. Available at: http://www.pedro.fhs.usyd.edu.au/index.html. Accessed February 20, 2006.
12. Maher CG, Sherrington C, Herbert RD, Moseley AM, Elkins M. Reliability of the PEDro scale for rating quality of randomized controlled trials. *Phys Ther.* 2003; 83(8):713–721.

13. Hooked on Evidence. American Physical Therapy Association Web site. Available at: http://www.hookedonevidence.com/. Accessed February 20, 2006.
14. International Classification of Diseases, Ninth Revision. National Center for Health Statistics. Centers for Disease Control and Prevention Web site. Available at: http://www.cdc.gov/nchs/icd9.htm. Accessed February 20, 2006.
15. Suomi R, Koceja DM. Postural sway characteristics in women with lower extremity arthritis before and after an aquatic exercise intervention. *Arch Phys Med Rehabil.* 2000; 81(6): 780–785.
16. Research. American Physical Therapy Association Web site. Available at: http://www.apta.org/AM/Template.cfm?Section=Research&Template=/TaggedPage/TaggedPageDisplay.cfm&TPLID=54&ContentID=12664. Accessed February 20, 2006.
17. Bandolier: "Evidence-based thinking about healthcare." Available at: http://www.jr2.ox.ac.uk/bandolier/index.html. Accessed February 20, 2006.
18. Netting the Evidence. The School of Health and Related Research Web site. Available at: http://www.shef.ac.uk/scharr/ir/netting/. Accessed February 20, 2006.
19. TRIP Database. Turning Research into Practice. Available at: http://www.updatesoftware.com/trip/logon.asp?Log=1&SrchEx=_SrchEx_. Accessed February 20, 2006.
20. Evidence in Motion. Available at: http://www.evidenceinmotion.com/index.asp. Accessed February 20, 2006.
21. EBM Online. Available at: http://ebm.bmjjournals.com/. Accessed February 20, 2006.
22. ACP Journal Club Web site. American College of Physicians. Available at: http://www.acpjc.org/. Accessed February 20, 2006.
23. Medscape. WebMD Web site. Available at: http://www.medscape.com/pages/homepages/splash?src=hdr. Accessed February 20, 2006.
24. MDConsult Web site. Elsevier. Available at: www.mdconsult.com. Accessed February 20, 2006.

Part II

Elements of Evidence

Chapter 4

Questions, Theories, and Hypotheses

It is better to know some of the questions than all of the answers.

—James Thurber

Objectives

Upon completion of this chapter the student/practitioner will be able to:

1. Discuss the purpose and characteristics of a well-worded research question or problem statement.
2. Discuss the purpose and characteristics of background information used to support the need for a study, including literature reviews and publicly-available epidemiological data.
3. Differentiate between the terms *theory*, *concept*, and *construct*.
4. Explain the use of theories and conceptual frameworks in clinical research.
5. Discuss the concept of biological plausibility and explain its role in clinical research.
6. Differentiate between the form and uses of the null and research hypotheses.

Terms in This Chapter

Biological Plausibility: The reasonable expectation that the human body could behave in the manner predicted.

Concept: A mental image of an observable phenomenon that is expressed in words.[1]

Conceptual Framework: A collection of interrelated concepts or constructs that reflect a common theme; may be the basis of a more formal theory; usually depicted in schematic form.[2]

Construct: A nonobservable abstraction created for a specific research purpose; defined by observable measures, such as events or behaviors.[2]

Disability: "The inability or restricted ability to perform actions, tasks, and activities related to required self-care, home management, work (job/school/play), community, and leisure roles in the individual's sociocultural context and physical environment."[4(p. 31)]

Functional Limitations: "Occur when impairments result in a restriction of the ability to perform a physical action, task or activity in an efficient, typically expected, or competent manner."[4(p.30)]

Impairment: "Alterations in the anatomical, physiological or psychological structures or functions that both (1) result from underlying changes in the normal state and (2) contribute to illness."[4(p. 31)]

Null Hypothesis: Also referred to as the "statistical hypothesis;" a prediction that the outcome of an investigation will demonstrate "no difference" or "no relationship" between groups (or variables) in the study other than what chance alone might create.[3]

Pathology: A disease, disorder, or condition that is "primarily identified at the cellular level" and is "(1) characterized by a particular cluster of signs and symptoms and (2) recognized by either the patient/client or the practitioner as abnormal."[4(p. 29)]

Research Hypothesis: Also referred to as the "alternative hypothesis;" a prediction that the outcome of an investigation will demonstrate a difference or relationship between groups (or variables) in the study that is the result of more than chance alone (i.e., statistically significant). May be written using directional language such as "more than," "less than," "positive," or "negative."[3]

Theory: An organized set of relationships among concepts or constructs; proposed to describe and explain systematically a phenomenon of interest, as well as to predict future behaviors or outcomes.[1,2]

INTRODUCTION

In the broadest sense, research is a quest for answers about the way the world works. Depending upon one's perspective, these answers are viewed either as absolute truths that are waiting to be revealed (the quantitative research view) or as constructions of reality that are relevant only to those involved (the qualitative research view).[1] Either way, a plan for obtaining the desired knowledge usually is developed and implemented by individuals or groups who have the motivation and resources to embark on the research quest. This plan, and its outcome, is documented in a variety of forms, the most common of which is the research article. Although the articles themselves may have different formats dictated by publishers' preferences, they usually contain information pertaining to a study's essential elements:

- Research question(s) or purpose statement(s);
- Background information;
- Theoretical or conceptual basis of the study;
- Hypothesis(es) about the study's outcome;
- Subjects used in the study;
- Research design;
- Variables and their measures;
- Method of statistical analysis
- Study results;
- Implications and importance of the study's findings.

Additional details may be provided related to limitations of the researchers' efforts, as well as suggestions for future research. This chapter will review the purpose, key features, and practical issues surrounding the first four bulleted items. Subsequent chapters will address the remaining research elements in the list.

THE RESEARCH QUESTION

Research is a serious and potentially complex endeavor that requires time and resources in support of the quest for answers. The desire to conduct a study may be stimulated by clinical experience and observation, a curious nature, or an interest in advancing knowledge for its own sake. In order to plan appropriately, an investigator must start with a specific objective toward which his or her research efforts will be directed. This objective may be expressed in the form of a question, a purpose statement, or a problem statement.[5] The content is more important than the form; in other words, the researcher should be clear about what he or she wants to know. Table 4–1 lists general questions that may serve as a study's objective, any of which can be tailored to address specific clinical concerns.

Washington *et al.* used research questions to describe their objectives in their study of neurologically impaired infants:[6(p. 1066)]

> The research questions were:
>
> 1. What are the effects of a CFS (contoured foam support) on postural alignment for infants with neuromotor impairments?
> 2. What are the effects of a CFS on the infants' ability to engage with toys?

Table 4–1 General research questions and their clinical focus.

Questions that Research May Answer	Clinical Focus
How does this work?	Background about a clinical technique or instrument
What does that look like?	Background about a clinical problem (pathology, impairment, functional limitation, disability)
How do I measure...?	Development of a clinical test
Which is the best test to determine if...?	Usefulness of a diagnostic test.
What is the risk of...?	Prediction about a future outcome
What happens when I do...?	Evaluation of treatment effects
How does my patient/client's life change when...?	Evaluation of outcomes from patient/client's point of view

3. How do parents perceive the use and effects of a CFS when used at home?

The first two questions address the effects of a specific intervention—contoured foam support—while the third question considers the impact of the device from the parents' point of view. Other authors have expressed their research objectives in purpose statement format, as illustrated in Table 4–2.[7–13] Whether formulated as a question or purpose statement, the research objective should be articulated clearly so that anyone reading will understand immediately what the study was about. The challenge for the investigators is to construct a research question or purpose statement so that it is not too broad to answer in a reasonable fashion, but not so small as to be insignificant.

BACKGROUND

A well-worded research question or purpose statement is necessary, but not sufficient by itself to define a useful study. Although knowledge may be important for its own sake to some individuals, evidence-based practice is best supported by research that is relevant and that advances knowledge in the professional field. These criteria also are used as part of the article review process required for publication in most scientific journals.[1] As a result investigators are obligated to demonstrate:

- Why the question or purpose statement is important to answer; and,

Table 4–2 Purpose statements from physical therapy research.

Citation	Purpose Statement
Systematic Review Milne S, Brosseau L, Robinson V, Noel MJ, Davis J *et al.* *Cochrane Database Syst Rev.* 2003; (2):CD004260.[5]	"The aim of this meta analysis is to determine the effectiveness of CPM following knee arthroplasty." (p. 2)
Randomized Clinical Trial Johansson KM, Adolfsson LE, Foldevi MOM. *Phys Ther.* 2005; 85:490–501.[6]	"The purpose of this study was to compare manual acupuncture and continuous ultrasound, both applied in addition to home exercises, for patients diagnosed with impingement syndrome." (p. 490)
Quasi-Experimental Study Kileff J, Ashburn A. *Clin Rehabil.* 2005 Mar; 19(2):165–169.[7]	"A pilot study to investigate the effect of aerobic exercise on the mobility and function of people with moderate disability multiple sclerosis." (p. 165)
Observational Study Kirk-Sanchez NJ. *Phys Ther.* 2004; 84:408–418.[8]	"The purpose of this study was to determine factors related to activity limitations in a group of Cuban Americans recovering from hip fractures." (p. 408)
Physiologic Study DeSimone NA, Christiansen C, Dore D. *Phys Ther.* 1999; 79:839–846.[9]	"The purpose of this in vitro study was to identify any possible bactericidal effects of the 0.95-mW He-Ne and 5-mW In-Ga-Al-PO_4 lasers on photosensitized *S. aureus* and *P. aeruginosa*." (p. 841)
Case Report Shrader JA, Siegel KL. *Phys Ther.* 2003; 83:831–843.[10]	"The purpose of this case report is to describe a patient with rheumatoid arthritis and functional hallus limitus who was managed with foot orthoses, footwear, shoe modifications, and patient education." (p. 831)
Summary Ciesla ND. *Phys Ther.* 1996; 76:609–625.[11]	"This article reviews how chest physical therapy is used with patients who are critically ill. A brief historical review of the literature is presented." (p. 609)

- How the results obtained will increase understanding of a particular phenomenon or situation.

In other words, they must provide sufficient background information to justify the need for their study. This background material usually comes in two forms—a literature review and citations of publicly-available epidemiological data. Either or both may be used to support the relevance of the research question or purpose statement.

Literature Review

Investigators often summarize and critique prior studies to clarify what is currently known and what remains to be answered about the research topic in which they are interested. These literature reviews may be brief in form and generally focus on previous works that have the closest relationship to the research question or purpose statement. Occasionally these reviews indicate the need to explore new frontiers in practice altogether, as may be the case when innovative technology is introduced to treat an established clinical problem in a new and different way. More often, limitations of prior research, such as insufficient numbers or types of subjects, supply the rationale for the current study. For example, an earlier work that evaluated a physical therapy intervention in five adult males may be offered as an argument for repeating the research with 200 adult males in order to verify that the first study's results were not a fluke related to such a small group. Similarly, the study of 200 men may be cited as justification for conducting the same research on a large group of adult women to evaluate potential gender differences in response to the experimental intervention. Other design problems related to measurement techniques, management of subjects during the study, and statistical analysis also may be identified as reasons for further study of a phenomenon or problem. In the end, the goal is to build a logical case supporting the necessity and importance of the current project.

A literature review must be comprehensive, but often must conform to the space restrictions a publisher imposes. As a result, investigators must select wisely the previous works they will include as part of their justification for their study. Evidence-based physical therapists then must decide whether the investigators considered, and accurately evaluated, the most relevant studies. A therapist with experience and/or expertise in a particular subject area usually will recognize whether a literature review is thorough and accurate. Less experienced practitioners, on the other hand, may rely on more superficial indicators such as 1) the age of the prior studies reviewed; 2) whether the review flows in a logical sequence toward the current research question; and, 3) whether the articles reviewed are related to the research question. This last point is tricky, however, because there are many occasions when an investigator has a question because there is no prior evidence available. In these cases, researchers may review studies from other disciplines (e.g., medicine, nursing, occupational therapy) or other practice settings (e.g., skilled nursing facilities, outpatient rehabilitation, home health). Alternatively, they may consider studies that look at diagnoses or clinical problems that have similar characteristics to the disease or disorder in which the researchers are interested. For example, if investigators want to study an exercise technique in patients with Guillain-Barré syndrome they may consider prior research on other remitting paralyzing diseases, such as multiple sclerosis or polio, because there is a limited body of evidence about rehabilitation for Guillain-Barré. Any of these tactics is reasonable as long as the researcher is able to use the information to demonstrate the relevance and significance of the current project.

Citations of Epidemiological Data

In addition to, or in lieu of, a literature review, researchers may cite routinely collected data about the phenomenon and/or about its impact upon society. Commonly used data in clinical research include health statistics[5] from: a) federal agencies, such as the Centers for Disease Control and Prevention,[14] the Occupational Health and Safety Administration,[15] the Department of Health and Human Services,[16] and the U.S. Census Bureau;[17] b) state agencies, such as departments of health and disability services, workers' compensation boards, and health care regulatory agencies; and, c) private organizations, such as the Pew Health Professions Commission[18] and the Robert Wood Johnson Foundation.[19] Academic centers also may collect and provide data about health-related issues in their community or data for which they have dedicated practice or research resources. Examples of data that physical therapy researchers might use include, but are not limited to:

- The incidence or prevalence of a pathology or impairment;
- The loss in productive work time due to injury;
- The cost of health care services provided to treat a problem that could have been prevented; and,
- Which segments of the population have the least access to health care services.

In rare instances, the need for a study is justified by the identification of a previously undiscovered clinical phenomenon. These events are more likely to be medical in nature, as was the case with polio, human immunodeficiency virus (HIV), and sudden acute respiratory syndrome (SARS). However, the onset of these events may stimulate the need for physical therapy research into examination and treatment techniques to manage their functional sequelae. Data in these situations may be incomplete at best, but still may provide support for pilot studies that explore the impact of physical therapy on these phenomena.

THEORIES, CONCEPTS, AND CONSTRUCTS

In addition to its clinical origins, a research study also may have a theoretical or conceptual basis that incorporates relevant concepts or constructs. A *concept* is a mental image of an observable phenomenon described in words.[2] For example, the concept "fatigue" refers to a collection of observable behaviors or states such as falling asleep in class, dark circles under one's eyes, and complaints of low energy. On the other hand, a *construct* is a nonobservable abstraction created for a specific research purpose that is defined by observable measures.[2] For example, the construct "readiness to change" describes an individual's openness to adopting a different behavior.[20] "Readiness" is not directly observable in the same way that one can detect an expression of fatigue or pain. However, "readiness" can be inferred from behaviors, such as gathering information about the proposed lifestyle changes, discussing the change with people from whom an individual will need support or guidance, and writing out a plan for implementing the change. Table 4-3 provides several examples of concepts and constructs used in physical therapy research.

A *theory* is an organized set of relationships among concepts or constructs that is proposed to describe and explain systematically a phenomenon of interest. A successful theory is one that is consistent with empirical observations and that, through repeated testing under various conditions, is able to predict future behavior or outcomes.[1,5] Comprehensive theoretical models, such as Einstein's theory of relativity and Darwin's theory of evolution, are referred to as "grand theories" because of their scope and complexity.[1] As the title implies, grand theories seek to explain as much as possible re-

Table 4-3 Examples of concepts and constructs used in physical therapy research.

Element	Example	Potential Measure
Concept	Age	Years since birth
	Pain	Visual scale with progressively grimacing faces
	Flexibility	Degrees of joint motion
Construct	Patient Satisfaction	Ratings of care and the clinical environment
	Health-Related Quality of Life	Ability to engage in physical, emotional, and social functions and roles
	Motivation	Attendance and active participation in a program

lated to their focus areas. Jean Piaget's theory of cognitive development in children is an example of a grand theory relevant to physical therapy.[21] Based on numerous empirical observations, Piaget proposed that children progress through four stages during which their understanding of the world develops from concrete perceptions and reflex-driven actions to abstract conceptualizations and purposeful choices. A child's interactions with his or her environment and social context, as well as the natural maturation of his or her physical and linguistic abilities, fuel the progression from one stage to another. Together these experiences result in the creation of new knowledge and understanding about the world that serves as the foundation for the next developmental stage. Figure 4–1 depicts Piaget's theory in schematic form. The diagram illustrates an important point about grand theories: they are comprehensive in detail, but often impractical to test in their entirety. The accumulation of evidence about various aspects of these theories usually is required to demonstrate their overall usefulness.

Smaller scale theories often are referred to as conceptual frameworks. *Conceptual frameworks* also describe relationships among concepts and constructs from which predictions may be made, but are not elaborate enough to explain the phenomenon of interest. An example of a conceptual framework relevant to physical therapy practice is Nagi's model of the disablement process.[22] As Figure 4–2 illustrates, the concepts in the model are active *pathology*, *impairment*, *functional limitation*, and *disability*. They are related to

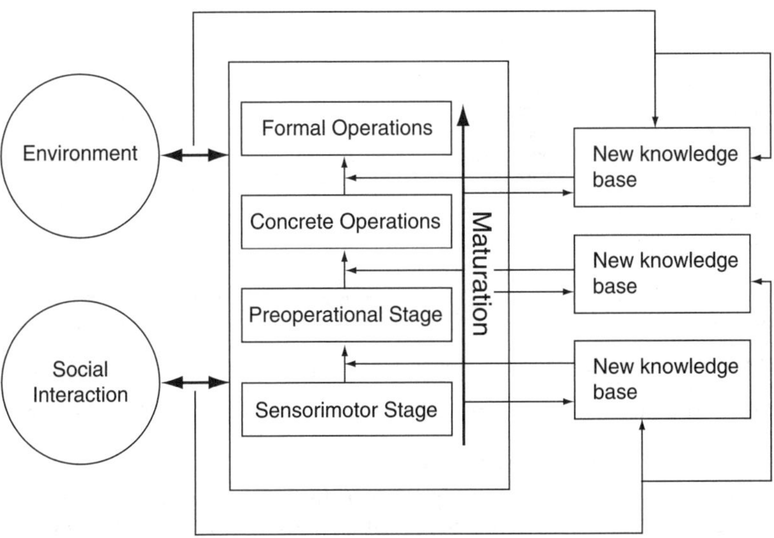

Figure 4–1 Piaget's Theory of Cognitive Development.[21]

one another in a unidirectional sequential fashion; in other words, an impairment may be predicted as the result of active pathology; a functional limitation may be predicted as the result of an impairment; and a disability may be predicted as a result of a functional limitation. In comparison to Figure 4–1, this model is simple and easy to interpret. Conceptual frameworks usually do not have the complexity of grand theories, making them easier to test in clinical research; however, frameworks with little detail may be criticized for their lack of sensitivity to environmental influences and individual subject variability.

Whether a clinical study of human behavior is based upon a theory or conceptual framework, it must also meet the test of *biological plausibility*—that is, the reasonable expectation that the human body could behave in the manner predicted. For example, a research question about the effect of a new therapeutic exercise technique on restoration of normal movement in adults following stroke might reasonably be based on observations about the developmental sequence of motor patterns in infants and children. Conversely, a study that examined the strengthening effects of a 3-day active-assisted exercise program fails to meet the biological plausibility test because of the insufficient time frame and intensity implemented for muscle adaptation to increased workloads. As was revealed by recent hormone replacement studies, approaches based on biological plausibility also must be tested by empirical research in order to avoid potentially harmful misdirection.[23]

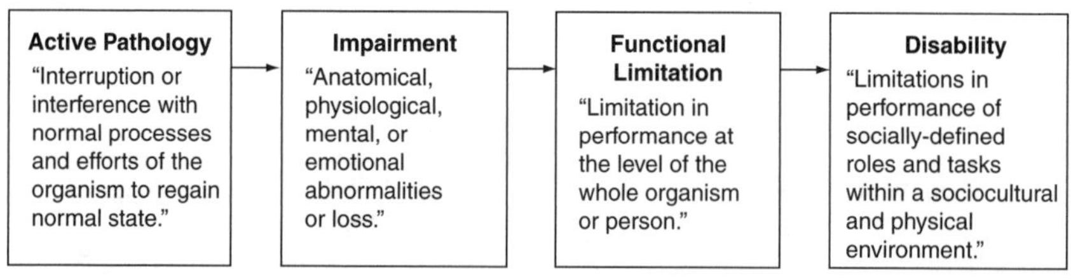

Potential Observable Measures:

Active Pathology: Data from lab tests, cell biopsies, radiographs, surgical exploration, etc.
Impairment: Limited degrees of motion in a joint, reduced torque in a muscle group, change in structure due to amputation or defect, etc.
Functional Limitation: Inability to move in and out of bed, rise from a chair, walk across a room, climb stairs, etc.
Disability: Inability to attend school, work, care for family, participate in leisure and social activities, etc.

Figure 4–2 Nagi's Model of Disablement[22]

Source: Reprinted from Jette AM with permission of the American Physical Therapy Association. Physical disablement concepts for physical therapy research and practice. *Phys Ther.* 1994; 74(5):380–386. This material is copyrighted, and any further reproduction or distribution is prohibited.

Many clinical studies do not have a formally stated theoretical or conceptual framework to test; their focus is much more pragmatic in terms of identifying the usefulness of a diagnostic test, predictive factor, intervention, or outcome. These studies are not intended to explain a phenomenon in an abstract way by developing or testing a theory. Nevertheless, researchers may "theorize" about phenomena they wish to study. Unless the investigators are proposing a formal theory of their own, their use of the term "theorize" is meant to indicate informed speculation and nothing more. Similarly, authors will interchange the terms theory, concept, and construct, as well as theoretical model and conceptual model. The key is to avoid being distracted by the terminology and focus on the content of what is proposed so that the remainder of the study may be evaluated based on this information.

HYPOTHESES

In addition to proposing a basis for the study, researchers also may offer predictions about its outcomes. When these statements are derived from theoretical or conceptual models they are called "hypotheses." Hypotheses usually are written as stand-alone statements that are structured in one of two ways. One version is the *null hypothesis* (H_0), the phrasing of which indicates that the researchers anticipate "no difference" or "no relationship" between groups or variables will be demonstrated by their study's results. This approach also is referred to as the "statistical hypothesis" because statistical tests are designed specifically to challenge the "no difference (no relationship)" statement.[1,2,3,5] The premise behind this approach is that a study's results may be due to chance rather than due to the experiment or phenomenon of interest. Jones *et al.* used a null hypothesis in their study of lung sound intensities recorded when subjects were placed in different positions:[24(p. 683-4)]

> We hypothesized that there would be no differences in the data recorded in corresponding regions between (1) the left and right lungs in the sitting position, (2) the dependent and nondependent lungs in the side-lying position (in side-lying positions, the upper hemithorax is "nondependent," and the side in contact with the bed is "dependent"), (3) the sitting position and the dependent position, or (4) the sitting position and the nondependent position.

In other words, these authors anticipated that values for lung sounds would be the same, on average, regardless of the position in which the subjects were placed. Any differences among the sounds would be due to chance—that is, these differences could not be reproduced systematically through repeated study. If the statistical tests investigators perform confirm their expectations, then the null hypothesis is "accepted." Researchers will identify this situation with phrases such as "we found no statistically significant difference (or relationship) between. . . ." On the other hand, if the tests indicate that the study's results are not due to chance, then the null hypothesis is "rejected." Researchers will indicate this situation with phrases such as "we found a statistically significant difference (or relationship) between. . . ."

The second form of hypothesis statement is referred to as a *research hypothesis* or "alternate hypothesis" (H_A). These statements predict that a difference or relationship between the groups or variables will be demonstrated by the study's results. Researchers even may provide directional language, such as "more than," "less than," "positive," or "negative," in order to make their predictions more specific.[1,2,3,5] Henry *et al.* used directional research hypotheses in their study of the effect of the number of home exercises assigned on performance and compliance with a home program for older adults:[25(p. 273)]

> Three hypotheses were formulated prior to this study: (1) Subjects who are prescribed two exercises will perform better than subjects who are prescribed eight exercises, (2) Subjects who are prescribed two exercises will comply on their self-report exercise log more than subjects who are prescribed eight exercises, and (3) Self-report percentage rates will highly correlate with performance assessment tool scores.

In other words, these authors predicted that a lower number of exercises would be related to greater success with the home program. In this example, if a statistical test demonstrates a significant difference or relationship, then the research hypothesis is "accepted." If the test indicates that the results likely occurred due to chance then the research hypothesis is "rejected." It is important to note that, regardless of form, hypotheses are tested *as stated* such that the statements are either accepted or rejected. Researchers may speculate about another possible outcome when their original hypothesis is rejected, but it would be inappropriate for them to claim that this alternate prediction has been "proven."

As is true with theories and conceptual frameworks, researchers may hypothesize about a result without stating their intentions in a formal way. An additional challenge for readers is that authors of physical therapy research often do not present any hypotheses at all. The presence or absence of hypothesis statements may be driven by publishers' formatting preferences, by the manner in which the researchers were trained to develop and communicate about their research, or by the nature of the research itself. The lack of hypothesis statements does not reduce the quality of the research in and of itself;

rather, it is the manner in which the authors interpret their results relative to these statements that may cause the reader to question the research quality.

SUMMARY

Research is a quest for answers about a question or purpose statement that investigators have identified through a variety of methods. The relevance and importance of the quest may be demonstrated through a review of prior literature, as well as by other data about the impact of a phenomenon on individuals or society. The quest may be guided or based upon formally stated relationships among ideas and observations that may be as elaborate as a grand theory or as simple as a conceptual framework. In all cases, proposals about human behavior must be based on biological plausibility. Finally, researchers may predict the outcome of their study using formal null or research hypotheses. Statistical tests are used to determine whether these hypotheses should be accepted or rejected as written; however, rejection does not prove that other possible explanations are true. Finally, the use of theories, models, or hypotheses will depend upon the investigator's research purpose and intent. Clinical studies may not have any of these elements, but authors may use the terminology in an informal way to convey their speculations or predictions. Readers should focus on the content of the material presented to determine the success with which the investigators have justified the need for their study and described the foundation upon which the project will be conducted.

Exercises

1. Think about a patient scenario or clinical situation in which you have been involved and ask yourself what more you would like to know about that situation.
   a. Write that thought in the form of a research question.
   b. Write that thought in the form of a purpose statement.
   c. Rewrite your statement from (a) or (b) to make it broader.
   d. Rewrite your statement from (a) or (b) to make it narrower.
2. Write a brief rationale justifying why your idea is relevant and important to study. Remember the issue of biological plausibility if it is appropriate to your question or statement.
3. Describe a plan for a literature review you would conduct in order to determine what is known about your research question or purpose statement. Include alternative strategies in case your first search attempt reveals no prior studies.

4. Identify sources of epidemiological data you would include (assuming they are available) to justify the need for your study.
5. Differentiate between a theory and a conceptual framework.
6. Differentiate between a concept and a construct. Give an example of each.
7. Differentiate between the null and the research hypothesis. Give an example of each based on your research question or purpose statement from Question #1 above.

References

1. Domholdt E. *Rehabilitation Research. Principles and Applications.* 3d ed. St Louis, MO: Elsevier Saunders; 2005.
2. Polit DF, Beck CT. *Nursing Research: Principles and Methods.* 7th ed. Philadelphia, PA: Lippincott Williams & Wilkins; 2003.
3. Portney LG, Watkins MP. *Foundations of Clinical Research. Applications to Practice.* 2d ed. Upper Saddle River, NJ: Prentice Hall Health; 2000.
4. American Physical Therapy Association, Guide to Physical Therapist Practice. 2d ed. *Phys Ther.* 2001; 81(1);9–746.
5. Batavia M. *Clinical Research for Health Professionals: A User-Friendly Guide.* Boston, MA: Butterworth-Heinemann; 2001.
6. Washington K, Deitz JC, White OR, Schwartz IS. The effects of a contoured foam seat on postural alignment and upper-extremity function in infants with neuromotor impairments. *Phys Ther.* 2002; 82(11):1064–1076.
7. Milne S, Brosseau L, Robinson V, Noel MJ, Davis J *et al.* Continuous passive motion following total knee arthroplasty. *Cochrane Database Syst Rev.* 2003; (2):CD004260.
8. Johansson KM, Adolfsson LE, Foldevi MOM. Effects of acupuncture versus ultrasound in patients with impingement syndrome: Randomized clinical trial. *Phys Ther.* 2005; 85(6):490–501.
9. Kileff J, Ashburn A. A pilot study of the effect of aerobic exercise on people with moderate disability multiple sclerosis. *Clin Rehabil.* 2005 Mar; 19(2): 165–169.
10. Kirk-Sanchez NJ. Factors related to activity limitations in a group of Cuban Americans before and after hip fracture. *Phys Ther.* 2004; 84(5):408–418.
11. DeSimone NA, Christiansen C, Dore D. Bactericidal effect of 0.95-mW helium-neon and 5-mW indium-gallium-aluminum-phosphate laser irradiation at exposure times of 30, 60, and 120 seconds on photosensitized *Staphylococcus aureus* and *Pseudomonas aeruginosa* in vitro. *Phys Ther.* 1999; 79(9):839–846.
12. Shrader JA, Siegel KL. Nonoperative management of functional hallux limitus in a patient with rheumatoid arthritis. *Phys Ther.* 2003; 83(9):831–843.
13. Ciesla ND. Chest physical therapy for patients in the intensive care unit. *Phys Ther.* 1996; 76(6):609–625.
14. Data & Statistics. Centers for Disease Control and Prevention Web site. Available at: http://www.cdc.gov/node.do/id/0900f3ec8000ec28. Accessed February 22, 2006.

15. Statistics & Data. Occupational Health & Safety Administration Web site. Available at: http://www.osha.gov/oshstats/index.html. Accessed February 22, 2006.
16. Reference Collections. U.S. Department of Health and Human Services Web site. Available at: http://www.hhs.gov/reference/index.shtml#statistics. Accessed February 22, 2006.
17. U.S. Census Bureau Web site. Available at: http://www.census.gov/. Accessed February 22, 2006.
18. Pew Health Professions Commission Web site. Available at: http://futurehealth.ucsf.edu/pewcomm/factsht3.html. Accessed February 22, 2006.
19. Robert Wood Johnson Foundation Web site. Available at: http://www.rwjf.org/index.jsp. Accessed February 22, 2006.
20. DiClemente CC, Schlundt D, Gemmell L. Readiness and stages of change in addiction treatment. *Am J Addict.* 2004; 13(2):103–119.
21. Jean Piaget's Stage Theory. School of Psychology, Massey University, New Zealand. Available at http://www.evolution.massey.ac.nz. Accessed September 24, 2005.
22. Jette AM. Physical disablement concepts for physical therapy research and practice. *Phys Ther.* 1994; 74(5):380–386.
23. Women's Health Initiative Participant Information. National Institutes of Health. Available at: http://www.whi.org/. Accessed February 15, 2006.
24. Jones A, Jones RD, Kwong K, Burns Y. Effect of positioning on recorded lung sound intensities in subjects without pulmonary dysfunction. *Phys Ther.* 1999; 79(7):682–690.
25. Henry KD, Rosemond C, Eckert LB. Effect of number of home exercises on compliance and performance in adults over 65 years of age. *Phys Ther.* 1999; 79(3):270–277.

Chapter 5

Research Design

Research is the act of going up alleys to see if they are blind.

—Plutarch

Objectives

Upon completion of this chapter the student/practitioner will be able to:

1. Differentiate between quantitative and qualitative research paradigms.
2. Differentiate among experimental, quasi-experimental, and nonexperimental research designs.
3. Discuss methods by which control may be imposed in the research process.
4. Describe research designs used for questions about diagnosis, prognosis, interventions, and outcomes.
5. Describe research designs for secondary analyses and qualitative studies.

Terms in This Chapter

Between-Subjects Design: A research design that compares outcomes between two or more groups of subjects.[1]

Bias: Results or inferences that systematically deviate from the truth "or the processes leading to such deviation."[2 (p. 251)]

Biological Plausibility: The reasonable expectation that the human body could behave in the manner predicted.

Case-Control Design: A retrospective epidemiological research design used to evaluate the relationship between a potential exposure (e.g., risk factor) and an outcome (e.g., disease or disorder); two groups of subjects—one of which has the outcome (the *case*) and one which does not (the *control*)—are compared to determine which group has a greater proportion of individuals with the exposure.[3]

Case Report: A detailed description of the management of a patient/client that may serve as the basis for future research.[4]

Case Series: A description of the management of several patients/clients for the same purposes as a case report; the use of multiple individuals increases the potential importance of the observations as the basis for future research.[5]

Cohort: A group of individuals in a study who are followed over a period of time; often the group is defined by a particular characteristic, such as age.[6]

Cohort Design: A prospective epidemiological research design used to evaluate the relationship between a potential exposure (e.g., risk factor) and an outcome (e.g., disease or disorder); two groups of subjects—one of which has the exposure and one of which does not—are monitored over time to determine who develops the outcome and who does not.[3]

Cross-Sectional Study: A study that collects data about a phenomenon during a single point in time or once within a defined time interval.[7]

Dose-Response Relationship: The magnitude of an outcome increases as the magnitude of an exposure or intervention increases.[3,7]

Effectiveness: The extent to which an intervention or service produces a desired outcome under usual clinical conditions.[2]

Efficacy: The extent to which an intervention or service produces a desired outcome under ideal conditions.[2]

Experimental Design: A research design in which the behavior of randomly-assigned groups of subjects is measured following the purposeful manipulation of an independent variable(s) in at least one of the groups; used to examine cause-and-effect relationships between an independent variable(s) and an outcome(s).[1,8]

Longitudinal Study: A study that looks at a phenomenon occurring over time.[2]

Masked (Blinded): 1) In diagnosis papers, the lack of knowledge about previous test results; 2) in prognosis papers, the lack of knowledge about exposure status; and 3) in intervention papers, the lack of knowledge about to which group a subject has been assigned.

Measurement Reliability: The extent to which repeated measurements agree with one another. Also referred to as "stability," "consistency," and "reproducibility."[6]

Measurement Validity: The degree to which a measure captures what it is intended to measure.[6(p. 61)]

Meta-Analysis: A statistical method used to pool data from individual studies included in a systematic review.[9]

Narrative Review (also referred to as a Summary or Literature Review): A description of prior research without a systematic search and selection strategy or critical appraisal of the studies' merits.[9]

Nonexperimental Design (also referred to as an Observational Study): A research design in which controlled manipulation of the subjects is lacking;[1] in addition, if groups are present, assignment is predetermined based upon naturally occurring subject characteristics or activities.[7]

Patient-Centered Care: Health care that "customizes treatment recommendations and decision making in response to patients' preferences and beliefs. . . . This partnership also is characterized by informed, shared decision making, development of patient knowledge, skills needed for self-management of illness, and preventive behaviors."[10 (p. 3)]

Placebo: "An intervention without biologically active ingredients."[3 (p. 682)]

Pretest: Application of an outcome measure at the start of a study for the purposes of obtaining baseline performance of the subjects prior to manipulation of the independent variable.[8]

Posttest: Application of an outcome measure at the conclusion of a study to determine whether a change occurred in response to manipulation of the independent variable.[8]

Prospective Design: A research design that follows subjects forward over a specified period of time.

Qualitative Research Approach: A research philosophy that assumes that multiple realities exist, the measurement of which is influenced by the interdependence of researchers and their subjects.[1]

Quantitative Research Approach: A research philosophy that assumes that an objective reality exists that can be measured through systematic methods conducted by researchers who are independent of the subjects.[1]

Quasi-Experimental Design: A research design in which there is only one subject group or in which randomization to more than one subject group is lacking; controlled manipulation of the subjects is preserved.[11]

Randomized Clinical Trial (also referred to as a Randomized Controlled Trial and a Randomized Controlled Clinical Trial)[RCT]: A clinical study that uses a randomization process to assign subjects to either an experimental group(s) or a control (or comparison) group. Subjects in the experimental group receive the intervention or preventive measure of interest and then are compared to the subjects in the control (or comparison) group who did not receive the experimental manipulation.[1]

Research Design: The plan for conducting a research study.

Retrospective Design: A study that uses previously-collected information in order to answer a research question.

Sample: A collection of individuals (or units of analysis, such as organizations) taken from the population for the purposes of a research study.

Single-System Design: A quasi-experimental research design in which one subject receives in an alternating fashion both the experimental and control (or comparison) condition.[1]

Subjects: Individuals, organizations, or other units of analysis about whom information will be gathered for the purposes of a research study.

Systematic Review: A method by which a collection of studies is gathered and critically appraised in an effort to reach a conclusion about the cumulative weight of the evidence on a particular topic.[9]

Within-Subjects Design: A research design that compares repeated measures of an outcome within the same individuals.[1]

INTRODUCTION

Chapter 4 describes research as a purposeful effort to answer a question or explore a phenomenon. In clinical care those questions relate to the human body and its responses to disease and injury, as well as to the methods by which providers attempt to prevent, reverse, or minimize any deleterious consequences resulting from these problems. In order to answer these questions in a meaningful and believable way, investigators should plan each step of the research process in careful detail. This plan is referred to as the *research design*. Research designs are analogous to the plans of care physical therapists develop for their patients/clients. Both include details about the methods by which the investigator (therapist) will interact with research *subjects* (patients/clients), the timing of these interactions, the length of time of the entire effort, and the type of outcomes that will be measured. In addition, research designs and plans of care are crafted to meet the needs of a specific research question or a specific patient/client. In their ideal form, research designs and plans of care both attempt to minimize the influence of unwanted factors or events that will interfere with the outcomes.

Physical therapists using evidence to inform their practice decisions must evaluate the strength of research designs in order to determine whether the research question was answered in a believable and useful way. As discussed in Chapter 2, research designs have been classified in evidence hierarchies to facilitate easier identification of their strength; however these hierarchies only serve as an initial screening process. A thorough reading of the research report is needed to identify specific strengths and weaknesses of an individual study before its conclusions can be accepted or rejected for use in patient/client management. This chapter discusses general approaches to research design that are used in health care research, along with their purposes, benefits, and limitations. Designs best suited for diagnosis, prognosis, intervention, and outcomes questions are described. Methods of controlling unwanted influences within these designs also are reviewed. Design issues specific to the selection and management of subjects and to measurement in research will be discussed in Chapters 6 and 7, respectively.

GENERAL FEATURES OF RESEARCH DESIGNS

There are several features of research designs that are important to recognize when reviewing evidence. First, designs usually will reflect one of two philosophies about how the world is understood—that is, either a quantitative or a qualitative perspective. A *quantitative research approach* assumes that there is an objective truth that can be revealed by investigators who are independent from their subjects.[1] This independence is reinforced by specific controls imposed by the investigators to minimize any unwanted (extraneous) influences. Implicit in the term "quantitative" is the use of standardized numerical measures that can be evaluated to determine cause-and-effect relationships. This view defines the traditional scientific method that is ubiquitous across many fields of research. A *qualitative research approach*, on the other hand, assumes that truth is subjective and relative to each individual.[1] Investigators and subjects are assumed to influence each other as the researchers gather information about subjects' thoughts, perceptions, opinions, and beliefs. Data are captured in words rather than numbers. Methods of control are irrelevant in this approach because it assumes that cause-and-effect relationships cannot be distinguished; rather, an emphasis is placed on description and interpretation of the information that is gathered.

Second, research designs are characterized by whether or not the investigators actively intervene with the research subjects. *Experimental designs* are those in which the researchers purposefully manipulate some of the subjects and then measure their resulting behavior.[1,8] These designs use at least two groups of subjects for comparison purposes and include a process for randomly placing individuals into each of these groups. The comparison allows investigators to determine whether there are differences in outcomes between the group(s) that is (are) manipulated and the group(s) that is (are) not. Random assignment to these groups is the method best suited to distributing individuals equally among them (details are discussed in Chapter 6). *Quasi-experimental designs* also involve purposeful manipulation of the subjects by the investigators, but lack either a second group for comparison purposes or a random assignment process, or both.[11] These designs often are used when the investigators have difficulty obtaining sufficient numbers of subjects to form groups or when group membership is predetermined by a subject characteristic, such as whether or not the subject received a particular medical or surgical intervention prior to physical therapy.[11] The inability to randomly assign subjects to groups or to make a comparison to a nontreatment group means that other influences may explain the outcome of the study, thereby potentially reducing the usefulness of its results. Finally, *nonexperimental designs* are those in which the investigators are simply observers who collect information about the phenomenon of interest; there is no purposeful manipulation of subjects in order to produce a change in behavior or status. In addition, if groups are present, assignment is predetermined based upon naturally occurring subject characteristics or activities. These designs also are referred to as observational studies.[3]

Third, research designs may be characterized by the number of groups of subjects used in the analysis. A study in which repeated measures of an outcome are compared for a single group of subjects is referred to as a *within-subjects design*.[1] In these designs each individual's baseline measure is compared to any of their own subsequent measures to determine if a change has occurred. Alternatively, a design in which outcomes are compared between two or more groups of subjects is referred to as a *between-subjects design*.[1] Typically the average outcome score for each group is used in these analyses.

A fourth design feature is the degree to which controls can be imposed upon the behavior of all participants in the study, as well as the conditions under which the project is conducted. The issue of control relates to the need to minimize bias in a study. *Bias* refers to results that systematically deviate from the truth,[2] a situation that is likely to occur when a research project is executed without detailed, thoughtful procedures related to:

a) Recruitment, assignment, communication with and management of subjects;
b) Calibration and use of necessary equipment;
c) Maintenance of the environmental conditions during study activities;
d) Administration of testing and/or training activities;
e) Collection and recording of data; and,
f) Communication among investigators and others involved in the project.

Experimental designs are the most restrictive in terms of the amount of control imposed on study participants and conditions, starting with randomization of subjects to two or more groups for comparison. This control is necessary to improve the believability of a study whose aim is to demonstrate a cause-and-effect relationship between the variable that is manipulated and the change in subject behavior.[6,8] Quasi-experimental designs lack either the control achieved by random placement of subjects into groups or the use of a comparison group, or both; however, they may still include procedures that manage participant behavior and environmental conditions pertinent to the study. Finally, the extent of control in nonexperimental studies is limited to protocols for measurement and collection of data. In all designs, additional control (or adjustment) may be achieved statistically.

Fifth, all designs incorporate a time element that has both duration and direction. With regards to the duration, investigators must decide whether they want data collected once during a single point in time or a limited time interval (a *cross-sectional study*) or whether they will take repeated measures over an extended period of time (a *longitudinal study*).[5] The choice is dictated by the research question to be answered, as well as by logistical issues that may limit the degree to which subject follow-up is possible. The time "direction" is determined by whether the investigators want to use historical information for data (a *retrospective design*) or whether they want to collect their own data in real time (a *prospective design*). Previously collected data often are attractive because they are readily available and may provide information about large numbers of subjects. Retrospective approaches have an important disadvantage, however; they lack control over the original measurement process and over the method by which a variable (or variables) is manipulated. Uncontrolled measurement may introduce inaccuracies into the data, while uncontrolled manipulation of the variable may cause excessive variation in the outcomes. The lack of randomization to groups in a retrospective study also means that the reason a subject is in a particular group cannot be determined. There may be underlying factors pertinent to the individual that may influence the outcomes beyond the intervention itself. These consequences make it difficult to determine whether an intervention "caused" a treatment effect. Prospective data collection allows the researchers to create and implement specific rules and methods by which the data are collected and the variables are manipulated so that other factors that may influence the study's outcome are minimized.

Which characteristics a particular study demonstrates depends on the type of question the investigators want to answer,[12] as well as on the logistical considerations with which each research team must contend. For example, a question about the effectiveness of joint mobilization on low back pain may be answered through an experimental design in which one group of randomly-assigned subjects receives specified mobilization techniques plus exercise, while another group of randomly-assigned subjects receives exercise alone. In this hypothetical study, the researchers are purposefully intervening (providing mobilization to one group and not to the other) and collecting outcome data in a prospective fashion according to the duration of the study. A significant logistical challenge in this design is the need to recruit a sufficient number of patients with low back pain to enhance the strength of subsequent statistical analyses. The availability of such patients often is out of the investigators' control and may result in a lengthy time frame for the execution of the study.

On the other hand, a more efficient approach may be to review medical records of patients with low back pain who have completed an episode of physical therapy care during which they received either mobilization and exercise or exercise alone. A potential advantage of this retrospective, nonexperimental approach is the immediate availability of data for many more subjects than it would be practical to recruit in real time. The disadvantage of this approach is the potential lack of standardized procedures for application of the mobilization techniques, the exercise, or the outcome measures. In this situation, the benefit gained from a large *sample* size may be undermined by the variability in the interventions such that it is difficult to determine the true impact of joint mobilization. Nevertheless, this study may provide information that serves as the basis for a more definitive experimental design.

Table 5-1 summarizes the general features and related options for research designs. As noted in Chapter 2, questions about diagnosis, prognosis, interventions, and outcomes are answered best by different research designs. The following sections discuss details of specific designs for each category of questions, as well as designs used to summarize a body of literature and designs used to explore subject experiences and perceptions.

Table 5-1 General features of research designs.

Feature	Options	Characteristics
Philosophical Perspective	• Quantitative	• Objective reality, measured in numbers
	• Qualitative	• Subjective reality, measured in words
Design Approach	• Experimental	• Purposeful manipulation of a variable(s); random assignment of subjects to two or more groups
	• Quasi-experimental	• Purposeful manipulation of a variable(s); no random assignment to groups; may have only one group
	• Non-experimental	• Observational without manipulation of a variable(s); no random assignment to groups; may have only one group
Degree of Control	• Maximal	• Experimental Design
	• Moderate	• Quasi-experimental Design
	• Minimal	• Nonexperimental Design
Time Frame	• Cross-sectional	• Data collected once from one point in time
	• Longitudinal	• Data collected repeatedly over a period of time
Time Line	• Retrospective	• Historical data
	• Prospective	• Data collected in real time

RESEARCH DESIGNS FOR QUESTIONS ABOUT DIAGNOSIS AND MEASUREMENT

Studies about diagnostic tests or measures usually are nonexperimental and cross-sectional in design. The goal of these projects is to determine the usefulness of the test of interest for correctly detecting or quantifying a pathology or impairment. Assignment to groups and purposeful manipulation of a variable is not relevant to these studies. Instead, the strongest research design is one in which individuals who appear to have a particular disorder are evaluated with the test of interest, as well as with a second test of which the usefulness already has been established.[7] The second test usually is referred to as the "gold standard" or "reference standard" because of its ability to correctly identify individuals with, and without, the disorder of interest. Comparison of the two sets of test results allows the investigators to determine if the test of interest provides accurate information about the presence or absence of a suspected pathology or impairment (i.e., *measurement validity*). Additional information about *measurement reliability*, or the stability of the results over repeated administrations, also can be obtained.

Control of unwanted factors in these studies can be achieved through several strategies. First, investigators can clearly delineate and apply criteria for identifying which individuals are suspected of having the disorder of interest. Second, protocols for performance of the test of interest can be implemented to ensure that each subject is examined using the same methods in the same sequence. These protocols also should identify criteria for determining a positive or negative result for the test of interest. Third, verification of the examiner's (or examiners') competence performing the test of interest and the "gold standard" test will reduce potential inaccuracies in the results. Fourth, criteria for verifying the presence or absence of the diagnosis via the "gold standard" test can be delineated. Finally, investigators can withhold the results of the test of interest from the examiners responsible for confirming the diagnosis and vice versa. Keeping the examiners *masked* will reduce the chance that they will introduce bias through their expectations about the outcome of the test they are administering.

Holtby and Razmjou used many of these methods of control in their study of the usefulness of the Speed's and Yergason's test for identifying individuals with biceps tendon and glenoid labrum pathologies.[13] In this study, arthroscopic surgery was used as the "gold standard" test; therefore, individuals with shoulder pain were required to meet established criteria for surgical eligibility in order to participate. The authors also defined the signs used to recognize a positive and negative result for the Speed's and Yergason's tests, as well as for diagnosis confirmation during the arthroscopy. However, the authors did not verify whether the examiners consistently performed the clinical tests, so some variation in results may have occurred. Finally, the surgeons conducting the diagnostic arthroscopy were unaware of the clinical tests' results prior to surgery. The use of these controls improves the credibility of this article's results by decreasing, although not eliminating, the chance that extraneous factors influenced the outcomes.

Methodological Studies of Impairment Measures

Research about the usefulness of diagnostic tests is complemented by studies in which new instruments are developed, or existing instruments are modified and tested for their usefulness. Collectively referred to as "methodological research,"[6] these studies usually focus on clinical measures used to quantify impairments, such as limited range of motion,[14] weakness,[15] and loss of balance.[16] Like studies for diagnostics tests, the designs for methodological studies are nonexperimental and usually, although not exclusively, cross-sectional in nature. Similarly, both types of studies evaluate an instrument's reliability and measurement validity. Details about these important measurement properties are discussed in Chapter 7. The usefulness of the instrument in different patient/client populations also may be explored. Methods of control in these designs focus on the procedures for identification and recruitment of subjects, protocols for the development and administration of the instruments, and statistical adjustment to account for extraneous factors that may influence subject performance, or for loss of information due to subject drop out.

RESEARCH DESIGNS FOR QUESTIONS ABOUT PROGNOSIS

Studies focusing on prognosis commonly have one of the following research designs used routinely in epidemiological research: 1) prospective cohort; 2) retrospective cohort; or, 3) case-control.[9] All of these designs assess the relationship between an exposure (i.e., risk factor, predictive factor) and an outcome. They also are descriptive in nature; therefore, control often is limited to methods by which the investigators identify eligible subjects and collect the data. Management of extraneous factors usually occurs through statistical adjustment. An important feature of these designs is that causal links between a risk factor or predictor and an outcome cannot be established directly. Causality may be inferred, however, when the following conditions are met:

- The exposure clearly preceded the outcome (demonstrated by longitudinal designs);

- The relationship between the exposure and the outcome was strong (as defined by the nature of its measurement);
- A *dose-response relationship* between the exposure and the outcome was demonstrated;
- The findings are consistent with results from previous (preferably well-designed) studies; and,
- The results are *biologically plausible*.[17]

Inferences about causality may be necessary in situations in which it would be inappropriate or unethical to perform an experiment to determine a cause-and-effect relationship.

Cohort Designs

The term *cohort* refers to a group of subjects who are followed over time and who usually share a common characteristic such as gender, age, occupation, the presence of a risk factor or diagnosis, and so forth.[6] *Cohort designs* have nonexperimental descriptive designs from which results are analyzed statistically to determine the relationship between risk (or predictive) factors and outcomes.

A prospective cohort design is one in which a group of subjects is identified and then followed over a specified period of time to see if, and when, the outcome of interest occurs.[9] Often more than one group is followed for the purposes of comparison. The second group usually does not have the risk factor or predictor of interest. Prospective cohort designs are the preferred research designs for prognosis questions because the authors have the best opportunity to control extraneous influences by collecting their own data in real time, rather than using historical information. In addition, starting with the risk or predictive factor and working toward the outcome is a necessary sequence to make a stronger case for a potential cause-and-effect relationship. An important challenge to this design is the time needed to ensure that the outcome could occur and be measured, as well as the resources necessary to follow subjects over long periods. Rainville *et al.* used a prospective cohort design to examine whether pain and disability in patients with chronic low back pain were related to financial compensation for the injury.[18] Patients from one spine rehabilitation center were divided into two groups based upon whether or not they were receiving (or pursuing) payment for their back pain. Procedures for the application of the pain and disability measures were defined in the study, thereby reducing the chances of variation due to inconsistent test performance. These authors collected follow-up measures at three and twelve months post completion of rehabilitation. These time frames were consistent with their study objective and certainly long enough for pain and disability to be minimized or corrected.

A retrospective cohort design is one in which data from medical records, outcomes databases, or claims databases are examined and a cohort or cohorts are identified during the review process.[9] This approach addresses the challenge of the prospective cohort design in that the outcomes already have occurred and can be identified. However, control over how the measures were collected during actual encounters with the subjects is lost. MacPherson *et al.* used this design to examine the relationship between the mechanism of injury and functional outcomes in children suffering trauma.[19] These authors identified a cohort of pediatric trauma patients admitted to one hospital and collected historical data regarding the injury's anatomic location, mechanism, and severity; patient age and gender; type of surgery; and rehabilitation services provided. Functional outcome data, measured using an instrument known as the WeeFIM,[20] also were collected from the medical records. The authors did not report the reliability or validity of any of these measures. In addition, they could not control for the fact that only 73 percent of the originally eligible subjects had six month follow-up data recorded—the time frame defined in the study's purpose. In this case, the logistical challenge of long-term follow-up of patients proved to be a problem that translated into a limitation for the researchers despite the use of a retrospective study design.

Case-Control Designs

A *case-control design* is a retrospective approach in which subjects who are known to have the diagnosis of interest are compared to a control group known to be free of the diagnosis.[9] The question investigated is the relative frequency of exposure to a risk factor or predictor in each group. The quintessential example here is the initial investigation into the relationship between smoking and lung cancer. Lung cancer takes years to develop so it was impractical to wait and see what happens once someone started smoking. Instead, researchers identified subjects diagnosed with lung cancer and subjects free of the disease and worked backwards to determine each individual's exposure to smoking. Eventually, results from both prospective and retrospective designs provided enough convincing evidence to conclude that smoking was a causal factor.[21]

A case-control design also is useful in physical therapy research. Riddle *et al.* used a case-control design to examine risk factors for the development of plantar fasciitis.[22] In this study each of the 50 subjects with plantar fasciitis was matched according to age and gender with two control subjects who did not suffer the condition. Potential risk factors then were measured in both groups and their relative proportions compared. Given that the etiology of plantar fasciitis is unknown in most cases, it may be logistically impractical to study the development of this disorder in a prospective fashion. Identification of risk factors through a retrospective design may provide useful information to fill the gap in knowledge.

Other Designs for Prognosic Indicators

Prognosic Indicators also may be gleaned from intervention papers including randomized controlled trials. Because prognostic information is not the focus of this type of research, readers will have to do some digging to determine what factors, if any, may be associated with the outcomes measured.[9] In light of the limited information available about prognostic indicators useful in physical therapy, any data about prognosis from clinical trials are important to evaluate.

RESEARCH DESIGNS FOR QUESTIONS ABOUT INTERVENTIONS

Studies of interventions are used to determine their beneficial effects, or harmful consequences, or both. Projects that measure the extent to which an intervention produces a desired outcome under ideal conditions focus on treatment *efficacy*. Studies that measure the impact of an intervention under usual clinical conditions focus on treatment *effectiveness*.[2] In both cases, these studies must be designed so that the treatment clearly precedes the outcome measured. In addition, the design should control or account for extraneous factors so that any treatment effect can be isolated and captured. Experimental research designs are promoted as the "gold standard" for determining the effects of interventions.[2,3,7,9,12] Increasing numbers of research articles pertaining to physical therapy interventions have experimental designs. However, numerous physical therapy research articles also have been published that are quasi-experimental in nature. Details of each of these design types are presented in the following sections.

Experimental Studies

The classic experimental study design used in clinical research is the *randomized clinical (or controlled) trial* (RCT). An RCT includes two or more groups to which subjects have been randomly assigned. The experimental intervention is provided to one of the groups and the resulting behavior in all of the groups is then compared. Campbell and Stanley described three experimental research formats that may be adopted for randomized clinical trials: the pretest-posttest control group design, the Solomon four-group design, and the posttest-only control group design.[8] Of these, the pretest-posttest control group design is the most commonly used in RCTs of interest to physical therapists.

In its simplest form the pretest-posttest format is composed of two groups—experimental and control. Performance on the outcome(s) of interest is measured in both groups at the start of the study (the *pretest*[s]). Then the intervention of interest is applied to the experimental group. Finally, subjects are remeasured at the conclusion of the experiment (the *posttest*[s]) to determine whether a change has occurred. Repeated posttest measures over time are used for longitudinal versions of this design. Figure 5-1 illustrates the pretest-posttest format. All else being equal, if the subjects in the experimental group change and the subjects in the control group do not, then it is likely that the intervention of interest was the change agent.

Randomized clinical (or controlled) trials are valued research designs because of their ability to control a number of extraneous influences that may interfere with a study's results. The typical methods of control in this design are outlined in Table 5-2. Control groups are the primary method by which investigators isolate the effects, if any, of the intervention of interest. A control group is differentiated from the experimental treatment group in one of several ways.[6] Subjects in the control group may receive no treatment at all and be instructed to behave as their usual routines dictate. Alternatively, they may be provided with a *placebo* or sham intervention that looks like the experimental treatment, but is inactive or inert. The classic ex-

R	O_1	X	O_2
R	O_3		O_4

R = Random assignment to the group

O_1 = Pretest for the experimental group

O_2 = Posttest for the experimental group

O_3 = Pretest for the control group

O_4 = Posttest for the control group

X = Experimental Intervention

Figure 5-1 Schematic representation of a pretest-post experimental design.

Source: Reprinted from *Experimental and Quasi-experimental Designs for Research.* Donald T. Campbell and Julian C. Stanley. Copyright 1963, with permission from Houghton Mifflin Company.

ample of the placebo in medical research is the sugar pill provided to control groups in drug trials. A third option commonly used in physical therapy research is to provide both groups with traditional (or "usual") care, but also to provide the intervention of interest to the experimental group. Finally, each group may be provided different treatments altogether, a situation that will challenge readers to remember which group is experimental and which is control. Often ethical issues related to withholding treatment from patients will dictate what type of control group is used.

Random assignment of subjects to groups is another method of control in experimental research. Randomization is used in an effort to create groups that are equal in size and composition. Equality of the groups is a necessary condition at the start of a study in order to protect its outcomes from the influence of extraneous factors inherent to the subjects. Characteristics commonly assessed for balanced distribution among groups in physical therapy research may include but not limited to: age, gender, ethnicity, baseline severity or function, and medication use, as well as sociodemographic factors such as education, employment, and social support.

Table 5–2 Methods of control in experimental designs.

Method of Control	Benefit
• Two (or more) groups to compare, one of which is a "control" group that does not receive the experimental treatment	• Effects of experimental treatment are isolated
• Random assignment of subjects to groups	• Subject characteristics that might influence the outcomes are distributed equally among the groups
• Efforts to mask (or "blind") subjects from knowledge of their group assignment	• Changes in subject behavior due to knowledge of group assignment are eliminated
• Efforts to mask investigators (or test administrators) from knowledge of subject group assignment	• Bias introduced because of investigator expectations about behaviors in different groups is eliminated
• Carefully delineated and applied protocols for subject testing AND subject treatment	• Consistency of techniques is ensured so that outcomes can be attributed to experimental intervention, not to procedural variation
• Stable environmental conditions during study activities	• Subject performance is unrelated to factors outside of the test or treatment procedure
• Complete and sufficient follow-up to determine the outcomes of treatment	• Adequate time is provided for outcomes of interest to develop and be measured

Masking of subjects and investigators helps to control bias by preventing changes in behavior as a result of knowledge of group assignment. Similarly, defined protocols for outcomes measurement and application of the intervention(s), as well as control of environmental conditions, are important to avoid unintended variation in the data that is unrelated to the intervention of interest. Finally, the time line for follow-up is important to ensure that an intervention's effects, if any, are not underestimated because they did not have sufficient opportunity to develop.

In addition to numerous methods for control within the study, an ideal RCT will enroll a large, representative group of subjects and suffer little attrition along the way. Higher numbers of subjects enhances the function of statistical tests and the ability to apply the findings to a large group from which the subjects were recruited. That said, clinical research with patients makes a representative selection of numerous subjects difficult except for the most well-funded and logistically-supported investigators. These studies are the multi-year investigations funded by large granting institutions, such as the National Institutes of Health and the Agency for Healthcare Research and Quality. Attrition, or loss of subjects during the study, often is out of the researchers' hands, but there are statistical methods with which to deal with the impact from those who drop out or who stop cooperating as the study proceeds.

An article by Houghton *et al.* illustrates the use of an RCT to investigate the usefulness of a physical therapy intervention.[23] These authors used a randomized pretest-posttest design to evaluate the effectiveness of high-voltage pulsed electrical current for chronic leg ulcer healing. An experimental group of subjects received high voltage current, while the control group received sham electrical therapy. Both groups also received "usual care" in the form of pressure relief, cleansing, debridement, and dressings for their wounds. The groups were equal in terms of subject age, gender, wound duration, initial wound size, sensory impairment, and wound location, as well as numerous other characteristics. Masking of all parties involved in the study was achieved by having the manufacturer deactivate some of the electrical stimulation units in a fashion that could not be detected by the patient or the therapist. The authors provided details regarding the standardized application of the interventions and outcome measures. Finally, a four-week time frame was utilized to provide adequate opportunity for healing to occur.

Only 29 individuals were enrolled in this study, a sample size that would be considered small but predictable for clinical research. In addition, two subjects chose to withdraw during the study. These low numbers are deceptive, however, because the focus of the study is on wounds, not on people. Houghton *et al.* wisely included individuals who had at least one wound, which means that some subjects had more than one.[23] In fact, the total count was 42 wounds, a sample size that likely enhances the ability of the statistical tests to find a difference between the groups if it is present.

Quasi-Experimental Studies

Quasi-experimental studies are projects in which there is a purposeful intervention with research subjects, but a comparison group and/or randomization to groups is missing.[8,11] However, other control methods used in experimental designs still may be imposed. There are several design options for quasi-experimental research including the time series design and the nonequivalent control group design. A simple time series format is one in which repeated measures are collected over time before and after the experimental intervention is introduced to a single group. If the measures are stable prior to the intervention but change following its introduction, then a cause-and-effect relationship might be inferred.[8] Unfortunately the lack of a control group reduces the certainty with which this causal connection can be stated because it is not possible to rule out natural subject improvement. Bhambhani *et al.* used a time series design to evaluate the effectiveness of circuit training in patients with traumatic brain injury.[24] The time line for the study was divided into three phases. During the first phase, the stability of the outcome measures was evaluated through repeated measures one week apart (T_1 and T_2). Routine rehabilitation was introduced during the second week. The experimental intervention–circuit training–was introduced to all subjects at the seventh week and continued for 14 weeks. Outcome measures were repeated at the conclusion of the rehabilitation (T_3), halfway through the circuit training (T_4) and at the conclusion of circuit training (T_5). Figure 5-2 provides a schematic representation of the design used in this study.

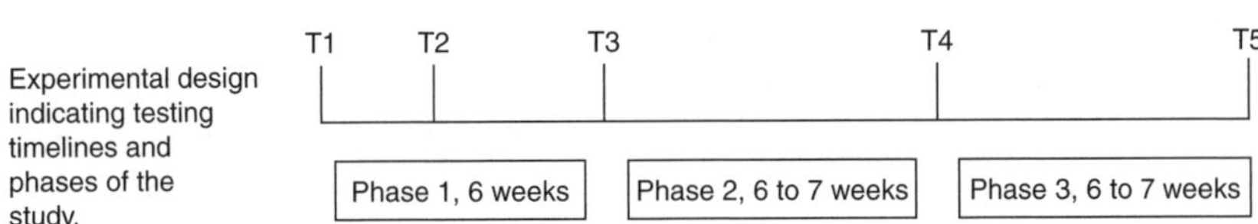

Figure 5-2 Schematic representation of a time series as performed by Bhambhani *et al.*[22]

Source: Reprinted from Bhambhani Y *et al. Archives of Physical Medicine and Rehabilitation*, volume 86. Effects of circuit training on body composition and peak cardiorespiratory responses in patients with moderate to severe traumatic brain injury, pp. 268-276, Copyright 2005, with permission from the American Congress of Rehabilitation Medicine and the American Academy of Medicine and Rehabilitation.

A nonequivalent control group format is similar to the experimental pretest-posttest design except that random assignment to groups is lacking. Instead, naturally occurring groups are identified with only one receiving the experimental intervention. Unlike the time series design, this format has a control group for the purposes of comparison; however, as the name implies, subject characteristics probably are not distributed equally at the start of the study.[11] Robitaille *et al.* used a nonequivalent control group design to evaluate the effectiveness of a group exercise program for improving balance in community-dwelling elderly individuals.[25] Two sets of community centers providing services to the elderly recruited potential participants. Subjects in one group of community centers received the experimental treatment, while subjects in the other centers had to wait for a period of time until the programs were initiated in their area. Although this study lacks randomized assignment of subjects to groups, it provides an example of a study conducted in typical community settings rather than in research labs or health care facilities.

Single-System Designs

Single-system designs are a type of quasi-experimental study that can be used to investigate the usefulness of an intervention. The distinguishing feature of these designs is their use of only one subject who undergoes, in an alternating fashion, an experimental treatment period and a control or comparison period. All of the controls used in quasi-experimental research can be imposed in this design. Studying only one individual is logistically easier for investigators as well. A single-system design is distinct from a *case report* or *case series* design in which the author simply describes the management of a patient/client.

Domholdt describes five variations of the single-system design, each of which is progressively more complex, as illustrated in Table 5-3.[1] Letters are used to represent the different phases of the design. "A–B designs" are the simplest version and reflect a control period followed by the experimental treatment period. "Withdrawal designs" add a second control period that is imposed following the withdrawal of the experimental treatment. This approach is preferable to the "A–B design" because it may be easier to detect a true treatment effect if the subject's condition reverts to baseline after the experimental intervention is removed. A "multiple baseline design" may be used with multiple individuals—each serving as their own single-system study—when investigators want to control for external events that may influence the outcomes of the study. Each individual may be assigned to baseline control periods that both vary in length and occur at different times, followed by the experimental intervention and subsequent

Table 5–3 Schematic representations of single-system designs.

Type of Design	Schematic Depiction
A-B Designs	A-B
Withdrawal Designs	A-B-A
Multiple Baseline Designs	A(1)-B-A A(2)-B-A A(1)-B-A
Alternating Treatment Designs	A-B-A-C-A
Interaction Designs	A-B-A-C-A – BC-A

A = Control phase
A(1) = Control phase with one duration
A(2) = Control phase with a different duration
B = Intervention phase with one experimental treatment
C = Intervention phase with a different experimental treatment
BC = Intervention phase with both experimental treatments combined

withdrawal periods. Results from all of the individuals then can be compared. This approach reduces the chance that a false conclusion will be drawn based on the response of one patient at one point in time. Finally, "alternating treatment designs" and "interaction designs" may be used to evaluate more than one experimental treatment and, in the latter case, the interaction of the two. In these designs investigators may randomize the order in which these interventions are applied. This approach is referred to as an "n-of-1 randomized controlled trial."[3]

The focus on one individual in a study may be useful for evidence-based physical therapists if that subject is very similar to the patient/client about whom the therapist has a clinical question. Any treatment effects detected are relevant to that person, not to an aggregate group in which the unique qualities of individuals are washed out in the averages. Guyatt and Rennie even go so far as to place an "n-of-1 randomized controlled trial" at the top of their evidence hierarchy for intervention studies.[3] Unfortunately, the need to withhold or withdraw a potentially beneficial treatment as part of the alternating sequence of the study design poses important ethical challenges that limit the extent to which this approach is used.

RESEARCH DESIGNS FOR QUESTIONS ABOUT OUTCOMES

Outcomes studies also focus on treatment effectiveness but use a nonexperimental, or observational, study design.[1] As a result, they lose much of the control that is imposed in experimental and quasi-experimental research. For example, they do not include randomization to groups, assuming there are groups to compare in the first place, and the researchers do not control the interventions applied to the subjects. Nevertheless, the motivation to conduct such studies stems from the desire to capture outcomes that are meaningful to patients based on treatments applied in real-world conditions. The benefits accrued from an intervention under controlled conditions may be mitigated by factors in the clinical environment, such as variability in medical or surgical management, that also should be considered in physical therapy clinical decision making.[1] In addition, these studies often focus on results that are meaningful to patients/clients in addition to, or in lieu of, pathology or impairment-based measures.

Outcomes studies often are retrospective in their approach; however, they may be cross-sectional or longitudinal depending upon the question to be answered and the nature of the data that are available. Retrospective studies usually rely upon large secondary administrative, insurance claims, or commercial outcomes databases for their data. For example, Jewell and Riddle used retrospective data maintained by Focus on Therapeutic Outcomes, Inc. on 1804 patients with sciatica to evaluate the likelihood of improvement in physical health based on the types of interventions provided.[26,27] The large sample size is an important statistical advantage for detecting differences if they exist. The primary disadvantage is that Jewell and Riddle did not have control over the application of the interventions nor the collection and recording of the data. In addition, a true cause-and-effect relationship could not be demonstrated with this study because of its cross-sectional design. Rather, this study provides the foundation for a future experimental design in which similar patients can be randomized into experimental and comparison groups and in which the provision of interventions can be controlled by the investigators in real time. Despite their limitations, retrospective single-group studies, such as the one performed by Jewell and Riddle[27] may be the only evidence available about outcomes in some physical therapy practice areas; therefore, they should still be evaluated to determine whether there is any information that would be useful during management of the individual patient/client.

Although less common, it is possible to conduct an observational outcomes study with more than one group of subjects. For example, a hypothetical investigator may want to answer the following research question:

> Which approach is more effective for restoring normal gait patterns after anterior cruciate ligament reconstruction—the addition of resistance training earlier or later in the rehabilitation program?

In this study the investigator could gather data to compare the gait patterns of patients from surgeon A, whose orders include resistance exercises at postoperative week three, with patients from surgeon B, who does not order resistance exercises until postoperative week six. This project could be conducted retrospectively through a medical records review or prospectively through standardized data recording methods. Again, the benefit of such a project is that it reflects real-world clinical conditions. However, because individuals are not randomized to the different surgeons there may be any number of inequalities between the two treatment groups (e.g., differences in medical history or preoperative activity levels) that may interfere with the outcomes of the study. In addition, the number of subjects in such a study is likely to be small unless both surgeons perform a high volume of anterior cruciate ligament surgeries over the time period in question. Both situations provide statistical challenges that must be addressed during the study.

Methodological Studies about Outcome Measures

For the purposes of this textbook, outcome measures refer to instruments or procedures that capture person-level endpoints such as functional limitations, disabilities, and quality of life. This distinction between impairment measures and outcome measures may seem arbitrary to some; after all, remediation of impairments in response to a physical therapist's intervention is a worthwhile result (i.e., "outcome"). Philosophically, however, defining outcome measures in this fashion is more consistent with the concept of *patient-centered care*, as well as with the disablement model upon which the *Guide to Physical Therapist Practice* is based.[10,28] Physical therapists also are encouraged by payers to write treatment goals that focus on functional performance meaningful to their patients/clients rather than emphasizing impairment-related targets.

The development of outcome measures is analogous to the development of impairment measures as discussed above. The designs for methodological studies about outcome measures also are nonexperimental in nature. A significant body of methodological research exists pertaining to the development and usefulness of outcome measures called "self-report instruments" that are used by patients/clients to provide information about their disability,[29] health status,[30,31] satisfaction,[32,33] or quality of life.[34] Health status, satisfaction, and quality of life are abstractions that cannot be observed in the direct way that we can "see" height or eye color. In addition, these constructs are based upon patient/client perceptions and experiences. As a result these phenomena require operational definitions that are measurable through a format that solicits the patient/client's assessment of his or her situation. The typical format for such an instrument is a survey with questions or statements serving as the direct measure of the phenomenon. For example, health status surveys may include items that ask a patient/client about symptoms experienced and their impact on physical and social activities, while satisfaction surveys may include items about the interpersonal and technical skill of the physical therapist and the comfort of the clinical environment.

Investigators developing new self-report measures start the process by crafting an initial set of operational definitions or survey items. The focus level of these definitions also is considered. Self-report measures with a general focus level, referred to as "generic instruments," can be applied to the widest variety of situations or with a variety of patients/clients. Other measures may focus on specific conditions, body regions, or satisfaction with particular aspects of the episode of care.[6] Methods used to develop operational definitions may include review of prior literature, consultation with content experts, focus groups of patients/clients and/or caregivers, or elaborations of theory. Once a list of survey items is generated, then testing and refinement with subjects of interest continues through a series of iterations designed to:[6]

1) Create the most complete, but efficient (parsimonious) set of items for the survey;
2) Establish the relationship among multiple items intended to measure one aspect of the phenomenon;
3) Establish the stability, interpretability, and meaningfulness of scores with a group of subjects for whom the survey is designed; and,
4) Establish the relationship between the survey and a previously, established instrument (or instruments).

If the research project is well-funded and has access to a large number of subjects, then the investigators also may explore the instrument's performance in a second group of individuals with the same diagnosis, clinical problem, or circumstances. In addition, the usefulness of the instrument measuring change over time may be demonstrated. Further studies are required to explore the measurement properties of the instrument using subjects with a related but distinct diagnosis or clinical problem, as well as versions of the survey in different languages.

SECONDARY ANALYSES

Secondary analyses are reports about individual studies. The motivation to conduct a secondary analysis stems from the reality that one single research study often does not provide a definitive conclusion about the usefulness of a diagnostic test, prognostic indicator, intervention, or outcome. The primary reasons for this limitation in clinical research are the difficulty locating and enrolling a large enough group of individuals in the study, as well as ethical and logistical challenges to testing, manipulating, and controlling patients who already are vulnerable based upon their diagnosis or disorder. Lack of funding of large-scale studies also poses a problem for many investigators. As a result, several smaller studies may exist addressing a specific topic that cumulatively may provide stronger evidence to answer a clinical question.

In their most basic form, secondary analyses have been referred to as "literature reviews" or, more recently, narrative reviews. A *narrative review* is a paper in which the authors describe prior research on a particular topic without using a systematic search and critical appraisal process. Current patient/client management also may be described in an anecdotal fashion. By definition, these articles are biased representations of a cumulative body of literature because standardized methods for article identification, selection, and review were not implemented.[9] Table 5-4 lists some narrative reviews relevant to physical therapy practice. Although these narrative reviews are lower forms of evidence, they may be useful in identifying other individual articles that have a true research design of some kind.

Systematic Reviews

As their name implies, *systematic reviews* are the antithesis of the narrative review and are located at the top of most evidence hierarchies. A systematic review is a true research paper with the following design elements and controls:

- A specific research question to be addressed;
- Detailed inclusion and exclusion criteria for selection of studies to review;

Table 5-4 Examples of narrative reviews pertinent to physical therapy.

Emery C. Conservative management of congenital muscular torticollis: a literature review. *Phys Occup Ther Pediatr*, 1997; 17(2):13-20.
Napolitano R Jr *et al.* The diagnosis and treatment of shoulder injuries in the throwing athlete. *J Chiropract Med*, 2002 Mar; 1(1):23-30.
Nyland J *et al.* Preserving transfer independence among individuals with spinal cord injury. *Spinal Cord*, 2000 Nov; 38(11):649-657.
Page JC. Critiquing clinical research of new technologies for diabetic foot wound management. *J Foot Ankle Surg*, 2002 Jul-Aug; 41(4):251-259, 273-275.
Stiller K *et al.* Respiratory muscle training for tetraplegic patients: a literature review. *Aust J Physiother*, 1999; 45(4):291-299.

- Elaborate and thorough search strategies;
- Standardized review protocols that often include trained reviewers other than the primary investigators;
- Standardized abstracting processes for capturing details about each study included in the review;
- Preestablished quality criteria with which to rate the value of the individual studies, usually applied by masked reviewers.

Systematic reviews look like typical research articles in the sense that they begin with an introduction and purpose statement, follow with methods and results sections, and conclude with a discussion and summary statement about what the cumulative weight of the evidence suggests. The most well-known and prolific source of systematic reviews is the Cochrane Collaboration;[35] however, similar methods for conducting systematic reviews are implemented by investigators independent of this international group.

Stuge *et al.* performed a systematic review of prospective randomized controlled trials evaluating the effectiveness of various physical therapy interventions for the prevention and treatment of back and pelvic pain in pregnant and postpartum women.[36] Both electronic and paper databases were searched and authors of primary studies were contacted. As is often the case, the review authors identified more studies (17) than they were able to include (nine) in their analysis because of the poor quality of many research designs, as well as the lack of other elements specified by the inclusion criteria. The total number of subjects from the studies they reviewed was 1350, whereas the number of subjects in the individual studies ranged from 26–407. Of the nine studies, only three were judged to be "high quality" according to preestablished criteria. The variety of treatments assessed and outcomes measured, coupled with the overall lack of quality of study designs, prevented the authors from making a definitive conclusion about the effectiveness of physical therapy for pregnant women with low back pain. However, the identification of individual high quality clinical trials may be a secondary benefit of systematic reviews even when the review itself results in equivocal conclusions.

Meta-Analyses

Whenever feasible, authors will conduct additional statistical analyses by pooling data from the individual studies in a systematic review. This approach requires that the interventions and outcomes of interest in individual studies be the same. When these criteria are met, authors can create a much larger sample size than any one study, thereby increasing the statistical power of the analysis and the representativeness of the sample. This form of a systematic review is referred to as a *meta-analysis.*

Main *et al.* performed a meta-analysis as part of their systematic review of conventional chest physical therapy compared to other airway clearance techniques for patients with cystic fibrosis.[37] Twenty-nine studies with a total of 475 subjects were included and reviewed. Once again, many of the individual trials were limited in their design quality. Data from pulmonary function test outcomes were pooled and revealed no statistically significant difference in treatment effect between conventional methods and any other technique utilized. It is important to note that the authors *did not* conclude that conventional chest physical therapy was "ineffective;" rather, they stated that there was no advantage to using conventional methods over other techniques. In other words, the pooled statistical results did not indicate that one method was more effective than another. This conclusion requires readers to use their clinical judgment regarding which treatment technique they will use based on this evidence, a common result of systematic reviews and meta-analyses of physical therapy research. Only when the individual studies are consistently high in quality will these types of reviews start to draw more definitive directional conclusions.

QUALITATIVE STUDIES

Qualitative studies focus on subjects' thoughts, perceptions, opinions, beliefs, and/or attitudes. Data are provided in words rather than in numbers through interviews, surveys, diaries, independent observations, or other mechanisms. The analyses focus on the identification of patterns or themes in the data that may be used for further exploration in a subsequent round of data collection. Domholdt refers to this step as "generating meaning" from the data.[1] Once data collection and analysis is complete, then the final set of verified themes is presented as the results of the study.

Qualitative studies often have one of the following three design orientations: a) ethnography; b) phenomenology; or c) grounded theory.[1,9] An ethnographic approach attempts to understand "what the subjects' lives are like." Data are collected directly from the subjects as well as from the investigator's observations of the subjects and their associates if pertinent to the topic area. Levins *et al.* used this design to explore the facilitators and barriers to physical activity in individuals with spinal cord injuries.[38] A phenomenologic approach addresses the question "what does this mean?" from the subjects' point of view. In this design, only the subjects provide information—there are no independent observers providing data. Miller and

Solomon used interviews and focus groups to determine how a shift in organizational structure affected physical therapists in one Canadian teaching hospital.[39] Finally, a grounded theory design is used to explain a phenomenon by repeatedly collecting and analyzing information from the subjects. These study designs are time consuming and usually involve multiple rounds of data analysis and collection of yet more data. Jensen *et al.* used this approach to develop a theory about expert practice in physical therapy.[40]

A detailed review of qualitative research methods is beyond the scope of this text. Readers with an interest in these designs are encouraged to obtain one of the qualitative methods resources listed at the end of this chapter.[41, 42] As more qualitative studies relevant to physical therapy practice are published, these research designs undoubtedly will become more familiar to readers and their results will be used more frequently to inform clinical decisions.

SUMMARY

Research designs describe the approach investigators will use (or have used) to answer their questions. They also reflect investigators' philosophical perspective regarding the inherent objectivity or subjectivity of the phenomenon of interest. Research designs provide details about the manner in which subjects will be selected and managed, how variables will be measured and/or manipulated, the timing of subject and investigator activities, the time frame of the study, and the means by which unwanted influences will be minimized or avoided. Each design has inherent strengths and weaknesses with which investigators must contend in order to have confidence in a study's findings.

Different research questions are answered best by specific research designs. The randomized clinical (controlled) trial is the most effective approach with regards to controlling unwanted influences and demonstrating cause-and-effect relationships between variables. As a result, this design is most appropriate for questions pertaining to interventions. Other designs that do not include randomization to groups are more useful when examining questions about diagnosis, prognosis, and patient/client outcomes; however, researchers must find additional means to control for extraneous factors that may interfere with the study's results. Evidence-based physical therapists must be able to identify and evaluate the strength of different research designs in order to determine whether the results provide important and useful information that should be considered during the patient/client management process.

Exercises

1. Differentiate between the quantitative and qualitative research perspectives and provide an example of a research question that might be answered in each approach.
2. Describe the general features of experimental research designs. Include important strengths and weaknesses. What type of question is best answered by this approach?
3. How is an experimental research design different from a quasi-experimental design? What additional challenges occur as a result of using the quasi-experimental approach?
4. Describe the general features of nonexperimental research designs. Include important strengths and weaknesses. What types of questions are best answered by this approach?
5. Discuss the primary methods of control for extraneous (unwanted) influences in experimental, quasi-experimental, and nonexperimental research designs. Give an example of each.
6. Differentiate between an impairment measure and an outcome measure.
7. Differentiate between narrative reviews and systematic reviews. Why are systematic reviews the preferred approach to answering questions about the cumulative weight of the evidence?
8. Describe the general approaches to qualitative research and the questions they answer.

References

1. Domholdt E. *Rehabilitation Research: Principles and Applications.* 3d ed. St. Louis, MO: Elsevier Saunders; 2005.
2. Helewa A, Walker JM. *Critical Evaluation of Research in Physical Rehabilitation: Towards Evidence-Based Practice.* Philadelphia, PA: W.B. Saunders Company; 2000.
3. Guyatt G, Rennie D. *Users' Guides to the Medical Literature: A Manual for Evidence-Based Clinical Practice*. Chicago, IL: AMA Press; 2002.
4. McEwen I. *Writing Case Reports: A How-To Manual for Clinicians.* 2d ed. Alexandria, VA: American Physical Therapy Association; 2001.
5. Batavia M. *Clinical Research for Health Professionals: A User-Friendly Guide*. Boston, MA: Butterworth-Heinemann; 2001.
6. Portney LG, Watkins MP. *Foundations of Clinical Research: Applications to Practice.* 2d ed. Upper Saddle River, NJ: Prentice Hall Health; 2000.
7. Straus SE, Richardson WS, Glaziou P, Haynes RB. *Evidence-Based Medicine: How to Practice and Teach EBM.* 3d ed. Edinburgh, Scotland: Elsevier Churchill Livingstone; 2005.

8. Campbell DT, Stanley JC. *Experimental and Quasi-experimental Designs for Research.* Boston, MA: Houghton Mifflin Company; 1963.
9. Herbert R, Jamtvedt G, Mead J, Hagen KB. *Practical Evidence-Based Physical Therapy*. Edinburgh, Scotland: Elsevier Butterworth Heinemann; 2005.
10. Knebel E. *Educating Health Professionals to be Patient-Centered.* Institute of Medicine Web site. Available at: http://www.iom.edu/Object.File/Master/10/460/Patient.pdf. Accessed February 15, 2006.
11. Cook TD, Campbell DT. *Quasi-experimentation: Design and Analysis Issues for Field Settings*. Boston, MA: Houghton Mifflin Company; 1979.
12. Sackett DL, Wennberg JE. Choosing the best research design for each question. *BMJ*. 1997; 315(7123):1636.
13. Holtby R, Razmjou H. Accuracy of the Speed's and Yergason's test in detecting biceps pathology and SLAP lesions: Comparison with arthroscopic findings. *Arthroscopy*. 2004; 20(3):231–236.
14. Reese NB, Bandy WD. Use of an inclinometer to measure flexibility of the iliotibial band using the Ober test and the modified Ober test: differences in magnitude and reliability of measurements. *J Orthop Sports Phys Ther*. 2003; 33(6):326–330.
15. Ford-Smith CD, Wyman JF, Elswick RK Jr, Fernandez T. Reliability of stationary dynomometer muscle strength testing in community-dwelling older adults. *Arch Phys Med Rehabil.* 2001; 82(8):1128–1132.
16. Wang CH, Hsueh IP, Sheu CF, Yao G, Hsieh CL. Psychometric properties of 2 simplified 3-level balance scales used for patients with stroke. *Phys Ther*. 2004; 84(5):430–438.
17. Grimes DA, Schulz KF. Bias and causal associations in observational research. *Lancet*. 2002; 359(9302):248–252.
18. Rainville J, Sobel JB, Hartigan C, Wright A. The effect of compensation involvement on the reporting of pain and disability in patients referred for rehabilitation of chronic low back pain. *Spine*. 1997; 22(17):2016–2024.
19. MacPherson AK, Rothman L, McKeag AM, Howard A. Mechanism of injury affects 6-month functional outcome in children hospitalized because of severe injuries. *J Trauma*. 2003; 55(3):454–458.
20. Research Foundation, State University of New York. *Guide for the Uniform Data Set for Medical Rehabilitation for Children (WeeFIM), version 1.5*. Buffalo, NY: State University of New York at Buffalo; 1991.
21. Sasco AJ, Secretan MB, Straif K. Tobacco smoking and cancer: A brief review of recent epidemiological evidence. *Lung Cancer*. 2004; 45(2):S3–S9.
22. Riddle DL, Pulisic M, Pidcoe P, Johnson RE. Risk factors of plantar fasciitis: A matched case-control study. *J Bone Joint Surg Am*. 2003; 85-A(5):872–877.
23. Houghton PE, Kincaid CB, Lovell M, Campbell KE, Keast DH *et al.* Effect of electrical stimulation on chronic leg ulcer size and appearance. *Phys Ther*. 2003; 83(1):17–28.
24. Bhambhani Y, Rowland G, Farag M. Effects of circuit training on body composition and peak cardiorespiratory responses in patients with moderate to severe traumatic brain injury. *Arch Phys Med Rehabil*. 2005; 86(2):268–276.

25. Robitaille Y, Laforest S, Fournier M, Gauvin L, Parisien M *et al.* Moving forward in fall prevention: An intervention to improve balance among older adults in real-world settings. *Am J Public Health.* 2005; 95(11):2049–2056.
26. Focus on Therapeutic Outcomes, Incorporate Web site. Available at: www.fotoinc.com. Accessed January 15, 2006.
27. Jewell DV, Riddle DL. Interventions that increase or decrease the likelihood of a meaningful improvement in physical health in patients with sciatica. *Phys Ther.* 2005; 85(11):1139–1150.
28. American Physical Therapy Association. Guide to Physical Therapist Practice. 2d ed. *Phys Ther.* 2001; 81(1);9–746.
29. Salaffi F, Bazzichi L, Stancati A, Neri R, Cazzato M *et al.* Development of a functional disability measurement tool to assess early arthritis: The Recent-Onset Arthritis Disability (ROAD) questionnaire. *Clin Exp Rheumatol.* 2005; 23(5):628–636.
30. Varni JW, Burwinkle TM, Katz ER, Meeske K, Dickinson P. The PedsQL in pediatric cancer: Reliability and validity of the Pediatric Quality of Life Inventory Generic Core Scales, Multidimensional Fatigue Scale, and Cancer Module. *Cancer.* 2002; 94(7):2090–2106.
31. Thompson DR, Jenkinson C, Roebuck A, Lewin RJ, Boyle RM *et al.* Development and validation of a short measure of health status for individuals with acute myocardial infarction: The myocardial infarction dimensional assessment scale (MIDAS). *Qual Life Res.* 2002; 11(6):535–543.
32. Beattie PF, Pinto MB, Nelson MK, Nelson R. Patient satisfaction with outpatient physical therapy: Instrument validation. *Phys Ther.* 2002; 82(8):557–565.
33. Beattie P, Turner C, Dowda M, Michener L, Nelson R. The MedRisk Instrument for Measuring Satisfaction with Physical Therapy Care: A psychometric analsyis. *J Orthop Sports Phys Ther.* 2005; 35(1):24–32.
34. Fang CT, Hsiung PC, Yu CF, Chen MY, Wang JD. Validation of the World Health Organization quality of life instrument in patients with HIV infection. *Qual Life Res.* 2002; 11(8):753–762.
35. The Cochrane Library. The Cochrane Collaboration. Available via Wiley Interscience Web site at: http://www3.interscience.wiley.com/cgi-bin/mrwhome/106568753/HOME. Accessed October 1, 2005.
36. Stuge B, Hilde G, Vøllestad N. Physical therapy for pregnancy-related low back and pelvic pain: A systematic review. *Acta Obstet Gynecol Scand.* 2003; 82(11):983–990.
37. Main A, Prasad A, van der Schans C. Conventional chest physiotherapy compared to other airway clearance techniques for cystic fibrosis. *The Cochrane Database of Systematic Reviews.* 2005; Issue 1. Article no. CD002011.pub2.DOI:10.1002/14651858.CD002011.pub2.
38. Levins SM, Redenbach DM, Dyck I. Individual and societal influences on participation in physical activity following spinal cord injury: A qualitative study. *Phys Ther.* 2004; 84(6):496–509.
39. Miller PA, Solomon P. The influence of a move to program management on physical therapist practice. *Phys Ther.* 2002; 82(5):449–58.

40. Jensen GM, Gwyer J, Shepard KF. Expert practice in physical therapy. *Phys Ther.* 2000; 80(1):28–43.
41. Denizen NK, Lincoln Y (eds). *Handbook of Qualitative Research.* 2d ed. Thousand Oaks, CA: Sage Publications; 2000.
42. Creswell JW. *Qualitative Inquiry and Research Design: Choosing among Five Traditions.* Thousand Oaks, CA: Sage Publications; 1998.

Chapter 6

Research Subjects

The tendency of the casual mind is to pick out or stumble upon a sample which supports or defies its prejudices, and then to make it the representative of a whole class.

—Walter Lippmann

Objectives

Upon completion of this chapter the student/practitioner will be able to:

1. Differentiate between a study population and sample.
2. Discuss the purpose and characteristics of inclusion and exclusion criteria used to identify potential subjects.
3. Describe probabilistic subject selection methods and discuss their strengths and limitations.
4. Describe nonprobabilistic subject selection methods and discuss their strengths and limitations.
5. Describe methods for assigning subjects to groups within a study and discuss their strengths and limitations.
6. Discuss methods for controlling extraneous influences related to subject participation in a study.
7. Discuss the role of sample size in the statistical analysis of a study's results.

Terms in This Chapter

Accessible Population: The pool of potential research subjects that are available for researchers to study.[1]

Assignment (Allocation): The process by which subjects are placed into two or more groups in a study.

Block Assignment: An assignment method in which the number of individuals in each group is predetermined; investigators randomly assign subjects to one group at a time until each quota is met.

Cluster Sampling: A probabilistic sampling method in which subjects are randomly selected from naturally occurring pockets of the population of interest that are geographically dispersed.

Convenience Sampling: A nonprobabilistic sampling method in which investigators select subjects who are readily available (such as students).

Exclusion Criteria: A list of characteristics that may influence, or "confound," the outcomes of a study; researchers use these criteria to eliminate individuals (or units of analysis such as an organization) with these characteristics as subjects in a study.

Extraneous Factors: Individual, organizational, or environmental characteristics other than the factor of interest (i.e., test, predictor, intervention) that may influence the outcome of a study.

Inclusion Criteria: A list of specific attributes that will make an individual (or a unit of analysis such as an organization) eligible for participation in a specific study.

Masked (Blinded): 1) In diagnosis papers, the lack of knowledge about previous test results; 2) in prognosis papers, the lack of knowledge about exposure status; and 3) in intervention papers, the lack of knowledge about to which group a subject has been assigned.

Matched Assignment: An assignment method in which subjects are first divided into subgroups based on a specific characteristic such as age, gender, and so forth; members of each subgroup are then randomly assigned to each group in the study in order to balance the characteristics across the groups.

Nonprobabilistic Sampling: Methods for choosing subjects that do not use a random selection process; as a result, the sample may not represent accurately the population from which it is drawn.

Power: The probability that a statistical test will detect, if present, a relationship between two or more variables or a difference between two or more groups.[1,2]

Primary Data: Data collected in real time from subjects in a study; used in prospective research designs.

Probabilistic Sampling: Methods for choosing subjects that use a random selection process to increase the chance of obtaining a sample that accurately represents the population from which it is drawn.

Purposive Sampling: A nonprobabilistic sampling method in which investigators hand select specific individuals to participate based on characteristics important to the researchers.

Random Assignment by Individual: An assignment method in which each subject is randomly allocated to a group based on which side of a coin lands upright or which number is pulled from a hat.

Sample: A collection of individuals (or units of analysis such as organizations) taken from the population for the purposes of a research study.

Sampling Error: Occurs when a sample has characteristics that are different from other samples and from the population from which the samples are drawn.

Sampling Frame: A list of potential subjects obtained from various public or private sources.

Secondary Data: Data that have been collected previously by others for non-research purposes that are used by investigators to answer a research question; used in retrospective research designs.

Selection (Sampling): The process by which subjects are chosen from a potential candidate pool.

Simple Random Sample: A probabilistic sampling method in which each potential subject has an equal chance of being selected.

Snowball Sampling: A nonprobabilistic sampling method in which the initial subjects in a study recruit additional participants via word-of-mouth communication.

Stratified Random Sampling: A probabilistic sampling method in which subgroups of a population are identified and randomly selected to ensure their inclusion in a study.

Subjects: Individuals, organizations, or other units of analysis about whom information will be gathered for the purposes of a research study.

Systematic Assignment: An assignment method in which subjects count off the group numbers until everyone is assigned.

Systematic Sampling: A probabilistic sampling method in which the first subject is randomly selected from a group organized according to a known identifier (such as a birth date) and then all remaining subjects are chosen based on their numerical distance from the first individual.

Target Population: The total aggregate of individuals to whom investigators wish to apply their research findings.[1]

Type II Error: A result from a statistical test that indicates no significant relationship or difference is present when in fact one exists (e.g., a false negative).[2]

INTRODUCTION

Clinical research requires data obtained from people. The research question or purpose will identify the general group of people from whom information is needed. In technical terms, this general group is referred to as the study's target population. The *target population* is the total aggregate of individuals to whom researchers wish to apply their study's findings.[1] All athletes who undergo anterior cruciate ligament (ACL) reconstruction or all children with asthma are examples of target populations that may be of interest to physical therapy researchers. Every member of these target populations may not be accessible to researchers because of their large number and geographic distribution. In addition, some members of these populations may not be identifiable. As a result, researchers will define the *accessible population* of individuals who are potential participants in their study. Athletes undergoing ligament surgery in hospitals in a large metropolitan area or children with asthma who are managed through community health centers in one state are examples of accessible populations.

Even though the accessible population is a smaller subset of the target population, it is often too large to study in its entirety; therefore, investigators must choose a smaller number of individual representatives.[2] The research design will specify the methods by which these individuals, referred to as *subjects*, will be selected from the accessible population, as well as in which activities they will participate during the study. A collection of subjects for a study is called a *sample*. Depending on the study's design, the sample may be composed of people from whom data will be collected in real time during the project (*primary data*) or it may be made up of people from whom data were previously collected (*secondary data*).

As noted in Chapter 5, evidence-based physical therapists must evaluate a study's design to determine if the results answer the research question in a useful and believable fashion. Three design steps pertaining to a study's subjects are essential ingredients of a successful project 1) identification of potential candidates for study; 2) selection of an appropriate number of individuals from the candidate pool; and 3) management of the subjects' roles and activities during the study. Appropriate subject identification, selection, and management will enhance a study's usefulness and believability, as well as the relevance of its results for similar individuals who were not study participants. In addition to these design considerations, a sufficient number of appropriate subjects are needed in order to increase the probability that a statistically significant result will be found. This chapter discusses commonly-used methods by which subjects may be identified, chosen, and handled during their participation in clinical research, as well as issues related to sample size.

SUBJECT IDENTIFICATION

The research question or purpose indicates in general terms the population of interest for a study. For example, in the studies itemized in Table 6–1, the populations of interest included "patients with rheumatoid arthritis,"[3] "patients diagnosed with impingement syndrome,"[4] "Cuban Americans recovering from hip fractures,"[5] and "patients who are critically ill."[6] Ideally, individuals who are candidates for each of these studies should have charac-

Table 6–1 Studies relevant to physical therapy.

Citation
Systematic Review Milne S, Brosseau L, Robinson V, Noel MJ, Davis J *et al.* Continuous passive motion following total knee arthroplasty. *Cochrane Database Syst Rev.* 2003; (2):CD004260.
Randomized Clinical Trial Johansson KM, Adolfsson LE, Foldevi MOM. Effects of acupuncture versus ultrasound in patients with impingement syndrome: Randomized clinical trial. *Phys Ther.* 2005; 85:490–501.
Observational Study Kirk-Sanchez NJ. Factors related to activity limitations in a group of Cuban Americans before and after hip fracture. *Phys Ther.* 2004; 84:408–418.
Summary Ciesla ND. Chest physical therapy for patients in the intensive care unit. *Phys Ther.* 1996; 76:609–625.

teristics that are consistent with the population's description while also being free of other attributes that may influence, or "confound," the results of the project. The characteristics of interest are referred to collectively as inclusion criteria, while the undesirable attributes are referred to as exclusion criteria.

Inclusion criteria define in more detail the characteristics that individuals from the population of interest must possess in order to be eligible for the study. These characteristics often are demographic, clinical, and/or geographic in nature.[1] For example, potential subjects in Johansson *et al.*'s study had to be between the ages of 30 and 65, have clinical signs of impingement syndrome for at least two months, and had to have sought care from a physician or physical therapist in one of three primary health care centers in one county in Sweden.[4] Similarly, potential candidates for Kirk-Sanchez's study had to identify themselves as Cuban Americans at least 50 years of age who were treated in one inpatient rehabilitation center in southern Florida following surgical repair for hip fracture.[5]

Inclusion criteria must be broad enough to capture all potentially eligible individuals without admitting too many *extraneous factors*. For example, Johansson *et al.* were interested in the effectiveness of two treatment techniques for remediation of impingement syndrome, but not for other pathologies of the shoulder.[4] Specifying which clinical signs will identify individuals with impingement syndrome is necessary to avoid also enrolling subjects with different problems, such as bursitis or cervical radiculopathy for whom the treatments might not be indicated or effective. On the other hand, had the authors made the inclusion criteria too narrow and enrolled only individuals with a mild form of impingement syndrome, they may have biased the study in favor of a positive treatment effect because these subjects may have recovered on their own even if the treatment did not work. In addition, the study's results would not be applicable to patients with more severe forms of the disorder. Support for selected inclusion criteria often is provided in the literature reviewed for the current study. Nevertheless, evidence-based physical therapists should judge for themselves whether the inclusion criteria are sufficient to make the study credible given the research question or purpose.

Exclusion criteria define in more detail characteristics that will make individuals ineligible for consideration as subjects. These criteria reflect extraneous factors that potentially will interfere with the study's outcome.[2] Exclusionary factors also may be demographic, clinical, or geographic in nature. For example, Johansson *et al.* listed twelve exclusion criteria, nine of which were indications of pathologies other than impingement syndrome, two of which were previous treatments to the affected shoulder and one that pertained to a person's ability to communicate.[4] Kirk-Sanchez also excluded individuals with cognitive deficits or language barriers that might interfere with their ability to complete surveys used for outcome measures.[5] The inability of potential study candidates to understand and respond consistently to directions provided or to answer questions consistently in oral or written form are common exclusion criteria because of the likelihood of unstable subject performance and inaccurate or incomplete data. As with inclusion criteria, support for exclusion criteria may be found in the background literature reviewed at the outset of the project. Evidence-based physical therapists must still determine for themselves whether extraneous factors were introduced because certain relevant exclusion criteria were not implemented in a study.

Once the inclusion and exclusion criteria are established, researchers must determine how they will locate potential subjects. Individuals who already belong to a specific group may be identified through records maintained by private or public organizations. For example, lists of potential subjects may be available from hospital medical records, insurance company beneficiary files, health care professional licensing boards, professional association membership rosters, or university registrars, to name just a few options. When such a list exists it is referred to as a *sampling frame*. The advantage of a sampling frame is that potential candidates are identified all at once, thereby expediting the selection process. If the investigators are interested in individuals at the time of their admission to a group, such as newly evaluated or diagnosed patients, then they will have to wait for these individuals to present themselves to participating clinicians because there will not be a preexisting sampling frame with which to identify them. Whether or not a sampling frame is used will be determined by the nature of the research question and the availability of records for use.

Additional methods for locating potential subjects include advertising in local media, direct solicitation or personal invitation, recruitment through clinical facilities, or recruitment through other organizations such as schools, churches, civic associations, colleges, and universities. The extent of the recruitment effort is dependent upon the definition of the accessible population, as well as practical issues related to cost and administrative requirements.

SUBJECT SELECTION

After potential candidates are identified, investigators must use a method for selecting individuals to participate in the study. Ideally, subjects will represent the population from which they are drawn so that any conclusions may be extrapolated to the larger group of people. There are two general approaches to subject selection: probabilistic sampling methods and nonprobabilistic sampling methods. Which approach is used often depends on a number of logistical factors including: the likelihood that a sufficient number of potential subjects exists and is available for study, the ability of subjects to get to researchers or vice versa, and the time frame in which the study is to be completed. The availability of sufficient funds often is a deciding factor.[2] Exploratory or pilot studies, as well as those that are self-funded, often use less involved sampling methods.

Probabilistic Sampling Methods

Probabilistic sampling refers to the use of a method for randomly selecting subjects for participation in a study. Random selection is the approach most likely (although not guaranteed) to capture a representative group of eligible individuals because the rules of probability suggest that repeated sampling will produce collections of similar individuals.[1] This potential similarity among samples is important because investigators want to attribute their study findings to the larger population from which subjects were selected. In order to do that, investigators either must demonstrate, or assume, that their study findings are reproducible every time they draw a sample from the population of interest. Samples from the same population that differ from one another, or from the population itself, reflect a problem referred to as *sampling error*. In addition to minimizing sampling error, a random selection process minimizes the opportunity for investigators to introduce bias into the study by using their own judgment or preferences to decide which individuals should serve as subjects.

The most basic probabilistic sampling method is referred to as the *simple random sample*. In this method, every subject that meets the inclusion criteria is assigned a number. Which individuals are selected is determined by identification of their numbers through methods as crude as drawing a piece of paper out of a hat or as sophisticated as using a random number generator. A simple random sample minimizes sampling error because each potential subject has an equal chance of being selected. This approach is useful when selecting from several hundred or fewer individuals, but may be impractical for application when the sampling frame or candidate pool numbers in the thousands.[2] An alternative method in this case is a *systematic sampling* approach in which potential subjects are organized according to an identifier such as a birth date, social security number, or patient account number. Only the first subject is selected randomly from this group and then all remaining subjects are chosen based on their numerical distance (e.g., every 10th person) from the first individual.

Stratified random sampling is a more complex probabilistic selection method used when investigators have an interest in capturing subgroups within the population. Subgroups often are based on naturally occurring differences in the proportion of a particular subject characteristic such as gender, race, age, disease severity, or functional level within a population. For example, imagine a study in which the researchers want to know whether risk factors for a disease differ depending upon the age of the individual. In this hypothetical study, the individuals in the population range in age from 18–65. Twenty percent of these individuals are 18–25 years old, 35 percent are 26–40 years old, and 45 percent are 41–65 years old. In order to answer their question, the investigators in this study might select a simple random sample from the entire population; however, doing so may result in such a small number of representatives from a particular age group that analyzing the differences in risk becomes difficult statistically. If the investigators wish to preserve the natural proportions of subjects' ages in their sample, then they will use the stratified sampling method. Table 6–2 provides a comparison of samples (100 subjects each) from this population selected using the simple random sample and stratified random sampling techniques. Researchers also may use stratified random sampling to ensure that certain members of the population are included in the study regardless of their proportion in the overall population.

Cluster sampling is a probabilistic selection method used when naturally occurring pockets of the population of interest are geographically dispersed. For example, imagine a prospective study in which investigators want to determine the effect of a new body mechanics education program for patients with lower back pain in the state of Virginia. The naturally occurring

Table 6–2 Number of hypothetical subjects selected from different age groups using different sampling techniques (total number of subjects = 100).

	Sampling Technique	
Age Group (% of total population)	**Simple Random Sample (% of total sample)**	**Stratified Random Sample (% of total sample)**
18–25 (20%)	33%	20%
26–40 (35%)	39%	35%
41–65 (45%)	28%	45%

clusters in this study might be major cities within the state and outpatient physical therapy clinics within these cities. Figure 6–1 illustrates this sampling technique using metropolitan areas with a population between 100,000 and 200,000 residents.[7] The cities highlighted in grey are randomly selected in the first step. Each city has a fictitious number of physical therapy clinics in which at least 50 percent of the patients served have low back pain. Three clinics in each city are randomly selected in the second step of the sampling process. Finally, each clinic has patients with low back pain who fall into one of four back pain categories. In the last step of the sampling process, the investigators randomly select 25 percent of the patients from each back pain category within each clinic. The primary benefit of cluster sampling is an improved ability to identify potential subjects when a sampling frame is not available. In addition, costs may be reduced if travel is required because only three clinics within three cities are involved rather than every physical therapy clinic in every city in Virginia.

Nonprobabilistic Sampling Methods

Nonprobabilistic sampling refers to methods for choosing subjects that do not involve a random selection process. These methods commonly are used in clinical research because they are easier to implement and cost less.[2] In addition, nonprobabilistic approaches may be needed when the length of time required to generate a large enough candidate pool will prevent the study's completion or when a potential sample size is already small (as in the case of a rare disorder).[8] These last two scenarios are common occurrences in clinical research, especially in those studies in which subject enrollment is dependent on new patients being identified and willing to participate. The absence of a random selection process means that the rules of probability

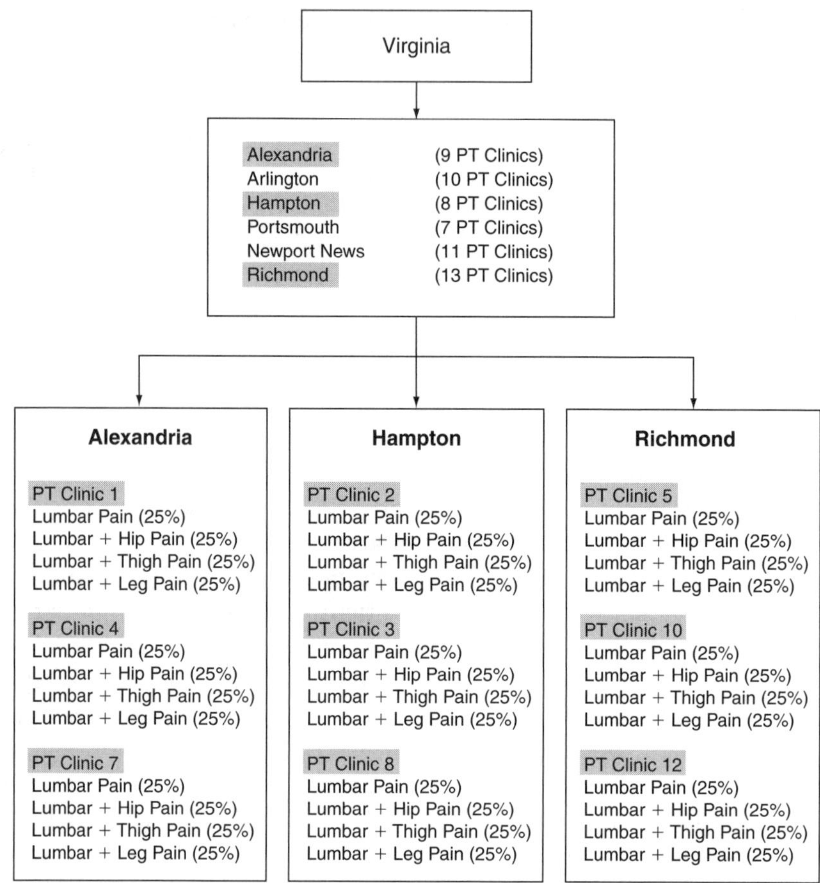

Figure 6-1 A cluster sampling plan in a hypothetical study of physical therapy visits in major cities in Virginia.

are not in effect; therefore, nonprobabilistic sampling methods increase the opportunity for sampling error. As a result, the sample drawn likely will not be representative of the population and may even be so different as to result in outcomes that cannot be reproduced with repeated study. In spite of this important limitation, nonprobabilistic selection methods are the most frequently used approaches in physical therapy research.

The most basic nonprobabilistic method is referred to as *convenience sampling*. In this approach, the investigators recruit easily available individuals who meet the criteria for the study. Common strategies for locating potential subjects include personal requests for volunteers to known assemblies of people (such as students) or direct invitation to passersby on a street or in a mall.[8] In effect, these individuals are "convenient" because of the ease of locating and contacting them. Often subjects are chosen consecutively as they become available or make themselves known. A challenge when using convenience sampling is the effect on study outcomes of potential dissimilarities between the individuals who volunteer and those who do not. For example, elderly residents of an assisted living community who sign up for a project about the effects of exercise on balance and falls may be more concerned about their safety than those who do not respond to the recruitment request. In this scenario, it is possible that these concerns will motivate the study participants to exercise in a way that is different than those who are not worried about their own safety. This differential in performance may result in a statistically significant beneficial effect of the program; in other words, balance improved and falls were reduced following participation in the exercise program. These results might not be reproducible in subjects whose lack of concern about their safety translates into minimal effort with exercise.

Snowball sampling is a nonprobabilistic technique in which the investigators start with a few subjects and then recruit more via word of mouth from the original participants. This approach is particularly useful when it is difficult to locate potential study candidates because their identity is unknown or purposefully concealed from public knowledge. For example, investigators interested in identifying risk factors for skin breakdown in homeless veterans may use snowball sampling to recruit other members of the street population who served in the military. Similarly, researchers examining the effectiveness of a treatment for repetitive motion injuries in undocumented farm workers might use snowball sampling because potential subjects may hide their immigration status for fear of criminal penalty or deportation.

The haphazardness of convenience and snowball sampling techniques *should not* be confused with random sampling methods. While it is true that the investigators do not have control over who responds to their invitations or who will be contacted via word of mouth, these processes lack the ability to give every individual within range an equal opportunity for selection. In the absence of an equal opportunity, the rules of chance cannot be applied; therefore, future samples from the same population are likely to be dissimilar.

Finally, *purposive sampling* is an approach in which the investigators make specific choices about who will serve as subjects in their study. This method is different from convenience sampling because the researchers do not rely simply on the availability of the potential subjects. Rather, the investigators hand-pick individuals with certain characteristics that are important to include and enroll them. This approach is commonly used in qualitative studies in which representatives from known groups are desired to ensure a variety of perspectives are obtained. For example, investigators studying the perceived value of a case management system with respect to the rehabilitation and return-to-work of injured shipyard employees might interview subjects specifically selected from the 1) shipyard executive staff; 2) the shipyard human resources staff; 3) employees with work-related injuries; 4) case managers; 5) physicians; and, 6) rehabilitation staff. These groups all have an interest in the outcomes of the injured workers' rehabilitation; therefore, their inclusion in the study is necessary to ensure that all perceptions of the usefulness of case management are considered. Unlike convenience and snowball sampling, purposive sampling may result in a reasonably representative sample as long as the researchers carefully consider all of the relevant characteristics before selecting their subjects.[2]

SUBJECT MANAGEMENT WITHIN THE STUDY

Subjects are enrolled in a study in order to collect data about them as they proceed through specified activities relevant to the research question. Which activities an individual subject will participate in is governed by the research design. If the design requires group comparisons, then the first issue to be determined is the group assignment for each subject. Ideally, the assignment process will lead to groups of equal size across which subject characteristics are evenly distributed. Balanced groups are important in order to isolate the effect of an experimental intervention on the study's outcome. If the groups are different at the outset of the study, then the outcome may be a result of these initial differences. As might be expected, a randomization process for subject assignment increases the likelihood of achieving group equality through the rules of chance.

Random Assignment Methods

The simplest approach among these methods is *random assignment by individual.* In this scenario each subject is *assigned*, or *allocated*, to a group according to which group number is randomly pulled from a hat or which side of a coin lands upright. The problem with this approach is that groups may be unequal in both number and distribution of characteristics, especially if the overall sample size is small.[2] An alternative strategy is to use *block assignment* in which the size of the groups is predetermined in order to ensure equal numbers. The investigators then randomly assign the identified number of subjects to the first group, then the second group, and so forth. Investigators implementing a third option, *systematic assignment*, will use a list of the subjects and repeatedly count off the group numbers until everyone is assigned. Table 6–3 illustrates this method for a hypothetical study with four groups. Based on the list in the table, Group 1 will contain subjects A, E and I, Group 2 will contain subjects B, F, and J, and so on. Finally, *matched assignment* is used when investigators want all groups to have equal numbers of subjects with a specific characteristic. Subjects first are arranged into subgroups according to attributes such as gender, age, or initial functional status. Then each member of the subgroup is randomly assigned to the study groups. Matching is a method of controlling for the potential effects of these specific characteristics on the outcome. Unfortunately, this approach is both time-intensive and expensive as investigators need to identify enough potential subjects with whom matching can be performed.[2]

Each of these assignment methods presupposes that all of the subjects have been identified and can be distributed to groups at one time. However, clinical research often deals with patients who are identified one at a time as they present with the relevant diagnosis or problem. This method of obtaining subjects may take months or years to complete depending on disease or problem prevalence. If researchers waited until all subjects were assembled to perform the assignment process, the study would be delayed unnecessarily. To avoid this problem, investigators will identify subjects based on their order of admission to the study—that is, the first subject enrolled, the second subject enrolled, and so on. If 50 subjects are needed for a study, then 50 consecutive enrollment numbers are randomly assigned to the study groups in advance of actual subject identification. As a result,

Table 6–3 Systematic assignment of subjects to four groups in a hypothetical study.

Subject Identification	Group Number
Subject A	Group 1
Subject B	Group 2
Subject C	Group 3
Subject D	Group 4
Subject E	Group 1
Subject F	Group 2
Subject G	Group 3
Subject H	Group 4
Subject I	Group 1
Subject J	Group 2
Subject K	Group 3
Subject L	Group 4

as each subject is enrolled, his or her group assignment already has been determined and the study can proceed without disruption.

Nonrandom Assignment

Nonrandom assignment to groups occurs when subjects are members of preexisting groups in which the investigators have an interest or when investigators make their own decisions about which subjects go in which groups. Nonrandom groups commonly are used in retrospective studies about prognostic factors or interventions. For example, a hypothetical study might compare shoe style preferences between a group of women who suffered ankle sprains and a group of women who did not in order to determine the risk of injury related to heel height. Group assignment in this study is determined by the presence or absence of the sprain, not by the investigators. Similarly, a hypothetical study about the effectiveness of rigid removable dressings following below knee amputations might compare limb girth and wound healing time in a group of patients whose surgeon requires the dressings postoperatively to a group of patients whose surgeon does not believe in or use them. In both examples, the lack of randomization reduces the likelihood that groups will be equal in size or in distribution of potentially confounding characteristics. As a result, the investigators may require statistical methods to adjust for extraneous influences introduced into the study.

Other Subject Management Issues

Assignment to groups is one of many methods investigators use to manage subjects in a study. Each of these tactics is intended to minimize the chance that an unwanted factor or factors will influence the outcome of the study. For example, investigators may follow preestablished protocols for dealing with subjects in order to reduce the possibility that variations in researcher behavior will result in changes in subject performance. Protocols may be written as scripts for instructions or as a specific sequence to follow for testing or providing the study interventions. Similarly, every subject is provided with the information necessary for appropriate participation in relevant study activities.[1] Training and practice sessions may be scheduled to ensure that individuals understand what is expected of them, can perform the tasks appropriately, and have time to overcome any learning curves that may result in an inconsistent performance.

Participation in a study usually means that subjects must avoid a change in their daily routine until the project is concluded. For example, subjects in an aerobic exercise effectiveness study may be instructed to maintain their usual activity levels and to postpone starting a new exercise program until after they have completed the project. This restriction is implemented in order to isolate the effect, if any, of the experimental intervention. A change in subjects' routines could influence their performance on the outcome measures and perhaps produce an inaccurate representation of the impact of the aerobics program.

Finally, subjects in studies with two or more groups may not be informed of their assignment in order to minimize changes in their behavior as a result of this knowledge. This strategy of keeping subjects in the dark about their group assignment is referred to as *masking* or *blinding*. Investigators also may ask subjects not to discuss the study's activities with other people during their participation. Conversations with individuals from other groups might result in subjects learning about their assignment and changing their behavior in response to this knowledge. Similarly, study personnel providing the treatment regimens or collecting outcome measures also may change their behavior upon learning to which group a subject has been assigned. Unfortunately, in physical therapy research it is often difficult to mask subjects or investigators to group assignment because of the movement-based nature of most interventions.

SAMPLE SIZE

An essential consideration with respect to study subjects is the number of them that will be required to ensure that important relationships between (or among) variables or differences between (or among) groups can be detected statistically if they are present. The probability that a statistical test will identify a relationship or difference if it is present is referred to as the *power* of the test. The concern is that an insufficient number of subjects will produce a result that incorrectly indicates that no significant relationship or difference exists. This false negative finding—failure to detect a relationship or difference when it is present—is called a *Type II error*.[2] Because of the many challenges in clinical subject recruitment and enrollment, investigators must be persistent in their efforts to achieve an adequate sample size. Fortunately, it is possible to calculate the minimum number of subjects needed prior to the start of the study. The details of this method are discussed in Chapter 9.

SUMMARY

Clinical research requires human subjects from whom to collect data to answer the research question. Identification of potential subjects starts with the establishment of specific inclusion and exclusion criteria. Once a candidate pool is determined, random selection of subjects is preferred because of the increased likelihood of drawing a representative sample from the population of interest. Unfortunately, random selection methods often are difficult to use when attempting to study patients who may be limited in number and availability. Nonrandom selection methods are used most commonly in physical therapy research, but may result in biased samples whose outcomes may not be reproducible. Once subjects are selected, they must be managed throughout the study to avoid any changes in their behavior that may affect the outcome. Studies that compare outcomes among two or more groups require a method for subject assignment to the groups. Random assignment methods are preferred because of the likelihood that they will distribute equally the subject characteristics that may influence the outcome. Finally, the statistical power of a study to detect relationships or differences when they exist is dependent in part on an adequate sample size, an estimate of which can be calculated prior to the start of a research project.

Exercises

1. Create a hypothetical research question you might pursue as a physical therapy researcher. From this scenario:
   a) Identify the target population of interest and explain why it might be difficult to study in its entirety;
   b) Identify an accessible population for study and explain why this group of individuals is easier to study; and
   c) Identify three inclusion criteria and three exclusion criteria you will use to identify eligible subjects; provide a rationale for each criterion.
2. Discuss the general strengths and weaknesses of probabilistic and non-probabilistic sampling methods. Pick one method from each sampling approach and explain how it would be used in your study from scenario in Question #1.
3. Discuss the benefits of random assignment of subjects to groups. Why do these benefits enhance the study's credibility?
4. Provide three examples of subject management during a study. Why is the control over subject and researcher behavior so important?
5. Explain the concept of statistical power. Why is a Type II error a concern in research?

REFERENCES

1. Portney LG, Watkins MP. *Foundations of Clinical Research: Applications to Practice.* 2d ed. Upper Saddle River, NJ: Prentice Hall Health; 2000.

2. Domholdt E. *Rehabilitation Research: Principles and Applications*. 3d ed. St Louis, MO: Elsevier Saunders; 2005.
3. Milne S, Brosseau L, Robinson V, Noel MJ, Davis J *et al.* Continuous passive motion following total knee arthroplasty. *Cochrane Database Syst Rev*. 2003; (2):CD004260.
4. Johansson KM, Adolfsson LE, Foldevi MOM. Effects of acupuncture versus ultrasound in patients with impingement syndrome: Randomized clinical trial. *Phys Ther*. 2005; 85(6):490–501.
5. Kirk-Sanchez NJ. Factors related to activity limitations in a group of Cuban Americans before and after hip fracture. *Phys Ther*. 2004; 84(5):408–418.
6. Ciesla ND. Chest physical therapy for patients in the intensive care unit. *Phys Ther*. 1996; 76(6):609–625.
7. Annual Estimates of the Population of Incorporated Places in Virginia. U.S. Census Bureau Web site. Available at: http://www.census.gov/popest/cities/tables/SUB-EST2004-04-51.xls. Accessed February 28, 2006.
8. Batavia M. *Clinical Research for Health Professionals: A User-Friendly Guide*. Boston, MA: Butterworth-Heinemann; 2001.

Chapter 7

Variables and Their Measurement

I have measured out my life with coffee spoons.

—T. S. Eliot

Objectives

Upon completion of this chapter the student/practitioner will be able to:

1. Differentiate among, and discuss the role of independent, dependent, and extraneous variables.
2. Identify the number of levels of independent variables in a study.
3. Differentiate among, and discuss the mathematical properties of nominal, ordinal, interval, and ratio levels of measurement.
4. Differentiate between norm-referenced and criterion-referenced measures.
5. Discuss the concept of measurement error and its implications for research findings.
6. Discuss the following forms of, and factors influencing measurement reliability, including:
   a) Test-retest reliability;
   b) Internal consistency;
   c) Parallel forms reliability;
   d) Split-half reliability;
   e) Intra-rater reliability; and
   f) Inter-rater reliability.
7. Discuss the following forms of, and factors influencing measurement validity, including:
   a) Face validity;
   b) Content validity;

c) Construct validity;
d) Convergent validity;
e) Discriminant validity;
f) Criterion validity;
g) Concurrent validity; and
h) Predictive validity.

8. Discuss the importance of, and potential barriers to responsiveness to change in measures.

Terms in This Chapter

Ceiling Effect: A limitation of a measure in which the instrument does not register a further increase in score for the highest scoring individuals.

Concept: A mental image of an observable phenomenon that is expressed in words.[1]

Construct: A non-observable abstraction created for a specific research purpose; defined by observable measures such as events or behaviors.[2]

Construct Validity: The degree to which a measure matches the operational definition of the concept or construct it is said to represent.[1]

Content Validity: The degree to which items in an instrument represent all of the facets of the variable being measured.[3]

Concurrent Validity: A method of criterion validation that reflects the relationship between a measure of interest and a criterion ("gold standard") measure, both of which have been applied within the same time frame.[1]

Continuous Variable: When the values of variables are on a scale with a theoretically infinite number of measurable increments between each major unit.

Convergent Validity: A method of construct validation that reflects the degree to which two or more measures of the same phenomenon or characteristic will produce similar scores.[2]

Criterion-Referenced: Measures the scores of which are compared to an absolute standard in order to judge an individual's performance.[1]

Criterion Validity: The degree to which a measure of interest relates to an external criterion measure.[2]

Dependent Variable: The outcome of interest in a study.

Dichotomous Variable: When only two values are possible for a variable.

Discrete Variable: When the value of a variable is a distinct category.

Discriminant Validity: A method of construct validation that reflects the degree to which an instrument can distinguish between or among different phenomena or characteristics.[2]

Face Validity: A subjective assessment of the degree to which an instrument appears to measure what it is designed to measure.[3]

Factorial Design: An experimental research design in which the effects of two or more independent variables, and their interactions with one another, are evaluated.[1]

Floor Effect: A limitation of a measure in which the instrument does not register a further decrease in score for the lowest scoring individuals.

Independent Variable: Traditionally defined as the variable that is purposefully manipulated by investigators in an effort to produce a change in outcome.

Internal Consistency: The degree to which subsections of an instrument measure the same concept or construct.[2]

Inter-Rater Reliability: The stability of repeated measures across two or more examiners.

Interval Level of Measurement: A measure that classifies objects or characteristics in rank order with a known equal distance between categories, but that lacks a known empirical zero point.

Intra-Rater Reliability: The stability of repeated measures by the same examiner.

Measurement: The process by which values are assigned to variables.

Measurement Error: "The difference between the true value and the observed value."[3(p. 62)]

Measurement Reliability: The extent to which repeated measurements agree with one another. Also referred to as "stability," "consistency" and "reproducibility."[3]

Measurement Validity: The degree to which a measure captures what it is intended to measure.[3]

Nominal Level of Measurement: A measure that classifies objects or characteristics, but that lacks rank order and a known equal distance between categories.

Norm-Referenced: Measures the scores of which are compared to the group's performance in order to judge an individual's performance.[1]

Ordinal Level of Measurement: A measure, that classifies objects or characteristics, in rank order, but that lacks the mathematical properties of a known equal distance between categories; may or may not have a natural zero point.

Parallel Forms Reliability: Reliability of a self-report instrument established by testing two versions of the tool that measures the same concepts or constructs.

Predictive Validity: A method of criterion validation that reflects the degree to which the score on a test predicts a future criterion score.[2]

Ratio Level of Measurement: A measure that classifies objects or characteristics in rank order with a known equal distance between categories and a known empirical zero point.

Responsiveness: The ability of a measure to detect change in the phenomenon of interest.

Split-Half Reliability: Reliability of a self-report instrument established by testing two versions of the tool that are combined into one survey that is administered at one time; investigators separate the items and compare results for the two forms after subjects complete the instrument.

Standard Error of Measurement: The extent to which observed scores are disbursed around the true score; "the standard deviation of measurement errors" obtained from repeated measures.[1(p.560)]

Variable: A characteristic of an individual, object, or environmental condition that may take on different values.

INTRODUCTION

Investigators require information to answer their research questions. The nature of the information is indicated by the question or purpose statement itself. For example, studies about diagnostic tests require information about the tests performed and the diagnoses obtained. Studies about interventions, on the other hand, require information about the treatments provided and their effects. The tests, diagnoses, treatments, and effects are referred to generically as variables. A research design should specify what variables will be included and how they will be measured. Ideally, instruments or techniques used will have established performance records that indicate their consistency and appropriateness for the measures of interest in the study. This chapter discusses different types of variables, as well as the characteristics of measures used in research.

VARIABLES

Variables are characteristics of individuals, objects, or environmental conditions that may have more than one value. Attributes of individuals commonly used in clinical research on patients include, but are not limited to: age, gender, race/ethnicity, type of pathology, degree of impairment, functional limitation, and disability. Functional performance characteristics, such as strength, flexibility, endurance, balance, and task-specific skill level, are analogous attributes that may be used in research of individuals who are healthy or who have stable chronic disease. Characteristics of objects often refer to the nature of diagnostic tests and interventions, whereas characteristics of environmental conditions describe the study's context. In nonexperimental research, information about variables of interest is gathered through investigator observation. Experimental or quasi-experimental research, on the other hand, is defined by the purposeful manipulation of some of the variables in the study. Different study designs, therefore, require different types of variables.

Independent Variables

An *independent variable* traditionally is defined as the variable that is purposefully manipulated by investigators in an effort to produce a change in an outcome. In clinical research, independent variables are the interventions that are evaluated through the use of experimental and quasi-experimental designs. For example, Seynnes *et al.* examined the impact of an exercise program on strength and function in frail elders.[4] The independent variable was a resistance training program that was implemented by the investigators according to a specific protocol under controlled conditions. Purposeful manipulation of the variable was achieved through the creation of a high-intensity exercise group, a low-moderate intensity exercise group, and a placebo group. These three groups reflect three "levels" of the independent variable. Investigators define levels when they determine what forms the independent variable will take in a study.

Intervention studies may have one or more independent variables, a situation that increases the complexity of the research design because of the potential interaction between the independent variables at their different levels. Studies in which this interaction is anticipated are referred to as *factorial designs*. For example, Bower *et al.* used a 2 × 2 factorial design in their study of the effects of physiotherapy in children with cerebral palsy.[5] The designation "2 × 2" refers to the number of levels in each of the independent variables: "goal setting" and "physiotherapy." Table 7–1 illustrates the interaction among the levels of each variable that results in the creation of four groups for study 1) aims-routine physiotherapy (AR); 2) aims-intense physiotherapy (AI); 3) goals-routine physiotherapy (GR); and 4) goals-intense physiotherapy (GI). Evidence-based physical therapists must be attentive to the number and

Table 7–1 Factorial design with two independent variables.

		Physiotherapies	
		Routine (R)	**Intense (I)**
Goal Setting	Aims (A)	AR	AI
	Goals (G)	GR	GI

Source: Reprinted from *Developmental Medicine and Child Neurology*, Randomized controlled trial of physiotherapy in 56 children with cerebral palsy followed for 18 months, Bower E, Michell D, Burnett M, Campbell MJ, McLellan DL, pp. 4–15. Copyright (2001), with permission from Blackwell Publishing.

definition of independent variables in a study in order to understand the potential cause(s) of change in the outcome of interest.

Investigators also may refer to the use of independent variables in prognosis studies. The usefulness of independent variables (also referred to as "factors" or "predictors") in these studies is determined based upon their ability to predict the outcome of interest. Although they are not purposefully manipulated interventions, they are variables that may assume different values that the investigators can measure. For example, Hulzebos *et al.* evaluated the role of 12 factors including patient age, presence of diabetes, smoking history and pulmonary function in predicting the development of pulmonary complications after elective coronary artery bypass surgery.[6] Independent variables in prognosis studies cannot be said to "cause" a change in the outcome; rather, they may be "related to" it depending upon the results obtained.

Some authors also may refer to interventions as independent variables when they are part of observational studies about outcomes. This designation is tricky, however, because clinicians apply these interventions beyond the control of the researchers. In other words, purposeful manipulation according to specific study protocols does not occur. Unless the clinicians already implement treatments in a standardized fashion, the application of the term "independent variable" is confusing more than helpful. Nevertheless, a statistical analysis of observed data in a pre-test/post-test format implies the application of an independent variable in these studies.

The term *independent variable* does not apply to purely descriptive studies or to studies in which relationships between variables are evaluated in the absence of a predictive model. A study characterizing the signs and symptoms of different forms of multiple sclerosis is an example of the first scenario. The investigator conducting this study does not manipulate anything nor is there an outcome of interest for which an independent variable might be responsible. Therefore, use of the term is irrelevant in this case. A study that evaluates the relationship between place of residence and the form of multiple sclerosis is an example of the second scenario. In this case, residence and form may be classified generally as variables, but the goal of the study is to determine simply the degree to which the value of one is aligned with the value of the other. Again, there is no active manipulation so identification of one variable as the independent variable is arbitrary.

Dependent Variables

A *dependent variable* is the outcome of interest in a study. In studies about interventions, the value of the dependent variable is presumed to occur as a result of the independent variable. Seynnes *et al.* evaluated the change in the dependent variables "strength," "function," and "self-reported disability," caused by different intensities of the independent variable "resistance training."[4] Similarly, Bower *et al.* examined effects of the independent variables "goal setting" and "physiotherapy" on the dependent variables "motor function" and "motor performance."[5] In studies about prognoses, on the other hand, investigators presume that the value of the dependent variable is predicted by, rather than caused by, the independent variable. This distinction is consistent with studies that examine differences versus studies that examine relationships. As noted in Chapter 5, studies of relationships cannot establish a causal connection between an independent and dependent variable. As a result, Hulzebos *et al.* could identify factors such as age and smoking history that increased the risk of postoperative pulmonary complications (the dependent variable), but they could not conclude that either of these independent variables caused the adverse outcome.[6]

Extraneous Variables

An extraneous variable is a factor other than the independent variable that is said to influence, or confound, the dependent variable.[1] The potential for extraneous variables is the principal reason why controls through study design and statistical adjustment are attempted in research. Subjects, investigators, equipment, and environmental conditions are just some of the sources of confounding influences in a study. For example, subject performance may wax and wane over the course of time due to fatigue or alertness levels. Investigators may have varying levels of experience with the outcome measure used. Equipment may lose accuracy with repeated use. Room temperature and lighting may influence a subject's ability to execute a task. Any of these problems may influence the outcome of the study resulting in misleading conclusions about the impact, if any, of the independent variables. Researchers must anticipate which of the many potential extraneous variables is/are most likely to be a threat to their study and try to control or adjust for them. Evidence-based physical therapists must determine the success with which this control or adjustment was performed, as well as whether any important factors were ignored or overlooked.

Table 7-2 itemizes different types of variables in the Seynnes *et al.* and the Hulzebos *et al.* studies.[4,6] Note that the extraneous variables are defined as "potential" because these were identified, but not controlled for, in these studies.

Table 7–2 Types of variables in selected intervention and prognosis studies.

Intervention Study: Seynnes *et al.*[4]		
Independent Variable	**Dependent Variables**	**Potential Extraneous Variables**
Training Intensity (3 levels)	Muscle strength	Overall subject health status
• Sham	Muscle endurance	Subject psychological status
• Low–moderate	Functional limitation #1	Subject emotional status
• High	Functional limitation #2	Environmental conditions during training
	Functional limitation #3	
	Disability	
Prognosis Study: Hulzebos *et al.*[6]		
Independent Variable	**Dependent Variable**	**Potential Extraneous Variables**
Gender	Postoperative pulmonary complications (4 grades)	Physician documentation
Body Mass Index (BMI)		Operation time
Age		Medications for cardiac conditions
History of cigarette smoking		Prior cardiac surgery
Coughing		Evidence of heart failure
Forced expiratory volume/sec		Previous myocardial infarction
Inspiratory vital capacity		Electrocardiographic changes
Maximal expiratory pressure		Anesthesiology classification
Maximal inspiratory pressure		
History of COPD		
Diabetes Mellitus		
Specific Activity Scale Score		

Other Terminology Related to Variables

In addition to the labels *independent*, *dependent*, and *extraneous*, variables may be characterized by the general methods by which they are measured. Variables whose possible values are distinct categories are referred to as *discrete variables*. Weight-bearing status characterized as "none," "toe-touch," "foot-flat," "as tolerated," and "full" is an example of a discrete variable. When only two values are possible—such as "male-female" or "disease present-disease absent"—then the variable is described as *dichotomous*. Investigators also may operationally define a quantitative variable in discrete terms, such as "number of hospitals in a region." In a practical sense, it is neither possible nor advisable to create a fraction of a patient! On the other hand, the values of variables which are on a scale with a theoretically infinite number of measurable increments between each major unit are referred to as *continuous*. Distance walked characterized in feet or meters is an example of a continuous variable.

MEASUREMENT

If investigators wish to gain an understanding of the role and behavior of variables in a study, then they must determine a method by which to assign values to them. Values may be qualitative or quantitative in nature; in both cases their assignment should be guided by clearly-defined rules that are consistently applied in a study.[1,3] The process of value assignment is referred to as *measurement*. Measurement of variables is a necessary step in order to perform descriptive or inferential statistical analysis of the information obtained by quantitative research.

Levels of Measurement

There are four levels of measurement that create a continuum from qualitative to quantitative value assignment: nominal, ordinal, interval, and ratio. A *nominal level of measurement* is one in which values are named categories without the mathematical properties of rank and a known equal distance between them. The variable "gender" is captured by the nominal measure whose values are "male" and "female." Instruments that have "yes" and "no" response options are nominal measures that are used commonly in clinical practice and research. In both cases, the categories are assumed to be equal—one is not greater than or less than the other (rank). As a result, any statistical analysis must be performed using the frequencies (e.g., numbers or percentages) with which these characteristics occur in the subjects in the study.

An *ordinal level of measurement* also classifies characteristics without a known equal distance between them; however, categories have a rank order relative to one another. Ordinal measures are used frequently in surveys in which subject opinion or perception is solicited. A common clinical example is a survey of patient satisfaction in which the response options are displayed with both word and numerical anchors (Figure 7–1). In this case, the numerals are symbols not quantities. The variable "weight-bearing status" progresses in value from "none" to "full" with categories in between reflecting increases in the amount of weight bearing allowed. These

Completely Dissatisfied	Somewhat Dissatisfied	Neutral	Somewhat Satisfied	Completely Satisfied
1	2	3	4	5

Figure 7–1 An ordinal scale used for responses in a hypothetical patient satisfaction survey.

increases are not measured with numbers, but are indicated with modifying words. The absence of a known distance between each level of these scales means that mathematical functions cannot be performed directly with the measure. As a result, quantities in ordinal levels of measurement are determined based on the number or percentage of each response or category selected.

An *interval level of measurement* is a scale that assigns quantitative, rather than qualitative, values to variables. These values are numbers that have rank and a known equal distance between them, but that do not have a known zero point. In other words, the value "0" does not reflect the absence of the characteristic. The classical example of an interval scale is the measurement of temperature in Fahrenheit or Celsius. Zero degrees on either scale represents an actual temperature, not the lack of temperature. Theoretically, the possible values extend to infinity on either side of both scales. The lack of a known empirical zero point means that the quantities identified with an interval scale may have positive and negative values. In addition, they may be added and subtracted from one another, but they are not appropriate for multiplication or division.

A *ratio level of measurement* has all of the necessary mathematical properties for manipulation with addition, subtraction, multiplication, and division. These quantities have rank order, a known equal distance between them, and a known empirical zero point. The presence of an empirical zero point means that these scales cannot have negative values. Height, weight, blood pressure, speed, and distance are just a few of the many clinical examples of ratio level measures.

Table 7–3 summarizes the four levels of measurement along with relevant clinical examples. Table 7–4 illustrates the application of these concepts using the dependent variables from Seynnes *et al.*[4]

Note that classifying a measure is not always a straightforward exercise. Consider the example "assistive device" in which the values are "cane," "walker," and "wheelchair." On the surface this would appear to be a nominal measure–classification without rank. Inherently, a cane has no more or less value than a walker or wheelchair. This would be an appropriate designation if the investigators were interested only in the type of device

Table 7–3 Levels of measurement.

Level	Clinical Examples
Nominal	Gender Race/ethnicity Religious affiliation Weight-bearing status Level of assistance required
Ordinal	Manual muscle test grades Patient satisfaction Temperature
Interval	Calendar year Height Weight
Ratio	Circumference Blood pressure Distance/Speed

for its own sake. On the other hand, if the researchers were interested in using "assistive device" as an indication of the level of assistance a subject requires for mobility, then the measure becomes ordinal based on the singular property of each device to provide more (or less) support. The point is that a level of measurement may be defined both by the qualities of the instrument itself and by the investigators' intention for its use. Evidence-

Table 7–4 Dependent variables and their measures in Seynnes *et al.*[4]

Dependent Variable	Measure	Type of Measure
Muscle strength	Maximal weight lifted one time (in kilograms)	Ratio
Muscle endurance	Number of repetitions lifting 90% maximal of maximal weight	Ratio
Functional limitation	Time required to rise from a chair (in seconds)	Ratio
Functional limitation	Stair-climbing power (in watts)	Ratio
Functional limitation	Distance walked in six minutes (in meters)	Ratio
Disability	Self-report on 0–3 scale (without difficulty, with some difficulty, with much difficulty, unable to do)	Ordinal

based physical therapists must discern both of these issues about a study in order to determine whether the measure is defined and used appropriately.

Reference Standards in Measurement

A measurement may be characterized not only by its level, but also by the standard against which its scores are evaluated. Investigators often wish to compare outcomes scores for individuals or groups with a previously-established performance level. When this performance standard is derived from the scores of previously-tested individuals, then the measurement is said to be *norm-referenced*. Growth curves for children are examples of clinical measurements that are norm-referenced. The values for the norms were gathered from a representative sample of healthy individuals characterized by different ages, heights, weights, and genders.[7] Figure 7–2 is the growth chart for boys from birth to 36 months. Investigators studying infant boys may use this chart to compare the growth of their subjects against these standards.

An alternative to norm-referencing a measurement is to compare the value obtained to a previously-established absolute standard. Measures evaluated in this manner are said to be *criterion-referenced*. Discharge criteria such as "transfers independently" or "ambulates 300 feet" are examples of clinical situations in which patient performance is judged against an absolute standard. Standardized license and specialist certification exams in physical therapy also use criterion referencing to determine the threshold for passing the test.

MEASUREMENT RELIABILITY

If measures were perfect, then every score obtained would be "true," or a precise reflection of the phenomenon of interest. Unfortunately, measures are not perfect which means that a portion of the value obtained is bound to be variability, or error, that is unrelated to the "true" score. If the error is large enough, then the results of the study may be questioned. In other words, it will be difficult to attribute a change in an outcome to an experimental intervention if the outcome scores are likely to be different simply because of measurement error. Investigators attempt to minimize *measurement error* through their choice of instruments and the methods for using them. Instruments with an established performance record are preferred, but not always available. Collection of measures usually is directed by protocols that are designed to minimize:

- The variability in investigator application of the device or technique;
- The variability in subject performance; and/or,
- The potential contribution of device malfunction or failure.

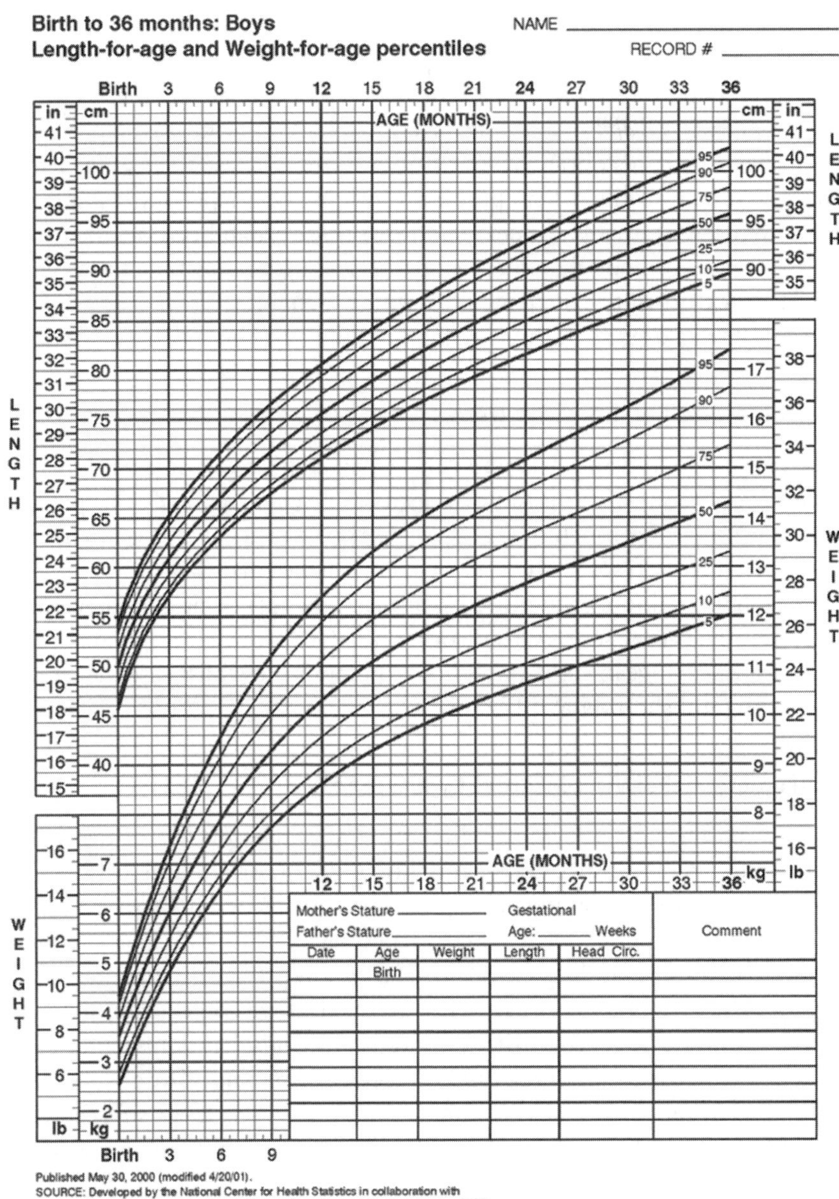

Figure 7-2 Boys birth to 36 months length-for-age and weight-for-age percentiles.

Source: Reprinted with permission from the Centers for Disease Control and Prevention.

If these choices are appropriate, then researchers and users of evidence should find that scores of the same phenomenon are stable with repeated measurement—that is, the measurement is reliable. There are several forms of *measurement reliability* that may be evaluated to determine the potential usefulness of scores obtained in a study. Some of these forms pertain to the instrument, while others pertain to the person or persons taking the measurements. Investigators may perform these reliability assessments as part of their study or they may refer to previous studies that have evaluated this feature of the instrument. Forms of reliability are discussed here; statistical tests used to evaluate reliability are discussed in Chapter 9.

Instrument Reliability: Test-Retest

Test-retest reliability may be established when an instrument is used on two separate occasions with the same subject(s). The challenge with this process is to determine how much time should pass between the two measurements. If the interval is too short, then subject performance may vary due to fatigue, change in motivation, or increased skill with practice—none of which are related to their "true" score. On the other hand, too long an interval may result in a real change in the variable being measured, in which case the second score will (and should be) different.

Instrument Reliability: Internal Consistency

Internal consistency is a form of reliability that is relevant to self-report instruments, such as health-related quality of life questionnaires. These surveys usually have several items or questions, groups of which are designed to measure different concepts or constructs within the instrument. For example, the Burden of Stroke Scale (BOSS) is a self-report instrument that assesses the consequences of stroke in terms of three constructs: "physical activity limitations," "cognitive activity limitations," and "psychological distress."[8] Each domain of the BOSS is measured by a number of subscales, each of which is comprised by several items (Figure 7-3). If the subscales are going to capture different aspects of each domain, then items must relate to one subscale and not to others. Similarly, the subscales should relate to one construct and not to the others. In other words, the instrument should demonstrate internal consistency for each construct.

Instrument Reliability: Parallel Forms

Parallel forms reliability also is relevant to self-report instruments. As the term implies, parallel forms reliability can be established only in cases where two

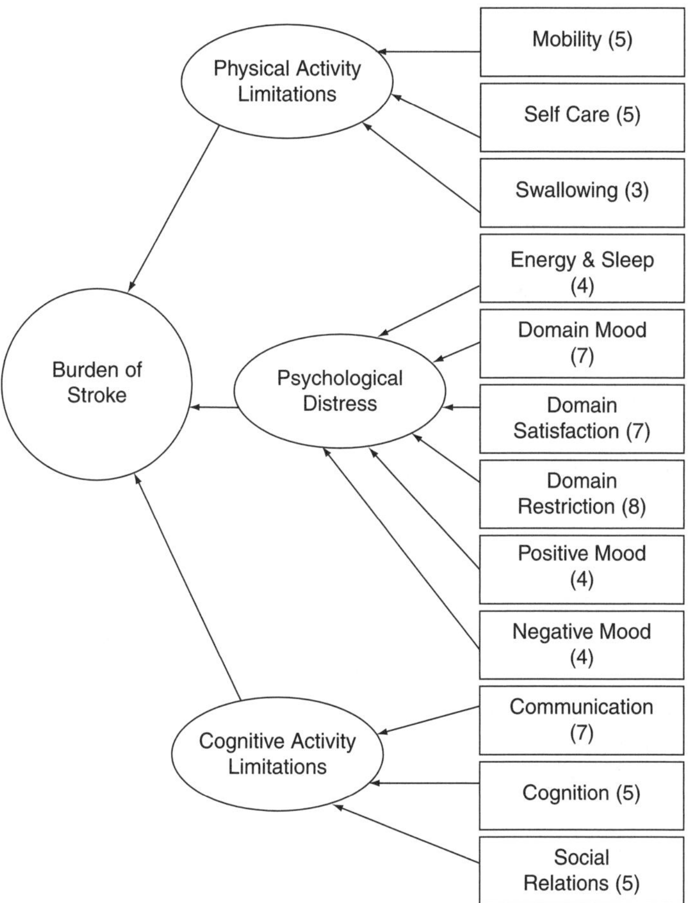

Figure 7–3 Conceptual model of the burden of stroke scale (BOSS).[8]
Source: Reprinted from *Journal of Clinical Epidemiology*, 57(10), Doyle PJ, McNeil MR, Mikolic JM, Prieto L, Hula WD *et al.*, pp. 997–1007. Copyright (2004), with permission from Elsevier.

versions of the instrument exist, both of which measure the same constructs or concepts. Each form of the test is administered on one occasion and the responses are compared to determine the degree to which they produce the same scores for the same items or concepts.

Instrument Reliability: Split-Half

Split-half reliability eliminates the need for two test administrations by combining the two forms of an instrument into one longer version. Subjects complete the entire instrument and then investigators separate the items for comparison to determine the degree to which scores agree for the same items or concepts.

Rater Reliability

Up to this point the forms of reliability discussed have pertained to the instrument; however, the stability of a measure also is dependent upon the person or persons collecting it. The consistency of repeated measures performed by one individual is referred to as *intra-rater reliability*. For example, a physical therapist responsible for measuring joint range of motion following an experimental stretching technique should be able to obtain nearly the same score for the same position each time the measure is taken. On the other hand, if several physical therapists from the same clinic take turns collecting data for this study, then the consistency of scores between raters—or *inter-rater reliability*—must be established.

MEASUREMENT VALIDITY

Another essential property of measurement is validity—the ability of a measure to capture what it is intended to capture.[3] In simple terms, a goniometer that measures joint position in degrees is a valid instrument for range of motion whereas a thermometer is not. Researchers usually are not choosing between two such nonsensical options; rather, they are making a decision between or among multiple instruments that purport to measure the same thing. As is the case with reliability, the selection of an instrument with previously-established validity is preferable. There are several forms of *measurement validity* that may be evaluated to determine the potential usefulness of scores obtained in a study. Forms of validity are discussed here; statistical tests used to evaluate validity are discussed in Chapter 9.

Face Validity

Face validity is both the simplest and most subjective form of measurement validity. Essentially, face validity is tested with the question, "Does this instrument appear to be the appropriate choice to measure this variable?" This is a "yes-no" question without a particular reference standard against which to make the judgment. As a result, investigators should look for instruments for which other forms of validity have been evaluated. However, keep in mind that an instrument that lacks face validity in the eyes of the investigators or subjects likely will not provide the desired information. Ordinal measures such as surveys, self-report instruments, and qualitative rating scales are most susceptible to this problem because of inadequate operational definition. Consider an employee performance rating system that does not define the labels "does not meet expectations," "meets expectations," and "exceeds expectations." Supervisors may apply these ratings inconsistently because they do not see the relevance of the labels to specific employee behavior. Similarly, employees may not feel compelled to change their behavior to achieve a higher rating because they do not believe the system adequately captures their performance. Despite the subjective nature of face validity, the lack of it may serve as a red flag regarding the potential usefulness of an instrument.

Content Validity

An instrument is said to have *content validity* when it represents all of the relevant facets of the variable it is intended to measure. In addition, the instrument should not contain elements that capture unrelated information. For example, a comprehensive balance test should include activities that challenge an individual's ability to maintain an upright position while sitting and/or standing, but should not include activities that require the subject to maintain a recumbent position. Similarly, a self-report instrument about the impact of a disease or disorder on lower extremity function should contain items that address the performance of the entire leg (not just the ankle), but should not include questions about upper extremity function.

Content validity is challenging to determine because there is no external standard or statistical criterion against which an instrument can be judged. The usual method for establishing content validity is to assemble a group of experts whose knowledge is deemed to be extensive enough to identify all of the types of activities or items an instrument should represent. This exercise becomes more challenging when the test is trying to measure multiple concepts or constructs, as is often the case with measures of health status and disability. A more complex instrument requires greater effort to ensure that all of the relevant facets of a variable are represented appropriately.

Construct Validity

The *construct validity* of an instrument is determined based on the degree to which the measure reflects the operational definition of the *concept* or *construct* it is said to represent.[1] Construct validity differs from content validity in that the emphasis is on the definition itself, rather than on the universe of characteristics or items that may comprise the definition. For example, "strength," "balance," and "level of dependence" are concepts that physical therapists measure routinely in clinical practice, each of which has more than one definition. Strength may be defined as an ability to lift a certain amount of weight a given number of times or an ability to move in relation to gravity. Balance may be defined as remaining upright while holding a position in space (static) or while moving (dynamic). Level of dependence may be defined in relation to the amount of effort required of the patient or the amount of effort required of the therapist. In order to assess the construct validity of a measure of each of these concepts, the definition must be specified.

"Patient satisfaction" is an example of a construct that is a challenge to define. If the patient survey only asks questions about the clinical environment—such as how clean it is, how well privacy is maintained, and how well the equipment is maintained—then the instrument reflects only satisfaction with the context of care, not the care itself. This definition may be sufficient depending upon what clinicians or administrators want to know. On the other hand, if the survey also asks questions about the behaviors and competence of the clinical and support staff, then the instrument reflects a broader definition of the construct "patient satisfaction." This holistic representation presumably increases the usefulness of the instrument in a wider variety of scenarios.

The BOSS illustrated in Figure 7-3 is an example of an effort to define a construct—"stroke burden"—in a comprehensive fashion. Construct validity is a moving target because definitions evolve over time through repeated testing that changes peoples' understanding of the theoretical basis underlying the concept or construct of interest. This is particularly true for newer instruments, such as the BOSS, that have been evaluated to a limited degree.

Convergent Validity

One method with which to evaluate the construct validity of an instrument is to assess the relationship between scores on the instrument of interest and scores on another instrument that is said to measure the same concepts or constructs. If the scores from both instruments yield similar results then they are demonstrating *convergent validity*.

Discriminant Validity

Construct validation also may be performed through the assessment of an instrument's discriminant validity. *Discriminant validity* reflects the degree to which an instrument can distinguish between or among different concepts or constructs. For example, if the patient satisfaction survey is able to differentiate appropriately between environment of care and delivery of care, then it is demonstrating discriminant validity. This form of validity also refers to an instrument's ability to differentiate among individuals with different levels of a characteristic of interest such as disease severity, functional level, or degree of disability.

Criterion Validity

The *criterion validity* of an instrument reflects the degree to which its scores are related to scores obtained with a reference standard instrument. If the instrument is a diagnostic test, then the reference standard is a superior test whose validity has been established previously. A common example is a comparison between the results of a clinical examination technique to detect soft tissue damage and a radiographic technique, such as a magnetic resonance imaging (MRI) scan. The MRI is the superior test because of its ability to capture images of the potentially-affected tissues. By comparison, clinicians must infer damage based on what they see, hear, and feel from the body's exterior. The clinical examination technique will have high criterion validity if it produces the same results as the MRI.

Criterion validity also applies to self-report instruments. For example, newly developed health status instruments frequently are compared to the Medical Outcomes Trust Short-Form 36 instrument because the latter has been tested successfully with a wide variety of patient populations in different settings and different countries.[9] Whether the instrument is a diagnostic tool or a paper survey, the challenge in both cases is to have a reference standard available in the first place. The validity of the criterion measure is dependent upon whether it measures the same thing as the instrument of interest, produces reliable results, and whether there is minimal evidence of bias.[3]

Concurrent Validity

Concurrent validity is a method of evaluating criterion validity that involves administering the test of interest and reference standard test at nearly the same time. The goal is to capture the same behavior, characteristic, or perception with each instrument because the passage of time may result in natural change that confounds the results. Concurrent validity is of particular interest when researchers wish to use a test of interest that is believed to be more efficient and/or less risky than the criterion test. For example, the use of a validated noninvasive method for measuring blood pressure may be preferable because it can be implemented in any setting and avoids the need for placement of a catheter in a peripheral artery.[10] Concurrent validity also is relevant to self-report instruments, although there may be logistical challenges to performing this assessment if one or both of the questionnaires is lengthy. Subject responses may be influenced by fatigue or loss of interest if an extensive amount of time is required to complete both instruments.

Predictive Validity

Predictive validity is another method for evaluating criterion validity that reflects the degree to which the results from the test of interest can predict a future outcome, preferably measured by a reference standard. Establishing predictive validity often requires a sufficient amount of time to pass before the outcome develops. For example, Werneke and Hart examined the ability of the Quebec Task Force Classification and Pain Pattern Classification systems to predict pain and disability at intake and discharge from rehabilitation, as well as work status one year following discharge for patients with low back pain.[11] Similar efforts are at work when colleges and universities attempt to predict the academic success of applicants to their programs based on performance on standardized test scores.

RESPONSIVENESS TO CHANGE

Change is a central theme in physical therapy practice. Remediation of impairments, functional limitations, and disabilities depends upon change that may reflect natural recovery, response to interventions, or both. Change also is the focus of experimental and quasi-experimental research as investigators watch for any effects produced when they manipulate the independent variable. Therapists and investigators alike need instruments that are reliable and valid, but also that are able to detect change in the phenomenon of interest. "Change" may be defined simply as the smallest amount of difference the instrument can detect. This interpretation is value-free; in other words, there is no preference for the amount of the change in the definition.

Responsiveness to change is dependent upon 1) the fit between the instrument and the operational definition of the phenomenon of interest; 2) the number of values on the instrument scale; and 3) the standard error of measurement associated with the instrument.[1] The first requirement for a responsive instrument is construct validity—the measure should match the operational definition of the phenomenon of interest. For example, if joint position is the construct of interest then the appropriate instrument would be a goniometer, rather than a strain gauge. Similarly, disease-specific health-related quality of life surveys address the nuances of specific conditions that are not otherwise captured by more generic instruments. Second, the more values on the scale of the instrument the greater the opportunity to detect change when it occurs. For example, a tape measure marked in millimeters will be more responsive to change in the dimensions of a wound bed than a tape measure marked in quarter fractions of an inch. Finally, the *standard error of measurement* is the extent to which observed scores are disbursed around the "true" score. The statistical basis for this concept is explained in Chapter 9. From a practical perspective, however, it makes sense that an instrument with a large standard error of measurement will be less responsive to change because the "true" values are lost in the inaccuracies produced each time a measure is repeated.

Floor and Ceiling Effects

Responsiveness also depends on the range of the scale utilized. *Floor and ceiling effects* occur when the scale of the measure does not register a further decrease or increase in scores for the lowest or highest scoring individuals, respectively. These problems are only relevant in situations in which the variable of interest has further room for change in the first place. For example, a hypothetical disability index for patients with a progressive neurological disorder would demonstrate a floor effect if the lowest score on the scale reflected individuals who required limited assistance for mobility despite anticipated further decline in function over time. Similarly, a disability index for patients with a reversible disorder would demonstrate a ceiling effect if the highest score reflected individuals who were not completely recovered. Floor and ceiling effects can be avoided with a thorough operational definition of the phenomenon to be measured and careful construction of the measurement instrument.

INTERPRETING CHANGE

The ability of an instrument to detect change in a phenomenon is complemented by the assignment of meaning to this new state. An ability to walk an additional 25 feet may be immaterial if the individual is still standing in the middle of the room. On the other hand, if that same improvement allows the individual to get to the bathroom or the kitchen table independently then this change makes an impact! The ability of an instrument to detect meaningful change often is an essential criterion for its selection.[12] Whether meaning is derived from the physical therapist or the patient/client also should be considered.

SUMMARY

Variables are characteristics of individuals, objects, or environmental conditions that investigators use in their research designs to find answers to their questions. Independent variables are the characteristics that are manipulated in intervention studies and the predictors of interest in prognosis studies. Independent variables in outcomes studies represent the interventions of interest that usually are applied out of the control of the researchers. Dependent variables are the outcomes of interest. Extraneous variables represent those factors that may influence a study's outcomes apart from the influence of the independent variable(s).

In addition to identifying relevant variables for study, investigators must identify methods for their measurement. Measurement assigns values that range from purely descriptive to quantitative in nature. The most useful measurement instruments are those that produce stable results over repeated measures (reliability) and that capture the phenomenon they are designed to measure (validity). Reliability may be assessed in relation to the performance of the instrument as well as to the person taking the measurement. Validity most frequently is established by the degree to which scores on the instrument of interest are related to scores on other instruments. Finally, a responsive instrument is one that detects change in the phenomenon of interest.

Exercises

1. Use your electronic database skills to locate an experimental or quasi-experimental study about a physical therapy intervention.
   a. Identify the independent and dependent variables in the study. Discuss the difference between the two types of variables.
   b. Identify 2–3 actual or potential extraneous variables in the study. Why are these variables problematic for the study's results?
   c. Identify the number of levels and their definition for each independent variable in the study.
2. Give one example each of a discrete and continuous variable.
3. Describe the differences between nominal, ordinal, interval, and ratio levels of measurement. Classify the type(s) of measurement(s) used for the outcome variable(s) in the study in Question #1.
4. Define measurement error and discuss its implications with respect to the usefulness of a study's results.
5. Discuss the difference between intra-rater and inter-rater reliability. What is the potential impact on a study's findings if rater reliability is not demonstrated?

6. Describe one method for establishing the reliability of self-report instruments.
7. Differentiate between the content and construct validity of an instrument.
8. Discuss two reasons why an instrument may not be sensitive to change. Provide a potential solution to each barrier identified.

REFERENCES

1. Domholdt E. *Rehabilitation Research: Principles and Applications.* 3d ed. St Louis, MO: Elsevier Saunders; 2005.
2. Polit DF, Beck CT. *Nursing Research: Principles and Methods.* 7th ed. Philadelphia, PA: Lippincott Williams & Wilkins; 2003.
3. Portney LG, Watkins MP. *Foundations of Clinical Research: Applications to Practice.* 2d ed. Upper Saddle River, NJ; Prentice Hall Health; 2000.
4. Seynnes O, Singh MAF, Hue O, Pras P, Legros P *et al.* Physiological and functional response to low-moderate versus high-intensity progressive resistance training in frail elders. *J Gerontol Biol Sci Med Sci.* 2004; 59(5):503–509.
5. Bower E, Michell D, Burnett M, Campbell MJ, McLellan DL. Randomized controlled trial of physiotherapy in 56 children with cerebral palsy followed for 18 months. *Dev Med Child Neurol.* 2001; 43(1):4–15.
6. Hulzebos EHJ, van Meeteren NLU, de Bie RA, Dagnelie PC, Helders PJM. Prediction of postoperative pulmonary complications on the basis of preoperative risk factors in patients who had undergone coronary artery bypass graft surgery. *Phys Ther.* 2003; 83(1):8–16.
7. *Overview of the CDC Growth Charts.* Centers for Disease Control and Prevention Web site. Available at: http://www.cdc.gov/nccdphp/dnpa/growthcharts/training/modules/module2/text/module2print.pdf. Accessed March 18, 2006.
8. Doyle PJ, McNeil MR, Mikolic JM, Prieto L, Hula WD *et al.* The Burden of Stroke Scale (BOSS) provides reliable and valid score estimates of functioning and well-being in stroke survivors with and without communication disorders. *J Clin Epidemiol.* 2004; 57(10):997–1007.
9. Short Form 36(v2). Medical Outcomes Trust. Available at: http://www.sf-36.org/tools/SF36.shtml#VERS2. Accessed March 18, 2006.
10. Brinton TJ, Cotter B, Kailisam MT, Brown DL, Chio SS *et al.* Development and validation of a noninvasive method to determine arterial pressure and vascular compliance. *Am J Cardiol.* 1997; 80(3):323–330.
11. Werneke MW, Hart DL. Categorizing patients with occupational low back pain by use of the Quebec Task Force Classification system versus pain pattern classification procedures: Discriminant and predictive validity. *Phys Ther.* 2004; 84(3):243–254.
12. Beaton DE, Bombardier C, Katz JN, Wright JG. A taxonomy for responsiveness. *J Clin Epidemiol.* 2001; 54(12):1204–1271.

Chapter 8

Research Validity

If we knew what we were doing, it would not be called research, would it?

—Albert Einstein

OBJECTIVES

Upon completion of this chapter the student/practitioner will be able to:

1. Discuss the concept of research validity of a study.
2. Discuss the general consequences of weak research validity of a study.
3. Recognize and discuss the consequences of the following threats to research validity in studies about interventions:
   a) Assignment
   b) Attrition
   c) History
   d) Instrumentation
   e) Maturation
   f) Testing
   g) Compensatory equalization of treatment
   h) Compensatory rivalry or resentful demoralization
   i) Diffusion or imitation of treatment, and
   j) Statistical regression to the mean.
4. Describe potential solutions researchers may apply to minimize threats to research validity in a study about interventions.
5. Discuss the relevance of threats to research validity for studies about diagnosis, prognosis, and outcomes.
6. Define the term "construct validity" and discuss its relevance and implications for studies.
7. Recognize and discuss the consequences of threats to the applicability of a study and describe potential solutions researchers may use to minimize these threats.

TERMS IN THIS CHAPTER

Assignment (Allocation): The process by which subjects are placed into two or more groups in a study; inadequate assignment procedures may threaten research validity (internal validity) by producing groups that are different from one another at the start of the study.

Attrition (also referred to as Drop Out or Mortality): A term that refers to subjects who stop participation in a study for any reason; loss of subjects may threaten research validity (internal validity) by reducing the sample size and producing unequal groups.

Bias: Results or inferences that systematically deviate from the truth "or the processes leading to such deviation."[1(p. 251)]

Compensatory Equalization of Treatments: A threat to research validity (internal validity) characterized by the purposeful or inadvertent provision of additional encouragement or practice to subjects in the control (comparison) group in recognition that they are not receiving the experimental intervention.

Compensatory Rivalry: A threat to research validity (internal validity) characterized by subjects in the control (comparison) group who, in response to knowledge about group assignment, change their behavior in an effort to achieve the same benefit as subjects in the experimental group.

Construct Validity: The degree to which a measure matches the operational definition of the concept or construct it is said to represent.[2]

Construct Underrepresentation: A threat to construct validity characterized by measures that do not fully define the variable or construct of interest.

Diffusion (Imitation) of Treatments: A threat to research validity (internal validity) characterized by a change in subject behavior that may occur as a result of communication among members of different study groups.

External Validity: The degree to which research results may be applied to other individuals and circumstances outside of a study.[2]

History: A threat to research validity (internal validity) characterized by events that occur during a study that are unrelated to the project, but may influence its results.

Instrumentation: A threat to research validity (internal validity) characterized by problems with the tools used to collect data that may influence the study's outcomes.

Internal Validity: In experimental and quasi-experimental research designs, the degree to which a change in the outcome can be attributed to the experimental intervention rather than to extraneous factors.[3]

Masking (Blinding): Prevention of knowledge about the groups to which subjects have been assigned.

Maturation: A threat to research validity (internal validity) characterized by the natural processes of change that occur over time in humans that may influence a study's results independent of any other factors.

Research Validity: "The degree to which a study appropriately answers the question being asked."[4(p. 225)]

Resentful Demoralization: A threat to research validity (internal validity) characterized by subjects in the control (comparison) group who, in response to knowledge about group assignment, limit their efforts in the study.

Statistical Regression to the Mean: A threat to research validity (internal validity) that may occur when subjects produce an extreme value on a single test administration;[2] mathematically the next test scores for these individuals mostly will move toward the mean value for the measure.

Testing: A threat to research validity (internal validity) characterized by a subject's change in performance due to growing familiarity with the testing or measurement procedure or to inconsistent implementation of the procedures by study personnel.

INTRODUCTION

Chapter 5 discusses a variety of research designs used to answer questions about diagnosis, prognosis, interventions, and outcomes. These designs have strengths and limitations that affect the extent to which the answers obtained in a study can be believed. "Believability" in research traditionally is referred to as *internal validity*; however, this term is defined specifically with reference to experimental and quasi-experimental designs that are used to study the efficacy or effectiveness of interventions. As a result, it is difficult to apply this concept to other types of research designs.[5] For the purposes of this text, the more general term *research validity* will be used to characterize the extent to which a study of any type produces truthful results.[4]

A number of factors may threaten a project's research validity. Investigators should anticipate and address through their research plan, the issues that may undermine the study's value. Furthermore, physical therapists reviewing evidence should make their own assessment about the degree to which research validity is supported by a study's design. This appraisal is a fundamental step in evidence-based physical therapy practice because weak research validity may suggest that a study's results cannot be trusted.

In addition to evaluating the accuracy of a study's results, therapists must also determine whether these findings are relevant to their patient/client. Relevance is established when the study includes subjects and circumstances that are similar to the therapist's patients/clients and clinical context. A study's relevance traditionally is referred to by the term *external validity*; however, "applicability" and "generalizability" are synonyms that are used routinely as well.

This chapter discusses factors that threaten a study's research validity, as well as potential design solutions investigators may apply to minimize the impact of these problems. The use of statistical adjustment to address some threats also is addressed. The chapter concludes with a brief discussion of potential threats to the external validity of a study.

RESEARCH VALIDITY

Research validity relates to the truthfulness, or accuracy, of a study's results and is determined based upon how well the research design elements a) focus on what the investigator wants to know; and, b) prevent unwanted influences from contaminating the study's outcomes. A quick way to evaluate the research validity of a study is to ask the following question:

- Can a "competing" (alternative) explanation for this study's results be identified?[3]

If the answer is "no," then it may be possible to conclude that the study has strong research validity. This conclusion should be verified by reviewing the research design elements in more detail to confirm that they are sufficient to achieve objectives (a) and (b) above. If the answer is "yes," however, then these follow-up questions should be asked:

- What are the specific problems with the research design elements?
- What unwanted influences are introduced into the study as a result of these design problems?
- What alternative explanation(s) of the study's results are possible due to the introduction of these unwanted influences?

The answers to these questions will help determine whether the research validity of the study has been so compromised that a physical therapist cannot (or will not) use this piece of evidence in his or her patient/client management process.

Threats to Research Validity

The design problems that introduce unwanted influences into a study are referred to collectively as "threats to research validity." There are a variety of ways in which a research design can be undermined. For evidence-based physical therapists the hope is that these threats have been anticipated by the investigator and addressed in such a way as to minimize their impact (keeping in mind of course that there is no such thing as a perfect research design!). The following sections of this chapter discuss the types of threats and potential solutions to avoid or minimize them, for which evidence-based practitioners should be watchful. Most of these threats are relevant only in intervention studies. Threats that also pertain to diagnosis, prognosis, and outcomes studies will be noted in a separate section along with possible solutions to minimize them.

THREATS TO RESEARCH VALIDITY OF INTERVENTION STUDIES

Imagine a study that is investigating the relative effectiveness of task-specific functional training versus a neurodevelopmental treatment (NDT)[6] approach for normalization of gait patterns in children with a form of cerebral palsy referred to as spastic paraplegia. Children with spastic paraplegia have excessive muscle tone in their lower extremities, but normal motor tone in their upper extremities.[7] There are four possible outcomes of this hypothetical study:

1. The two techniques are equally effective;
2. The functional training approach is more effective than the NDT approach;
3. The NDT approach is more effective than the functional training approach; or,
4. Neither approach improves the subjects' gait patterns.

No matter which answer is identified, a physical therapist reading this study should think about whether any of the following factors interfered with its accuracy.

Threat #1: Assignment

The Problem

Assignment is a threat to research validity that occurs when the process of placing subjects into groups results in differences in baseline characteristics between (or among) the groups at the outset of a study. Characteristics commonly of interest in clinical studies include: subject age, gender, ethnic and racial background, education level, duration and severity of the clinical problem(s), presence of comorbidities, medication regimen, current functional status, and current activity habits, among others. In the gait study it is possible to envision that children might be different in their age, gender, number and effect of other disease processes, current motor control abilities, and severity of spasticity. If the group allocation process is successful, then these characteristics will be distributed equally between the functional training group and the NDT group before either intervention is applied.

At a minimum, authors will provide descriptive statistics about the relevant characteristics of each group. A more sophisticated approach is to test statistically for differences in these descriptive characteristics. Whether differences are identified by visual inspection of descriptive data or by statistical inference, the concern is the same: if the groups are unequal before the functional training and NDT is provided, then the investigators will have difficulty attributing any change to the intervention of interest. In other words, the study's outcome may be due to baseline differences between groups rather than to either treatment approach.

Study Design Solutions

The most important solution to the assignment problem is to use a randomization technique to put the subjects into groups. As discussed in Chapter 6, randomization techniques help to distribute characteristics and influences equally to avoid extraneous influences created by the presence of imbalances between or among study groups. When randomization is not possible, then statistical adjustment for baseline differences should be implemented.

Threat #2: Attrition

The Problem

Attrition (also referred to as "drop out" or "mortality") refers to the loss of subjects during the course of a study. Subjects may leave a study for any number of reasons including: recurrent illness, injury, death, job or family demands, progressive loss of interest in study participation, or a change of mind about the value of participating in the first place. In the gait study, children may withdraw because of competing school demands, boredom or frustration, a change in a parent's availability to bring them to the treatment session, and so on. When subjects withdraw from a study they reduce the sample size and, in the case of multiple groups, introduce the possibility of group inequality in terms of relevant characteristics. The reduction in sample size has implications for statistical analysis because of mathematical assumptions about the number and distribution of data points in a sample. The group inequality issue is the same as described when assignment is a threat.

Study Design Solutions

In well-funded studies with the necessary administrative infrastructure and the availability of more study candidates, replacement of lost subjects may be possible. Absent that opportunity, investigators should at least document the characteristics and reasons for withdrawal of the subjects lost. A comparison of characteristics between the lost and remaining subjects might reveal that they were similar (a desirable result) or that they were somehow different and are now not represented in the sample (a less desirable result). In addition, a reexamination of the remaining groups would be warranted to determine if they are now, in fact, different from each other. Investigators should not arbitrarily remove subjects to equalize the numbers between groups because this step introduces additional bias into the study. Statistical estimation of missing data is another strategy that may be used. Finally, an "intention-to-treat" analysis may be performed in cases when it is possible to collect outcomes data on study dropouts. Both of these techniques are discussed in more detail in Chapter 12.

Threat #3: History

The Problem

History refers to events that occur outside of an intervention study that are out of the investigators' control. This threat can be remembered with the phrase "life goes on." In other words, the events and activities of daily life proceed whether or not a research project is underway, thereby producing extraneous influences that may interfere with the study. The opportunity for a history effect to occur grows as the length of time between measures of the outcome increases. For example, children in the functional training versus NDT study may have changes in their physical education activities over the course of a school year that may enhance or diminish their ambulatory abilities during the study. If the investigators cannot control the timing of the study to avoid this natural alteration in a child's school agenda, then they will have to find another way to deal with this situation. Otherwise, any differences (or lack thereof) in gait performance noted might be attributed to changes in the schedule rather than to the interventions provided during the study.

Study Design Solutions

Investigators have a couple of design options to deal with the threat of history to their study. First, they might use a control or comparison group in addition to their treatment group and then randomly assign subjects to each. Random assignment should distribute subjects most susceptible to "history threats" equally between the groups, thereby minimizing the influence of any changes as a result of the events occurring outside of the study. This would be a workable solution in the gait study as it already has two groups in its design.

Second, the investigators can try to schedule the study to avoid a predictable external event altogether. In this example, the researchers might contact the schools attended by their subjects and inquire as to the nature and timing of their physical education activities. The information provided by the schools may allow the investigators to organize the intervention and data collection timetable in such a way as to miss the changes in activity that are planned for physical education over the course of the school year.

Threat #4: Instrumentation

The Problem

The research validity of an intervention study may be challenged by problems with the tools used to measure the variable(s) of interest. Examples of *instrumentation* problems include selection of the wrong measurement approach or device, inherent limitations in the measurement, malfunction of the device, and inaccurate application of the device. For example, gait analysis of children with spastic paraplegia might be performed through visual inspection by the physical therapist (less accurate) or it might be performed by progressively sophisticated technological means including a video and computer (more accurate). In the former case, the potential for inaccuracy rests in the normal variability that is part of all human activity. What one physical therapist sees in terms of a child's ability may not be what another therapist sees. On the other hand, use of technology requires an understanding of how to use it properly and how to calibrate it (if possible) in order to ensure that the measures are reliable and valid. There also is a possibility for equipment malfunction (sometimes in subtle ways) that are not detected immediately by the researcher. Finally, instruments that are applied incorrectly may produce inaccurate measures. As a result of these issues, improvement of gait patterns may be an artifact of measurement rather than a true change in the subjects.

Study Design Solutions

First and foremost, investigators should consider carefully what it is they want to measure and the techniques available to do so. As discussed in Chapter 7, reliability, validity, responsiveness, and other important measurement properties, (e.g., floor and ceiling effects) should be evaluated with an effort toward obtaining the most useful device or technique known.

Any technological equipment should be calibrated against a known measure prior to use in the study. Similarly, the authors should describe an orientation and training process during which individuals collecting data for the study learned and demonstrated the proper use of the measurement device (technique). Protocols for collection of measures also should be implemented. Statistical comparisons of their results may be offered to demonstrate stability of these measures within and across raters. Finally, the conditions under which the measurements are taken (e.g., temperature, humidity) should be maintained at a constant level throughout the study if possible.

Threat #5: Maturation

The Problem

Whereas history considers events external to the study, *maturation* refers to changes over time that are internal to the subjects. A person's physical, psychological, emotional, and spiritual status progresses and declines as a result of, or in spite of, the events in the "outside world." These changes are reflected by age, growth, increased experience and familiarity with a particular subject or skill, healing, development of new interests and different motivations, and so on. Any of these situations may alter subjects' performance in a study and thereby introduce a competing explanation for the study's results. In other words, the results might indicate a change due to the variable of interest when in fact the change was due to maturation of the subjects. The length of time between measures will increase the possibility of a maturation effect occurring.

The children with spastic paraplegia certainly will be changing as a result of their natural growth process. How that growth affects their muscle length and tone, their coordination, their understanding of the interventions applied to them, and so on, may influence their ability and desire to improve their gait patterns. If the investigators cannot account for the reality of the children's growth, how can they conclude which, if either, intervention facilitated the subjects' normalization of gait?

The timing of events in a study also may result in maturation effects. Subjects may have a greater or lesser ability to perform a study-related task based on when the task is scheduled and/or how frequently it is performed. For example, fatigue may play a role in performance in children who receive their functional training followed by gait assessment later in the day as compared to children who participate earlier in the day. Similarly, if the study requires repeated measures of gait, then performance may decline over time as children lose energy (or interest). Finally, subject familiarity with the study's procedures is a form of maturation that may influence the results. Children who practice standing activities at the end of every session may feel more relaxed and comfortable walking than children who work on trunk control in sitting prior to the gait activity.

Study Design Solutions

As with the history threat, investigators may randomly assign subjects to a treatment and a control (comparison) group in order to equally distribute the effects of subjects' natural change over time, such that their impact is washed out. In this example, children would be assigned randomly to the functional training and NDT groups. In addition, the investigators may take several baseline measures of each subject's performance (e.g., gait) before starting the experiment. Baseline measures that are similar to one another would suggest that maturation is not occurring. Finally, investigators can reduce problems related to the timing and sequencing of interventions through a protocol designed to ensure that:

- The time of day for study participation is consistent;
- Adequate rest is provided in between repeated measures;
- Specific intervention techniques are provided in random order to avoid the practice or familiarity effect.

Threat #6: Testing

The Problem

Testing can threaten a study's research validity because subjects may appear to demonstrate improvement based upon their growing familiarity with the testing procedure or based upon different instructions and cues provided by the person administering the test. For example, children in the gait study may demonstrate improvement because of practice with the gait assessment process rather than because of the functional training or NDT. Similarly, investigators who encourage some children during their test, but not others (e.g., "Come on, you can walk a little farther") may introduce the potential for performance differences due to extraneous influences rather than the interventions.

Study Design Solutions

In studies in which increasing experience with the testing procedures is the concern, investigators may give the subjects several practice sessions with a particular test or measure before collecting actual data, on the assumption that subjects' skill level will plateau. This leveling off would eliminate the practice effect once the actual data collection started. Alternatively, the authors might average the scores of multiple measures from one testing session in order to reduce the effect of changing skill level through a mathematical aggregation technique. To avoid introducing unwanted influences during the testing procedure itself, the investigators should describe a clearly articulated protocol for administering the test, including a script for instructions or coaching if indicated. Finally, competence performing the test to specification also should be verified in all test administrators prior to the start of the actual data collection.

Threat #7: Compensatory Equalization of Treatments

The Problem

Compensatory equalization of treatments occurs when the individuals providing the interventions in the study purposefully or inadvertently supplement the activities of subjects in the control (comparison) group in order to "make up for" what subjects in the experimental group are receiving. The potential for this situation may be stronger in studies in which multiple physical therapists are providing treatments outside the supervision of the investigator. In their quest to do the best for their patients, these therapists may feel compelled to work them a little harder, give them extra opportunities to practice, provide more encouragement, and so on. This extra effort by the physical therapists may dilute the differences in performance attributable to the intervention of interest. Put in the context of the gait study, children in the functional training group may walk just as well as children in the NDT group because the physical therapists provided additional training opportunities to the children who were performing task-specific skills.

Study Design Solutions

The most direct method for dealing with compensatory equalization of treatments is to *mask* (or "*blind*") the investigator(s) or the therapist(s) such that they do not know what the interventions are in each group. This is a standard approach in drug trials, but often is not practical in studies of physical therapy interventions. In the gait study it will not be possible to "disguise" the treatments so that therapists do not know if they are providing task-specific training or NDT. A second step is to provide a clear and explicit protocol for intervention administration, including a script for instructions if indicated. A third step is to ensure that communication about the interventions between investigators or therapists is minimized or eliminated. In effect, the physical therapists in the gait study would know simply that they are to perform NDT techniques or task-specific skills according to the protocol provided to them. The details of the other intervention would be unavailable. If enough therapists in different clinics are involved in the study, then it may be possible to avoid cross contamination by keeping children receiving NDT treatment in one clinic and children receiving functional training in another.

Threat #8: Compensatory Rivalry or Resentful Demoralization

The Problem

If communication among study participants is not tightly controlled, then subjects may acquire knowledge about the different groups' activities. If members of the control (comparison) group learn details about the interventions in the experimental group, and if they perceive that these interventions are significantly better than what they are receiving, then these subjects may react in one of two ways:

1. *Compensatory rivalry,* or the "we'll show them" attitude; or,
2. *Resentful demoralization,* or the "we're getting the short end of the stick so why bother" attitude.[2(p. 96)]

In both cases, the control (comparison) group's knowledge about the experimental group results in an alteration in behavior such that potential differences due to the intervention might be diminished (rivalry), eliminated, or inflated (demoralization). Consider the children in the gait study. If they all attend the same school or special education class then they will have natural opportunities to interact with one another. A perception of inequality among members of one or the other group may trigger one of the responses described, thereby resulting in a change in behavior or effort by children in one of the groups.

Study Design Solutions

One method by which investigators may avoid compensatory rivalry or resentful demoralization is to keep the subjects in each group separated such that communication is not possible. A second method is to mask the subjects and the investigators so that they do not know to which group the subjects belong. A third option is to provide thorough, explicit instruction to subjects (or their caregivers) about the importance of adhering to their current routine or regimen by not adding or changing anything. In the case of the gait study the first two options may be difficult, if not impossible to achieve. As noted above, it is hard to disguise or hide the treatment in the traditional way that a placebo is created. Children going to the same school or class are bound to interact. The most reasonable alternative would be to approach parents, teachers, and the children themselves, about the need to avoid changes in behavior during the study.

Threat #9: Diffusion or Imitation of Treatment

The Problem

Diffusion or *imitation of treatment* may occur when subjects in different groups have contact with one another during the study. Either purposefully or unintentionally, these individuals may share aspects of the treatment in their group that prompts changes in behaviors by members in a different group. If the children in the functional training group describe the tasks they perform as part of their treatment, then children in the NDT group might start performing these same tasks at home in an effort to copy or try out these alternative activities. If this situation occurs, it will be difficult to attribute any changes to the NDT approach.

Study Design Solutions

The solutions for diffusion of treatment are the same as those applied to compensatory rivalry and resentful demoralization.

Threat #10: Statistical Regression to the Mean

The Problem

Statistical regression to the mean occurs when subjects enter a study with an extreme value for their baseline measure of the outcome of interest. For example, a few children in the gait study may have a crouched gait pattern comprised of hip and knee flexion in excess of 100 degrees when compared to the majority of children in the sample whose flexion at the same joints exceeds normal by only 10–25 degrees. As a result, the children with the crouched gait pattern may show improvement simply because a second measure of their hip and knee position is likely to show decreased flexion. This situation will cloud the true effects, if any, of the interventions.

Study Design Solutions

Investigators have two options to help avoid statistical regression to the mean. Option one is to eliminate outliers from the baseline scores so that the sample is limited to a distribution that is closer to the mean (i.e., within one standard deviation). The second option is to take repeated baseline measures and average them to reduce the extremes through the aggregation process. This solution is preferable when small samples must have their size and composition preserved.

Table 8–1 summarizes the threats to research validity, along with possible remedies, for studies about interventions physical therapists use.

Table 8–1 Threats to research validity of intervention studies and possible solutions.

Threat	Nature of Threat	Possible Solutions
Assignment	• Unequal baseline characteristics of groups that might influence the study's outcome	• Adequately defined inclusion and exclusion criteria • Random assignment to groups • Statistical adjustment
Attrition	• Loss of subjects resulting in reduction of sample size and/or inequality of group baseline characteristics	• Replacement, if appropriate and feasible • Statistical adjustment
History	• Events occurring outside the study that influence the study's outcome	• Random assignment to groups • Timing of study to avoid the event(s) • Statistical adjustment
Instrumentation	• Inappropriate selection, application, or function of techniques or instruments, used to collect data in a study	• Select appropriate technique or instrument • User training and practice • Specific protocols for use by testers • Instrument calibration
Maturation	• Natural change in human behavior or function over the course of time that may influence the study's outcome	• Random assignment to groups • Time the study to minimize the effect • Randomize testing or treatment order • Statistical adjustment
Testing	• Change in the outcome that occurs as a result of a subject's increased familiarity with the testing procedure, or as a result of inappropriate cues provided by the tester	• Provide subjects with practice sessions • Specific protocols, including scripts, for use by testers
Compensatory Equalization of Treatments	• Purposeful or inadvertent supplementation of the control or comparison group's activities that influences these subjects' performance	• Mask the investigators to prevent knowledge of group assignment • Ask all study participants to avoid discussing their activities to anyone
Compensatory Rivalry or Resentful Demoralization	• Changes in behavior that occur as a result of subjects learning they are members of the control or comparison group	• Mask the subjects to prevent knowledge of group assignment • Mask the investigators to group assignment • Keep subjects separated • Ask all study participants to avoid discussing their study activities with anyone

Table 8-1 Threats to research validity of intervention studies and possible solutions *(continued)*.

Threat	Nature of Threat	Possible Solutions
Diffusion of Treatments	• Changes in behavior that occur in the control or comparison group as a result of communication with subjects in the experimental group	• Mask the subjects to prevent knowledge of group assignment • Keep subjects separated • Ask all study participants to avoid discussing their study activities with anyone
Statistical Regression to the Mean	• Subjects who start the study with extreme scores for the outcome measure change as a result of the mathematical tendency for scores to move toward the mean value	• Trim extreme data values from the study • Aggregate repeated baseline measures

THREATS TO RESEARCH VALIDITY IN DIAGNOSIS, PROGNOSIS, AND OUTCOMES STUDIES

Many of the threats to research validity described above, as well as their potential solutions, are relevant only to intervention studies. Assignment, diffusion or imitation of treatment, compensatory rivalry, resentful demoralization, and compensatory equalization of treatments, do not apply to diagnosis, prognosis, or outcomes studies, either because there is only one group in the study or because purposeful manipulation of one group differently from another group does not occur.

On the other hand, attrition is a concern in any study because loss of subjects reduces the sample size and may interfere with statistical analyses of the data. In addition, if groups are present in prognosis or outcomes studies, then attrition may exaggerate a preexisting imbalance in the distribution of subject characteristics. Similarly, instrumentation as a threat is applicable to any type of study because it refers to the devices and methods used to collect data. Inadequacies in a measurement device or technique will produce inaccurate information. Instrumentation problems can undermine completely the usefulness of a study about diagnostic tests or measures. History and maturation are time-related threats that may be at work in prospective studies about prognosis and outcomes; however, these problems are unlikely to be relevant in cross-sectional diagnosis studies unless there is a significant delay between administration of the clinical test of interest and the reference standard test used to confirm the diagnosis. Testing threats, on the other hand, will have greatest relevance to diagnosis and outcomes studies because the issue is change in subject performance based upon familiarity with the testing

Table 8–2 Threats to research validity of diagnosis, prognosis, and outcomes studies and possible solutions.

Threat	Present (+)/Absent (−)
Assignment	−
Attrition	+
History	+
Instrumentation	+
Maturation	+
Testing	+
Compensatory Equalization of Treatments	−
Compensatory Rivalry or Resentful Demoralization	−
Diffusion of Treatments	−
Statistical Regression to the Mean	+

procedure. Finally, selection of subjects with extreme values (e.g., "too healthy" or "too sick") may produce a skewed representation of the usefulness of a diagnostic test, prognostic factor, intervention, or outcome.

Strategies to minimize the threats to research validity in diagnosis, prognosis, and outcomes studies include:

- Obtaining a sufficient sample size to minimize the effects of attrition should it occur;
- Timing the study to avoid or minimize history or maturation effects;
- Implementing clear protocols for testing and measurement of subjects;
- Defining inclusion and exclusion criteria to obtain as representative a sample as possible, given the lack of a random selection process.

Table 8–2 summarizes threats to research validity of intervention studies that are relevant to diagnosis, prognosis, and outcomes projects.

THE ROLE OF INVESTIGATOR BIAS

Assignment, instrumentation, testing, and compensatory equalization of treatment are threats that reflect the potential role of investigator *bias* in a study. Investigator bias results when investigators purposefully or inadvertently design, or interfere with, the study's procedures such that the results systematically deviate from the truth. Two additional sources of investigator bias in intervention studies relate to knowledge of subject status in the study. First, individuals responsible for enrolling subjects may respond to additional information by placing (or allocating) subjects into groups rather than following the preestablished assignment protocol. This purposeful interference undermines the benefits achieved from a randomization process and adds to the threat of "assignment." Second, individuals responsible for application of tests and measures may produce inaccurate results due to their knowledge of subjects' group assignment or prior test results, or both. Prior knowledge of subject status may produce an expectation for a particular result that influences investigator interpretation of the measurement they are taking, a situation that adds to the "testing" threat to research validity. In both instances, the strategy to minimize these threats is to conceal the information from the study personnel so that they are not tempted to respond to, or influenced by, knowledge about the subjects.

Investigator bias also may threaten the validity of studies about diagnosis, prognosis, and outcomes. For example, bias may be introduced into any study if the investigators specify selection criteria that result in subjects that are defined too narrowly relative to the question of interest. Issues with subject testing with the reference standard are another potential source of investigator bias in diagnosis studies. First, investigators evaluating the usefulness of a diagnostic test may decide to apply a superior comparison test only to subjects who have a positive finding on the test of interest. As a result, the actual diagnosis cannot be verified in subjects who tested negative, a situation that may overestimate the usefulness of the test of interest. Second, investigators (or participating clinicians) may have prior knowledge of the results of the test of interest that influences their interpretation of the comparison test (or vice versa). For example, knowledge of a positive test result may prompt the investigator to "look for" confirmation in the second test. Bias due to investigator knowledge about test results also applies to prognosis and outcomes studies because of the potential to "see" the desired outcome, if it is known by the person taking the measure. Table 8-3 summarizes threats related to investigator bias, as well as possible design solutions, in all studies.

ADDITIONAL SOLUTIONS TO RESEARCH VALIDITY THREATS

When investigators do not have a study design solution available to them to protect against threats to research validity, they do have two alternatives. First, they can statistically compensate for the threats through the use of control variables in their analyses. For example, "time" might be used as the control variable to reduce the effects of history or maturation. Problems with testing and instrumentation might be addressed by adding

Table 8–3 Threats to research validity from investigator bias.

Threat	Type of Study Affected	Nature of Threat	Possible Solutions
Allocation	• Intervention	• Individuals responsible for enrolling subjects interfere with group assignment process • May create unbalanced groups prior to the start of the study	• Create predetermined subject assignment list and conceal information about subject allocation
Selection	• Diagnosis	• Use of subjects that do not represent the population of interest defined by the research question • Limits the ability to determine how well diagnostic test differentiates between or among different stages of the disorder of interest	• Adequately defined inclusion and exclusion criteria to create a sample that represents the spectrum of the disorder of interest
Selection	• Prognosis	• Use of subjects that are "too healthy" or "too sick" • May result in misrepresentation of timetable to recovery or adverse outcome, thereby undermining the usefulness of a prognostic factor(s)	• Enroll subjects at a common early point in their condition
Selection	• Interventions • Outcomes	• Use of subjects that do not represent the population of interest defined by the research question • Limits ability to determine usefulness of intervention for individuals with different levels of condition and/or different prognostic profiles	• Adequately defined inclusion and exclusion criteria to create a sample that represents the spectrum of the condition of interest
Testing	• Diagnosis	• Investigators apply the superior comparison test to subjects who test positive on the diagnostic test of interest	• Apply the superior comparison test to all subjects regardless of result of diagnostic test of interest

Table 8–3 Threats to research validity from investigator bias *(continued)*.

Threat	Type of Study Affected	Nature of Threat	Possible Solutions
		• May overestimate the usefulness of the diagnostic test	
Testing	• Diagnosis • Prognosis • Interventions • Outcomes	• Individuals responsible for measurement of subjects are influenced in their interpretation by knowledge of current subject status or prior test results • May produce inaccurate results due to investigator expectations	• Conceal information about subject status or prior test results from individuals collecting measures

control variables, such as the people administering the test or using the instrument. When groups differ at the outset of a study, then specific subject characteristics, such as age or baseline functional status, might be used as control factors. An alternative statistical method to address unbalanced groups—the "intention to treat analysis"—is discussed in Chapter 12. The point is that there may be a mathematical way to isolate the effects of these unwanted influences so that the investigators can more accurately determine the contribution of their intervention or other variable(s) of interest.

Second, the investigators can simply acknowledge that threats to research validity were present and need to be recognized as a limitation to the study. Reasons for the inability to control these issues at the outset of the study usually are presented in order for the reader to understand the logistical challenges the researchers faced and to help future investigators avoid similar problems.

THREATS TO CONSTRUCT VALIDITY

The "believability" of research results also depends upon a clear and adequate definition of the variables used in the study. "The meaning of variables within a study" is characterized by the term *construct validity*.[2(p. 96)] An evidence-based physical therapist assesses the integrity of construct validity by comparing the variable(s) with their measures to determine if the latter truly represent the former. For example, investigators may wish to examine the relationship between patients' socioeconomic status and their attendance in outpatient physical therapy. The researchers must decide how to measure the variable "socioeconomic status" in order to determine a result through statistical analysis. There are several options from which to choose in this example including, but not limited to, a patient's:

- Salary;
- Assets (e.g., home, car);
- Investments; and
- Family income.

All of these measures have a monetary basis that is consistent with the word "socioeconomic." To enhance the construct validity of their study, researchers may select one or more of these measures to define this variable.

There are frequent occasions when the measure desired for a particular variable is not available to the researchers. Study design problems also may result in threats to construct validity of an independent, dependent, or control variable. One construct validity threat is the lack of sufficient definition of the variable, also referred to as *construct underrepresentation*. For example, a study of patient satisfaction with physical therapy may involve questions that ask patients for their perceptions about their experience. If the questions only focus on issues related to making appointments, then an argument could be made that "satisfaction with physical therapy" was not completely addressed. Instead, the variable measured was satisfaction with the appointment-making process.

Another threat to construct validity occurs when subjects change their behavior in response to the perceived or actual expectations of the investigators; this is referred to by Domholdt as "experimenter expectancies."[2(p. 96)] In this situation, subjects respond to what they anticipate the investigator wants (also known as the "Hawthorne effect")[3] or to subtle cues provided by the investigator as they perform a test or measure. Consider a hypothetical study in which the method of instruction is being evaluated for its effectiveness in teaching the safest way to rise from a chair to patients following total hip replacement. Left to their own devices, some subjects may try to rise from the chair by increasing their hip flexion beyond the prescribed 60-degree limit, while others would comply with the motion restriction. If the investigator frowns as subjects start to lean forward, then the subjects may modify their movement in response to this facial cue, especially if the investigator then smiles as a result of the correction. The variable "safest way to rise from a chair" is now being measured as "patient's response to investigator cues when rising from a chair," a situation that undermines the construct validity of the variable.

Additional threats to construct validity occur when there are interactions between multiple treatments or when testing itself becomes a treatment. In the former case, independent variables initially defined as one treatment may in actuality reflect a combination of treatments that study subjects undergo. For example, a study looking at the effects of oral vitamin supplementation on aerobic exercise capacity may experience a construct validity problem if additional vitamins are obtained through subtle changes in diet not recognized by the subjects or the investigator. In the latter case, a study examining the effects of several stretching techniques on hamstring flexibility may experience a construct validity threat because the process of measuring the knee or hip range of motion also produces a stretching effect on the muscle group of interest.

Avoidance of construct validity problems starts with providing clearly stated operational definitions of all variables in the study. To the degree it is feasible, investigators should then select measures that are direct representations of these variables. In addition, masking investigators who are collecting measurements so as to minimize the effect of cues, as well as clearly differentiating and documenting treatments, are design steps to be considered. If all else fails, researchers should acknowledge where construct validity is in jeopardy and provide potential explanations for these problems so that future research may address these issues and readers may consider them when appraising the evidence for use with patients/clients.

EXTERNAL VALIDITY

External validity of a study refers to its usefulness with respect to the "real world." In other words, a study has strong external validity when a reader can apply its results across groups (or individuals), settings, or times specific to his or her clinical situation. Threats to external validity include:

1. Biased sample selection—subjects are different than, or they comprise only a narrowly defined subset of, the population they are said to represent;
2. Setting differences—the environment requires elements of the study to be conducted in a manner different than what would happen in another clinical setting; and,
3. Time—the study is conducted during a period with circumstances considerably different from the present.[2]

To a certain extent, the logistics and resource (e.g., money) limitations with which all investigators must cope will introduce external validity threats to every study. For example, it may not be possible to recruit a diverse and large enough sample or to conduct the study in "real time" particularly when patients are the subjects. Individuals only become patients when they are affected by pathology or injury, the incidence and prevalence of which will determine the potential availability of subjects. On the other hand, the quest for a reasonable sample size may result in such a diverse subject pool that it cannot be said to represent anyone to any extent.

Researchers may try to control for external validity threats by randomly selecting a large sample, conducting a study under "real world" conditions, and studying a recent phenomenon and publishing the results as quickly as possible. As with threats to research and construct validity, evidence-based practitioners must assess the extent and impact of threats to external validity of a study to determine whether its results can be applied to their patients/clients.

SUMMARY

Research validity addresses the extent to which a study's results can be trusted to represent the truth about a phenomenon. Construct validity refers to the degree to which variables are clearly defined and measured in a study. External validity of a study reflects the relevance of its results. A variety of threats to research and construct validity may result in competing explanations for the study's results, while limitations to external validity may restrict the degree to which the results can be applied to patients/clients outside of the study. Numerous design and statistical solutions are available to researchers to minimize threats to these three forms of validity. Evidence-based physical therapists must be aware of these threats and the solutions used to decrease their impact when determining if evidence is useful and appropriate for their patients/clients.

Exercises

1. Define research validity, construct validity, and external validity. What is the focus of each of these terms? Why are they important to a study's integrity?
2. Pick three threats to research validity and identify one cause and one design solution for each. Provide an example of a study scenario to support your answers.
3. Explain how investigators may introduce bias into a study. Provide an example of a study scenario to support your answer.
4. Pick one threat to construct validity and identify one cause and one design solution. Provide an example of a study scenario to support your answers.

5. Pick two threats to external validity and identify one cause and one design solution for each. Provide an example of a study scenario to support your answers.

References

1. Helewa A, Walker JM. *Critical Evaluation of Research in Physical Rehabilitation: Towards Evidence-Based Practice.* Philadelphia, PA: W.B. Saunders Company; 2000.
2. Domholdt E. *Rehabilitation Research: Principles and Applications.* 3d ed. St Louis, MO: Elsevier Saunders; 2005.
3. Portney LG, Watkins MP. *Foundations of Clinical Research: Applications to Practice.* 2d ed. Upper Saddle River, NJ; Prentice Hall Health; 2000.
4. Guyatt G, Rennie D. *Users' Guides to the Medical Literature: A Manual for Evidence-Based Clinical Practice.* Chicago, IL: AMA Press; 2002.
5. Herbert R, Jamtvedt G, Mead J, Hagen KB. *Practical Evidence-Based Physical Therapy*. Edinburgh, Scotland: Elsevier Butterworth Heinemann; 2005.
6. Neuro-developmental treatment. Neuro-developmental Treatment Association Web site. Available at: http://www.ndta.org/. Accessed March 5, 2006.
7. Cerebral Palsy—Hope through Research: Glossary. National Institute of Neurologic Disorders and Stroke Web site, National Institutes of Health. Available at: http://www.ninds.nih.gov/disorders/cerebral_palsy/detail_cerebral_palsy.htm#52163104. Accessed March 5, 2006.

Chapter 9

Unraveling Statistical Mysteries

Not everything that counts can be counted, and not everything that can be counted counts.

—Albert Einstein

Objectives

Upon completion of this chapter the student/practitioner will be able to:

1. Differentiate between:
   a. Descriptive and inferential statistical tests;
   b. Parametric and nonparametric statistical tests;
   c. Tests of differences and tests of relationships; and
   d. Independent and dependent data.
2. Discuss the following characteristics of selected statistical tools:
   a. Purpose;
   b. Indications for use;
   c. Method for use;
   d. Information provided by the tests; and
   e. Limitations or caveats to their use.
3. Interpret information provided by:
   a. The statistical tests reviewed in this chapter; and
   b. p-values and confidence intervals.
4. Distinguish between statistical significance and clinical relevance.
5. Discuss the concept of statistical power.

Terms in This Chapter

Alpha (α) Level (also referred to as Significance Level): A threshold set by researchers used to determine if an observed relationship or difference between variables is "real" or the result of chance.[1]

Coefficient of Variation: The amount of variability in a data set expressed as a proportion of the mean.[2]

Confidence Interval: A range of scores within which the true score for a variable is estimated to lie within a specified probability (e.g., 90 percent, 95 percent, 99 percent).[3]

Data Transformation: A mathematical method by which researchers can convert their data into a normal distribution as required for parametric statistical tests.

Effect Size: The magnitude of the difference (or the relationship) between two mean values.[3]

Inferential Statistics: Statistical tests that permit estimations of population characteristics based on data provided by a sample.

Interpercentiles: Division points in the data, such as quartiles or tertiles, that are used to identify where a certain percentage of the scores lie.[1]

Mean: The sum of the data points divided by the number of scores (e.g., the average).

Median: The middle score in a data set.

Mode: The score that occurs most frequently in the data set.

Multicollinearity: The degree to which independent variables in a study are related to one another.[4]

Negative Likelihood Ratio: The likelihood that a negative test result was found in a patient with, as compared to a patient without, the disease or disorder of interest.[5]

Negative Predictive Value: A diagnostic test's ability to correctly identify the proportion of patients with a negative test result who do not have the disease or disorder of interest.[5,6]

Nonparametric Tests: Statistical tests that are used with nominal and ordinal level data; also may be used with interval and ratio level data that are not normally distributed.

Number Needed to Treat: The number of subjects treated with an experimental intervention over the course of a study required to achieve one good outcome (i.e., cure).[6]

Odds Ratio: The odds that an individual with a risk (prognostic) factor will develop the problem of interest as compared to the odds for an individual without the risk (prognostic) factor.[6]

Parametric Tests: Statistical tests that are used with interval and ratio level data that are normally distributed.

Positive Likelihood Ratio: The likelihood that a positive test result was found in a patient with, as compared to a patient without, the disease or disorder of interest.[5]

Positive Predictive Value: A diagnostic test's ability to correctly identify the proportion of patients with a positive test result who have the disease or disorder of interest.[6]

Power: The probability that a statistical test will detect, if it is present, a relationship between two or more variables or a difference between two or more groups.[1,3]

p-value: The probability that a statistical finding occurred due to chance.

Range: The spread of data points from the lowest to the highest score.

Risk Reduction: The degree to which the risk of disease is decreased as a result of an intervention; can be calculated in absolute and relative terms.[6]

Sensitivity: A diagnostic test's ability to correctly classify patients with the disease or disorder of interest.[6]

Skew: A distortion of the normal bell curve that occurs as the result of extreme scores in the data set.

Specificity: A diagnostic test's ability to correctly classify patients without the disease or disorder of interest.[6]

Standard Deviation (SD): The average absolute distance of scores from the mean score of a data set.[7]

Standard Error of the Estimate: "The standard deviation of the difference between individual data points and the regression line through them."[3(p. 560)]

Standard Error of the Mean: An estimate of the standard deviation of the population of interest; indicates the degree of error associated with repeated samples from the population.[1]

Standard Error of Measurement: The extent to which observed scores are disbursed around the true score; "The standard deviation of measurement errors" obtained from repeated measures.[3(p. 560)]

Type I Error: A result from a statistical test that indicates a significant relationship or difference exists when one does not exist (e.g., a false positive).[1]

Type II Error: A result from a statistical test that indicates a significant relationship or difference does not exist when one does exist (e.g., a false negative).[1]

Variability: The degree to which scores in a data set are dispersed.[2]

INTRODUCTION

The word "statistics" is intimidating to many researchers and clinicians alike, perhaps because of the often complex mathematical formulas used to create them, as well as the cryptic way in which they provide information. Yet statistics are simply a collection of tools that researchers use in the same way that physical therapists use clinical tools. For example, therapists can measure aerobic capacity with walking tests, treadmill tests, and cycle ergometer tests. Similarly, they can measure range of motion with manual goniometers, electronic goniometers, or inclinometers. All of these tools are meant to capture a particular phenomenon in an objective (unbiased) manner. In addition, they quantify what is measured so that changes in performance can be computed over the episode of physical therapy.

The tools physical therapists use in the clinic have the following features in common with statistics:

a) A purpose for which they were specifically designed;
b) Indications for their use;
c) A defined method for their use;
d) A specific set of information they provide when used; and,
e) Limitations beyond which the instruments cannot perform properly and/or important caveats to their use.

For example, a manual goniometer:

a) Is designed to measure angles;
b) Is used when a physical therapist needs to quantify joint position and available range of motion during a physical examination;
c) Is applied with the pivot point over the axis of joint motion and the arms aligned with relevant bony landmarks;
d) Provides information in degrees; and,
e) Has a standard error of measurement of plus or minus four degrees.

When a physical therapist uses the goniometer properly, then information about joint position and range of motion is obtained and can be interpreted based on normative data about the way the human body performs given age and gender. A physical therapist's interpretation of the value indicated by the goniometer may be expressed with terms like "normal," "limited," "excessive," "improved," or "worsened."

When reading a study it is helpful to think about the statistical tests the authors used in the same way that we think about the features of a goniometer. An evidence-based physical therapist's job is to consider whether the investigators selected the right statistical tools for their research question and applied the tools appropriately. A therapist then has to consider what information the statistics have provided (e.g., the results of the study) and what he or she thinks about that information (e.g., whether the results provided are important and useful).

This chapter contains information about statistics commonly used in clinical research: descriptive statistics, parametric statistics, and nonparametric statistics. The intent is to help the reader understand how these statistics are used and how to interpret the information they provide. A discussion about additional statistical methods relevant to evidence-based physical therapy follows. Finally, methods to determine the importance of statistical results are reviewed. Calculation of specific statistics and their practical application in research projects is beyond the scope of this textbook. Readers with a desire to learn more should start with the sources itemized in the reference list at the end of the chapter to obtain additional details about these procedures.

DESCRIPTIVE STATISTICS

Descriptive statistics do what their name implies: describe the data collected by the researchers. Researchers describe data for several reasons. First, they will use descriptive statistics when the sole purpose of their study is to summarize numerically details about a phenomenon of interest. Common focus areas in these circumstances include, but are not limited to: the incidence and prevalence of a disease or disorder, characteristics of individuals with this problem, and associated diagnostic and intervention utilization rates. Second, researchers use descriptive statistics in studies about relationships and differences to determine whether their data are ready for statistical testing. This step is necessary because statistical tests are developed based on assumptions about the nature of the data and the patterns in which the data points lie. Violation of these assumptions likely will undermine the investigators' results. Finally, investigators use descriptive statistics in studies about relationships or differences in order to provide information about relevant subject and/or environmental characteristics.

Distribution of the Data

Readiness for statistical testing is determined by examining the distribution of scores within the data set. Specifically, a researcher wants to know 1) the central point around which some of the data tend to cluster; and 2) how far away from the central point all of the data lie. The first feature is referred to as a "measure of central tendency"[3] and may be characterized by the mean, the median, or the mode of the data. The most commonly used descriptive statistic is the *mean* (noted with the symbol $\bar{x}$), which represents the average of all of the data points. The mean traditionally is calculated with ratio or interval level data. The *median* represents the score that is in the middle of the data points, while the *mode* is the score that occurs most frequently in the data set. Both the median and the mode can be used with ratio, interval, and ordinal level data; however, the mode is the only measure of central tendency used to describe nominal data.[3]

The second feature of a data set is its *variability*, that is, the degree to which scores are distributed around the central value. Variability most commonly is characterized by the the range, the standard deviation, and/or interpercentiles. The *range* identifies the lowest and highest score in the data set and may be expressed either by providing these values (e.g., 20–100) or by calculating the difference between them (e.g., 80). The limitation of using the range is that it does not provide information about each score. On the other hand, the *standard deviation* (SD) is a value that summarizes the average absolute distance of all of the individual scores from the mean score.[7] Investigators typically report a mean value along with its standard deviation to provide the most complete picture of the data. Bigger standard deviations indicate greater variability in the data set. *Interpercentiles* are used to divide the data into equal portions (i.e., tenths, quarters, thirds, and so on) in order to determine where an individual score lies relative to all of the other scores.[1] This approach often is used to divide subjects into smaller groups for further comparison.

Researchers also may have an interest in comparing the variability among different measures of the same phenomenon or among the same measure from different samples. The descriptive statistic commonly used in these circumstances is the coefficient of variation. The *coefficient of variation* divides the standard deviation by its mean to create a measure of relative variability expressed as a percentage. The units of measurement cancel each other out in this calculation allowing comparisons between or among different types of measures.

The measures of variability described to this point typically are used to evaluate data that have been collected a single time. Researchers also may evaluate the variability that occurs when measures are performed, or samples are drawn, multiple times. Every measure is associated with some degree of error; the standard deviation of errors from multiple measures is a value referred to as the *standard error of measurement.*[3] This statistic indicates by how much a measurement will vary from the original value each time it is repeated. The known variability in measurement error helps researchers and clinicians alike determine whether "true" change has occurred from one measure to the next. The *standard error of the mean*, on the other hand, provides an assessment of the variation in errors that occurs when repeated samples of a population are drawn. This value also may be referred to as an estimate of the variability around the mean for the population of interest in a study.[1] Unfortunately, both measures of variability have the same abbreviation–SEM–which can be confusing when reading or listening to a research report. Evidence-based physical therapists should be mindful of the definition of the abbreviation, as well as of the context in which it is used, in order to avoid misinterpretation of the information provided. Table 9-1 summarizes the descriptive statistics commonly used in clinical research.[1,2,3,4,7]

In addition to obtaining measures of central tendency and variability, researchers can quickly determine if data are ready for statistical testing by examining a visual display of the scores. Commonly used graphic displays include histograms (Figure 9-1) and line plots (Figure 9-2). Specifically, investigators want to know whether a plot of the data points results in a symmetrical bell-shaped curve (Figure 9-3).

Data that create a bell curve are said to be "normally distributed"[3] around a central value (usually the mean) for the group of scores. In addition, a predictable percentage of the scores can be located within one, two, or three standard deviations away from the mean score of normally distributed data. This feature of a bell curve is the foundation for a group of tests referred to as parametric statistics.

In the case of interval or ratio level data, extreme scores for the group can distort the curve or make it asymmetrical in one direction or the other. Scores that pull the end (or "tail") of the curve farther out to the right result in a distribution that is "positively *skewed*," while scores that pull the end of the of the curve farther out to the left result in a distribution that is "negatively skewed" (Figure 9-4).[7]

Note that extreme values also result in a shift in the mean toward the elongated tail, a situation that occurs because the mean is calculated using all values in the data set (including the extreme ones). The mode remains stationary because it is the value that occurs the most frequently; it is not a mathematical summary of all of the data set values. Finally, the median moves between the mean and mode because it is the value in the middle of a distribution that is now shifted in one direction or the other.

Subject Characteristics

An important feature of all clinical research is the description of subjects included in the study. This information is essential to the evidence-based physical therapist in order to determine how closely the subjects resemble the individual patient/client about which the therapist has a question. A summary of subject characteristics also is important to investigators for two reasons. First, researchers wish to know the degree to which their sample represents the population of individuals from which it was drawn. Extreme differences between the sample and the population will limit the extent to

Table 9–1 Descriptive statistics.

Statistic	Purpose	Indications for Use	Method for Use	Information Provided	Limitations or Important Caveats
Frequency	• To count things, such as numbers of subjects, their characteristics, etc.	• In epidemiological papers, to describe phenomena and their characteristics • In all other papers, to describe subjects, test results, and/or outcomes	• May be used with any level of data	• Numbers (counts) • Percentages	• None
Mean	• To summarize data • To determine the central point around which most of the data cluster	• In epidemiological papers, to describe phenomena and their characteristics • In all other papers, to describe subjects, test results, or outcomes	• May be used with ratio and interval level data • Often used with ordinal data despite their lack of mathematical properties	• Average of all the values in the data set	• Influenced by extreme data values because all of the data points are used in the calculation
Median	• To summarize data • To determine the central point around which most of the data cluster	• Same indications as with the mean, especially when data set is skewed	• May be used with ratio, interval, and ordinal level data	• The middle value in the data set	• Not influenced by extreme values because no math is performed
Mode	• To summarize data • To determine the central point around which most of the data cluster	• Same indications as with the mean	• Best used with any level of data • Only summary statistic that may be used with nominal data	• The value(s) occurring most frequently in the data set	• Not influenced by extreme values because no math is performed • May have more than one mode in a data set

Range	• To describe the variability in a data set	• Often used to supplement information about the mean or median	• May be used with ratio, interval, or ordinal data	• The highest and lowest data values, or the difference between them	• Represents only two scores out of the entire data set; they may be outliers • The least helpful descriptor of variability
Standard Deviation (SD)	• To describe variability in the data set around the mean	• In papers that are purely descriptive in nature • In all other papers, to describe subjects	• Calculated as deviation of data from the mean	• Summary of individual data point deviations from the mean	• When data are normally distributed (bell shaped): ◦ 68% of data lie within ±1 SD ◦ 95% of data lie within ±2 SD ◦ 99% of data lie within ±3 SD
Percentiles	• To describe the variability in a data set	• Often used to supplement information about the median	• Can use with any level of data • Division points may be tertiles, quartiles, etc.	• Ranges that contain a certain % of scores (e.g., the 25th percentile)	• Not greatly influenced by extreme values
Coefficient of Variation (CV)	• To measure variation relative to the mean (rather than variation "around" it)	• To compare variation among subject groups when units of measure are different between each group	• Calculated as a ratio of the standard deviation over the mean	• % variation	• None
Skewness	• To describe the shape of the curve created by the data points	• To determine whether the values in the data set are normally distributed	• Calculated as part of the summary description of the data	• Positive (right) or negative (left) value	• Skew will occur when there are outliers in the data set

continues

Table 9–1 Descriptive statistics *(continued)*.

Statistic	Purpose	Indications for Use	Method for Use	Information Provided	Limitations or Important Caveats
Standard Error of Measurement (SEM)	• To determine the variability in repeated measures of an individual	• To differentiate between true change and error when measures are repeated in a study	• Estimated mathematically because it is logistically impractical to perform enough repeated measures to obtain this value	• Standard deviation of measurement errors	• Measurement errors are assumed to be normally distributed ◦ 68% of data lie within ±1 SEM ◦ 95% of data lie within ±2 SEM ◦ 99% of data lie within ±3 SEM • SEM is also the abbreviation for "standard error of the mean"
Standard Error of the Mean (SEM)	• To determine the variability in repeated samples from the same population	• May be reported in addition to, or instead of, the standard deviation	• Estimated mathematically because it is logistically impractical to draw repeated samples	• Standard deviation of the population mean (or sampling distribution)	• The larger the sample the smaller the SEM • Sampling errors are assumed to be normally distributed ◦ 68% of data lie within ±1 SEM ◦ 95% of data lie within ±2 SEM ◦ 99% of data lie within ±3 SEM • SEM is also the abbreviation for "standard error of measurement"

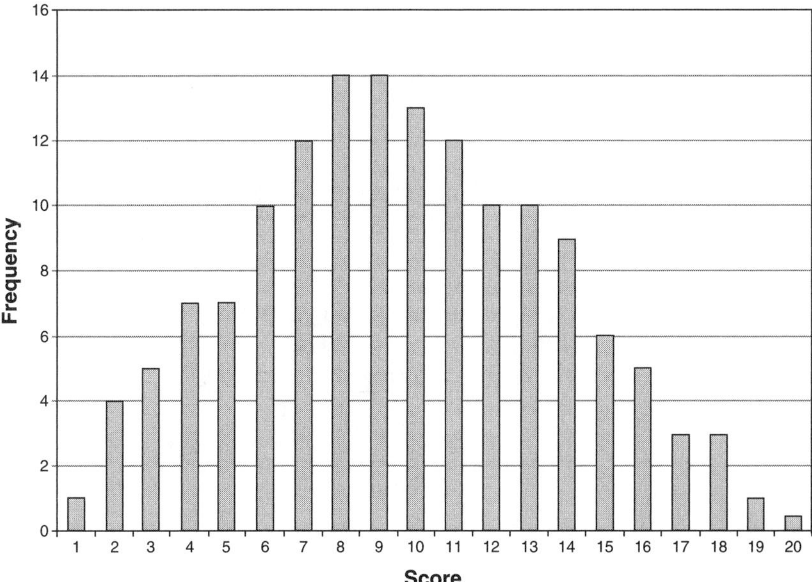

Figure 9–1 A histogram for a hypothetical set of data.

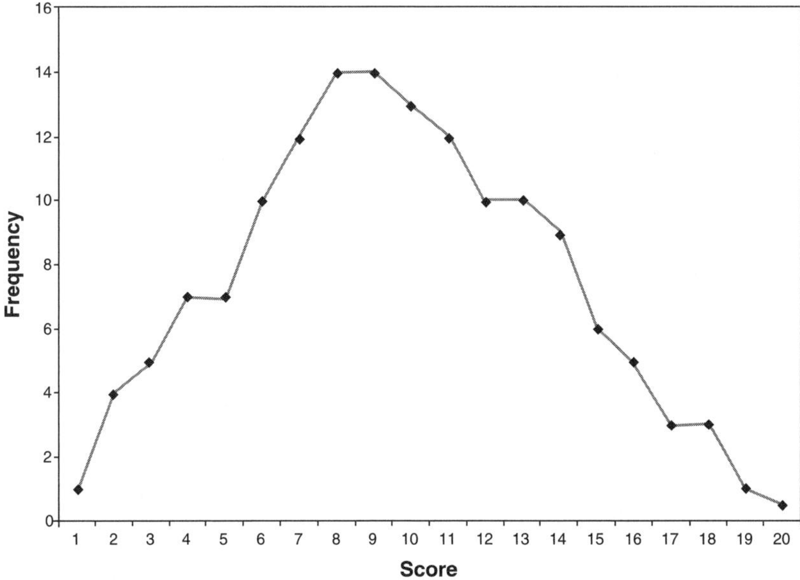

Figure 9–2 A line plot for the same hypothetical set of data as above.

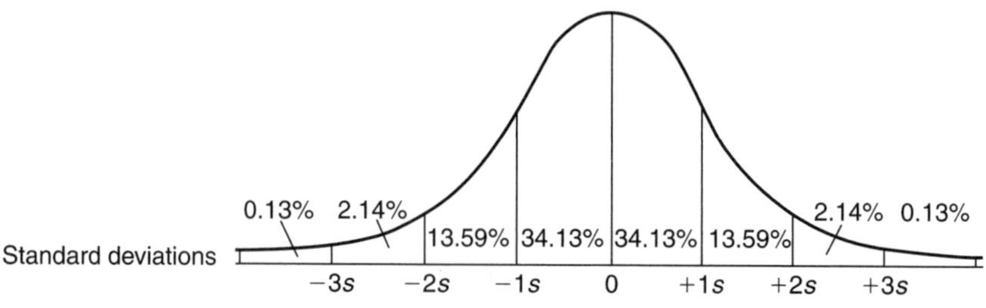

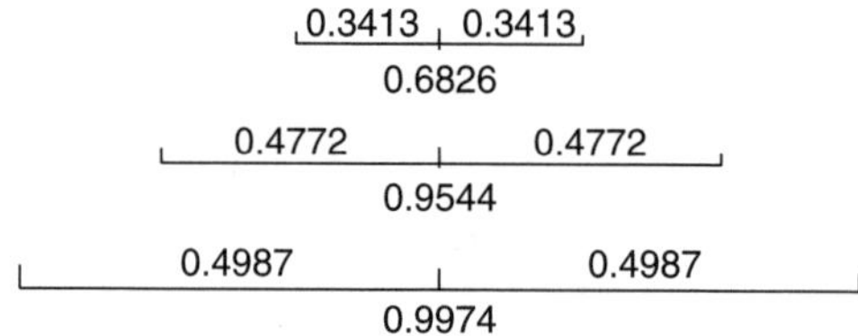

Figure 9–3 Normal distribution of data (bell curve) with 1, 2, and 3 standard deviations.

Source: Reprinted from Leslie Gross Portney & Mary P. Watkins, *Foundations of Clinical Research: Applications to Practice*, 2nd edition, Chapter 17. Copyright (2000), with permission from Prentice-Hall, Inc.

which the results can be applied beyond the study itself. Second, investigators interested in comparing the outcomes of an intervention between two or more groups need relevant subject characteristics to be equally distributed among the groups at the start of the study. Unbalanced groups may undermine the research validity of a study as discussed in Chapter 8.

Patient/client characteristics commonly summarized using descriptive statistics include, but are not limited to:

1. demographic information
   a) Age;
   b) Gender;
   c) Race/ethnicity;
   d) Education level;
   e) Socioeconomic status;
   f) Employment status;
   g) Marital status; and
   h) Presence and/or type of insurance coverage.
2. Clinical information
   a) Height;
   b) Weight;

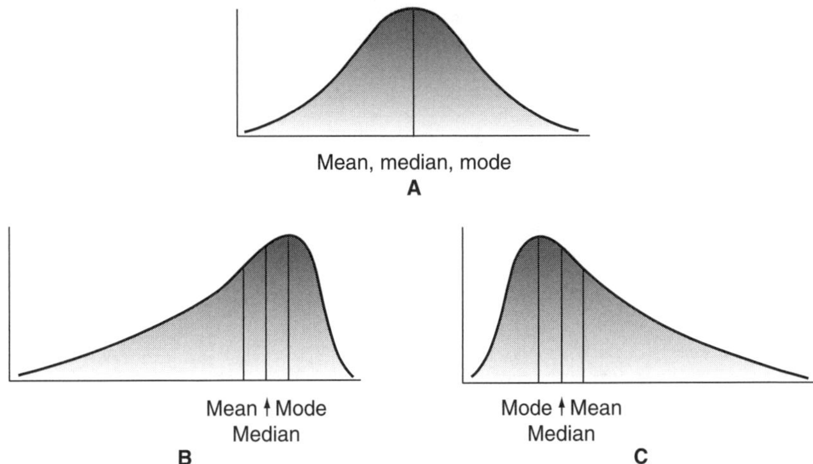

Figure 9–4 Data distribution: (A) normal, (B) skewed left, and (C) skewed right.
Source: Reprinted from Leslie Gross Portney & Mary P. Watkins. *Foundations of Clinical Research: Applications to Practice*, 2nd edition, Chapter 17. Copyright (2000), with permission from Prentice-Hall, Inc.

c) Diagnosis;
d) Number and/or type of risk factors for disease or adverse event;
e) Number and/or type of comorbidities;
f) Health or functional status;
g) Mental or cognitive status;
h) Type of assistive device required for mobility;
i) Number and/or type of medications;
j) Number and/or type of diagnostic tests;
k) Number and/or type of surgeries;
l) Number and/or type of diagnostic tests; and
m) Type of referring physician.

Table 9-2 displays descriptive statistics for subject characteristics in a hypothetical study about risk factors for development of knee flexion contractures in elderly nursing home residents.[8] Means, standard deviations, and ranges are presented for the variables that are ratio level measures. On the other hand, the values for "gender" and "prior knee surgery" are recorded as percentages because these are nominal measures that require mathematical expression through frequencies. Frequencies may be stated as the actual number of subjects or as a proportion of the total number of subjects who have the characteristic.

Table 9–2 An example of descriptive statistics in a hypothetical study of risk factors for knee flexion contracture development in elderly nursing home residents

Characteristic	Mean or %	Standard Deviation	Range
Age	84.4	4.5	77–92
Gender (% Female)	72	—	—
Mini Mental State Exam Score[8]	20.7	2.8	16–27
# of Comorbidities	2.75	1.2	1–5
# of Medications	3.75	1.1	2–6
Prior knee surgery (% yes)	31	—	—

PARAMETRIC STATISTICS

Parametric statistics are a form of *inferential statistics* that do more than describe; they help investigators and evidence-based physical therapists make decisions about what the data indicate. Traditionally, these statistics are used for ratio or interval level data. An advantage of these tests is that detailed information can be derived from this type of data because it is continuous in form.[7] Investigators also use these tests with ordinal level data.[1] This practice is somewhat controversial, but is becoming more prevalent especially in social sciences research. Remember that ordinal level measures use symbols (e.g., numerals) that are ordered in rank; however, the distance between each symbol is not known so technically there is no way to "do math" with this data. For example, imagine a ruler with no hash marks on it and the numerals 1–12 written at random intervals along the face. In the absence of equal distances between each symbol, it would be impossible to quantify what is being measured. Despite these issues, parametric tests are viewed as "robust" enough to withstand their use with ordinal level data.[1]

A key assumption in parametric statistical tests is that the data are normally distributed.[3] If the distribution is not normal, then a number of methods are available to transform the data to fix the problem. Options include logarithmic transformation, squaring the data, and taking the square root of the data, among others.[1] The decision to transform depends upon how skewed the distribution is and whether *data transformation* will permit interpretation of the results. Authors will indicate which transformation technique they used, if any. An alternative to transformation is to use a nonparametric statistical test instead.[1]

Parametric tests can be categorized into one of two groups: tests of differences and tests of relationships. The following sections describe frequently-encountered statistical tests in each category.

TESTS OF DIFFERENCES

Tests of differences are used when an investigator wants to compare two or more groups of subjects or sets of scores from the same subjects. Comparisons are indicated to evaluate whether the groups have equally-distributed characteristics at the start of the study and in studies where a treatment approach is tested for its ability to produce a difference in one group as compared to the other(s).

Before conducting a parametric test of differences, investigators must determine whether the data points in each group are independent of one another. In other words, data either came from distinctly separate individuals or were gathered upon repeated measures of the same subjects. Comparisons made using distinct groups of subjects are referred to as "between-group" tests, while comparisons made using repeated measures on the same subjects are referred to as "within group" tests.[7] Table 9-3 illustrates a "between-group" comparison at the start of a hypothetical study examining the outcome (Disability of the Arm, Shoulder, and Hand [DASH] score)[9] between one group of individuals who received body mechanics training plus exercise and another group of individuals who received exercise training alone.

A "within-group" version of this study would be to compare the DASH score at the end of the study with the score at the beginning of the study for individuals in only one of the groups (e.g., the body mechanics training plus exercise group). Data points between groups are said to be independent of one another because they are obtained from different subjects. Data points within a group are said to be dependent on one another; in other

Table 9-3 A comparison of group characteristics in a hypothetical study investigating the use of body mechanics training plus exercises versus exercise alone for the management of shoulder pain in hair salon workers.

Characteristic	Body Mechanics Plus Exercise Group Mean (SD) or %	Exercise Alone Group Mean (SD) or %	p-value
Age	35.8 (3.6)	29.2 (2.2)	0.04
Gender (% Female)	73	64	0.01
Income	$31,456.00	$30,598.00	0.48
DASH[9] score at start of study	73.4 (3.8)	71.6 (3.1)	0.27
# of Medications	1.8 (0.4)	2.0 (0.6)	0.34
Prior surgery (% yes)	15	16	0.15

words, the disability score a subject gets at the end of the study is related to the disability score a subject produced at the start of the study because it came from the same person. This dependency must be acknowledged mathematically for statistical purposes. As a result, there are independent and dependent versions of the same tests of differences available for use.

Selection of the appropriate statistical test of differences also depends upon several other factors. First, the number of groups to be compared must be considered. The most simplistic versions of these tests are designed to compare two groups only, whereas more sophisticated tests compare three or more groups. A related issue is the number of variables utilized. Factorial study designs in which two or more variables are of interest, require analysis of the main effects resulting from each variable, as well as analysis of the effects that occur as a result of the interaction between or among variables. Second, the ability to control for extraneous variables may be desired. Only certain forms of difference tests permit this adjustment. Third, more than one dependent variable or outcome will require yet another test. Table 9-4 itemizes parametric tests of differences commonly used in clinical research:

- The t-test and its dependent measure counterpart, the paired t-test;
- The analysis of variance (ANOVA) test and its dependent measure counterpart, the repeated measures ANOVA test;
- The analysis of covariance (ANCOVA) test, used to adjust for confounding variables; and,
- The multiple analysis of variance (MANOVA) test, used when there is more than one dependent variable.[1,3,4,7]

TESTS OF RELATIONSHIPS

Tests of relationships are used when an investigator wants to determine whether two or more variables are associated with one another. These tests have several functions in clinical research. First, association tests may be used in methodological studies to establish the reliability and validity of measurement instruments. Second, investigators perform these tests to examine the intra- and/or inter-rater reliability of data collectors prior to the start of a study. In both cases, the preferred outcome of the tests is to show a strong correlation or relationship indicating that the measures are stable and are capturing what they propose to capture. Third, association tests are used to evaluate whether all variables under consideration need to remain in the study. Variables that have overlapping qualities can add redundancy to statistical models, thereby causing some difficulties with the

Table 9–4 Parametric statistical tests of differences.

Statistical Test	Purpose	Indications for Use	Method for Use	Information Provided	Limitations or Important Caveats
Independent t-test	• To answer the question "Is there a difference between 2 groups?"	• Comparisons of characteristics between groups at start of study • Comparison of outcomes due to risk factor or treatment	• Examines differences between the means of two groups only • Designed for use with parametric data (interval, ratio)	• t-statistic • p-value	• Assumes: ◦ Normally distributed data ◦ Equal variance between groups ◦ Independence of scores from one another
Paired t-test	• To answer the question "Is there a difference within the same group?"	• Pretest /Posttest designs in which subjects act as their own controls	• Examines differences in mean values between the experimental condition and control condition • Designed for use with parametric data (interval, ratio)	• t-statistic • p-value	• Assumes: ◦ Normally distributed data
Analysis of Variance (ANOVA)	• To answer the question "Is there a difference between 2 or more groups?"	• Designs in which the independent variable (e.g., the treatment) has 2 or more levels • Factorial designs with ≥ 2 independent variables • Used when there is only 1 dependent variable (outcome)	• Examines differences between or among the means of each group • Designed for use with parametric data (interval, ratio) • Factorial designs ◦ 1 independent variable = 1-way	• F-statistic • p-value • For tests with ≥ 2 independent variables: ◦ Main effects for each variable ◦ Interaction effects between each variable	• **All assumptions listed under** t-test **apply** • Will only indicate that a difference exists—will NOT indicate where the difference is (e.g., which groups are different)

continues

Table 9–4 Parametric statistical tests of differences *(continued)*.

Statistical Test	Purpose	Indications for Use	Method for Use	Information Provided	Limitations or Important Caveats
ANOVA			• 2 independent variables = 2-way ANOVA		• Requires additional ("post hoc") statistical tests to determine which groups are different from one another
Repeated Measures Analysis of Variance (ANOVA)	• To answer the question "Is there a difference among repeated measures on subjects within the same group?"	• Repeated measures designs in which the independent variable (e.g., the treatment) has 2 or more levels AND subjects act as their own controls • Factorial designs with ≥ 2 independent variables • Used when there is only 1 dependent variable (outcome)	• Examines differences in mean values among repeated measures • Designed for use with parametric data (interval, ratio)	• F-statistic • p-value • For tests with ≥ 2 independent variables: ◦ Main effects for each variable ◦ Interaction effects between each variable	• **All assumptions listed under** t-test **apply** • Will only tell you that a difference exists—will NOT indicate where the difference is (e.g., which groups are different) • Requires additional ("post hoc") statistical tests to determine which groups are different from one another
Analysis of Covariance (ANCOVA)	• To answer the question "Is there a difference among 2 or more groups while controlling for covariates (extraneous variables)?"	• Designs in which the independent variable (e.g., the treatment) has 2 or more levels • Used when there is only 1 dependent variable (outcome)	• Uses the covariate(s) to adjust the dependent variable, then examines differences among the means of each group	• F-statistic • p-value	• **All assumptions listed under** t-test **apply**, plus: • Covariates are not correlated with each other

			• Designed for use with parametric data (interval, ratio)		• Covariates are linearly related to the dependent variable • Covariates may be nominal, interval, or ratio level measures
Multivariate Analysis of Variance (MANOVA)	• To answer the question "Is there a difference in 2 or more outcomes among 2 or more groups?"	• Designs in which the independent variable (e.g., the treatment) has 2 or more levels • Factorial designs with ≥ 2 independent variables • Used if > 1 dependent variable (outcome)	• Accounts for the relationship among multiple dependent variables during group comparisons • Designed for use with parametric data (interval, ratio)	• Wilks's lambda • F-statistic • p-value	• **All assumptions listed under** t-test **apply** • Will only tell you that a difference exists—will NOT indicate where the difference is (e.g., which groups are different) • Requires additional ("post hoc") statistical tests to determine which groups are different from one another

analysis. In cases where this interrelationship is strong, the variables in question are said to demonstrate *multicollinearity*.[4] Often researchers will eliminate one variable in the associated pair to reduce this problem. Finally, the most sophisticated tests of association are used to model and predict a future outcome as is required in prognosis studies.

Basic parametric association tests evaluate the relationship's strength, direction, and importance. "Strength" refers to how closely the values of one variable correspond to the values of the other variable(s) and is expressed by a correlation coefficent with a scale from −1 to +1. A coefficient that equals one indicates perfect association while a coefficient that equals zero indicates no association at all. Portney and Watkins offer the following criteria by which to judge the strength of the correlation coefficient: [1(p. 494)]

- 0.00–0.25 "little or no relationship"
- 0.26–0.50 "fair degree of relationship"
- 0.51–0.75 "moderate to good relationship"
- 0.76–1.00 "good to excellent relationship"

"Direction" is noted via the (−) or (+) sign in front of the correlation coefficient. The (−) indicates a negative or inverse relationship and is illustrated by the statement "bone density decreases as age increases." The (+) indicates a positive relationship and is illustrated by the statement "alertness decreases as caffeine levels decrease." In other words, a negative correlation means that the values of the two variables change in opposite directions, while a positive correlation means that the values of the two variables change in the same direction.

Finally, the importance of the association is indicated by the amount of variability in the outcome (expressed as a percentage) that can be explained by the relationship and is indicated by the coefficient of determination. For example, although age may account for some of the reduction in bone density over time, other factors such as diet, exercise, heredity, and smoking also may play a role. If age only explains 30 percent of the variability in bone density, then 70 percent is left over to explain with these other factors. On the other hand, if age explains 85 percent of the variability in bone density, then there are fewer factors to search out and evaluate.

More sophisticated tests of association are used to predict the value of the dependent variable based on the value(s) of the independent variable(s). The dependent variable usually is referred to as the "outcome," while the independent variables may be called "predictors," or "factors." Collectively known as regression equations or models, these tests provide information about the strength and direction of the relationship between the predictors and outcome, as well the proportion of variability in the outcome explained by each individual factor. Regression equations also calculate the extent to which individual data points vary from the predicted model, a value referred to as the *standard error of the estimate*.[3] Consider again the question about factors related to bone density in the example above. A regression equation could be used to determine whether, and to what degree, age, diet, exercise, heredity, and smoking predict the actual bone density values of individuals suspected of having osteoporosis. A regression equation also may be tested statistically to help a researcher determine whether it is an important method with which to model a particular phenomenon.

Table 9-5 itemizes parametric tests of association commonly used in clinical research:

- The Pearson's Product Moment Correlation;
- The Intraclass Correlation Coefficient (ICC);
- Multiple correlation;
- Linear regression; and
- Multiple linear regression.[1,3,4,7]

Effect Size

The detection of differences or relationships between or among groups is an important discovery for researchers, but this result in and of itself may be insufficient for clinical use. The decision to apply the evidence to an individual patient/client is further enhanced when investigators also indicate the magnitude of the difference or the relationship. Statistically, this information is conveyed via calculation, in absolute or relative terms, of the *effect size*. For example, if the DASH[9] scores at the conclusion of the hair salon study in Table 9-3 differ by 15 points, then the absolute magnitude of the effect is 15. The relative magnitude of the effect is derived when the variability in the data is included in the calculation. Often these relative effect sizes have values between zero and one. Several authors provide the following criteria for evaluating relative effect sizes:[1,3,7]

- 0.20 minimal effect
- 0.50 moderate effect
- 0.80 large effect

Effect sizes that exceed one are even more impressive using these standards.

NONPARAMETRIC STATISTICS

Nonparametric statistical tests are designed to deal with nominal and ordinal level data. As such, they cannot extract as much information as para-

Table 9–5 Parametric statistical tests of relationships.

Statistical Test	Purpose	Indications for Use	Method for Use	Information Provided	Limitations or Important Caveats
Pearson Product Moment Correlation (Pearson's r)	• To answer the question "Is there a relationship between 2 variables?"	• Designs used to assess the reliability of measures • Designs used to assess the association between 2 variables	• Designed for use with ratio or interval level data	• Correlation coefficient (r); indicates the strength of the association from −1 to +1 (negative to positive) • Coefficient of determination (r^2); indicates the % variation in one variable that can be explained by the other variable • p-value • Confidence interval (CI)	• Synonyms = correlation, association, relationship • Assumes the data are linearly related • Association does not equal causation
Intraclass Correlation Coefficient (ICC)	• To answer the question "Is there a relationship among 3 or more variables?"	• Designs used to assess the reliability of repeated measures • Designs used to assess the association among 3 or more pairs of variables	• Designed for use with ratio or interval level data • 6 formulas to choose from depending upon purpose of analysis	• Reliability coefficient (ICC); indicates the strength of the association from −1 to +1 ◦ a value of 0 means the variation in the scores is due to measurement error • p-value • Confidence interval (CI)	• Assumes the data are linearly related

Multiple Correlation	• To answer the question "Is there a relationship among 3 or more variables?"	• Designs used to assess the association among 3 or more variables	• Designed for use with ratio or interval level data	• Correlation coefficients; indicate the strength of the association from -1 to $+1$ (negative to positive) • Coefficient of determination; indicates the % variation in one variable that can be explained by the other variable • p-value • Confidence interval (CI)	• Assumes the data are linearly related • Association does not equal causation
Linear Regression	• To answer the question "Can an outcome (y) be predicted based on the value of a known factor (x)?"	• Prognosis studies	• Dependent variable (y) is ratio or interval level data	• β = the amount of change in y per unit change in x • SE = standard error of the estimate • r = the strength of the relationship between x and y (-1 to $+1$) • r^2 = the percent of variance in y explained by x • F-statistic to determine if $r^2 > 0$ • p-value for r^2 • Confidence interval for the predicted value of y	• Works best when the independent variable is highly correlated with the dependent variable

continues

Table 9–5 Parametric statistical tests of relationships *(continued)*.

Statistical Test	Purpose	Indications for Use	Method for Use	Information Provided	Limitations or Important Caveats
Multiple Linear Regression	• To answer the question "Can an outcome (y) be predicted based on the value of 2 or more known factors (x_1, x_2, etc.)?"	• Prognosis studies	• Predictions performed with 2 or more independent variables • Dependent variable (y) is ratio or interval level data • Independent variables (x) may be nominal, interval, or ratio level data • Independent variables may be entered into the regression equation in several ways: ◦ All together in a block ◦ One at a time (forward step-wise) ◦ All together with removal one at a time (backward step-wise)	• β= the amount of change in y per unit change in x • SE = standard error of the estimate • R = the strength of the relationship between x and y • R^2 = the percent of variance in y explained by x • Beta = standardized regression coefficient that explains the percent of variance in y attributable to x; calculated for each independent variable • F- or t-statistic to determine if Beta> 0 and/or $R^2 > 0$ • p-value for Beta and R^2 • Confidence interval for the predicted value of y	• Works best when the independent variable is highly correlated with the dependent variable • Assumes independent variables are not correlated with one another

metric tests because the data are no longer continuous. An advantage to these tests is that they do not rely as heavily on normal distributions of the data; therefore, they also may be an appropriate choice when interval or ratio data are severely skewed and are not appropriate for transformation. Finally, these statistics do not depend on large sample sizes in order to have their assumptions met, so they may be an appropriate choice for interval or ratio data for small groups.[1]

Nonparametric tests parallel their parametric counterparts in that there are tests of differences and tests of relationships. In addition, there are considerations related to the independence of the scores, the number of groups to be compared, the need to control extraneous variables, and the number of dependent variables included. Table 9-6 itemizes nonparametric tests of differences, while Table 9-7 itemizes nonparametric tests of relationships.[1,3,4,7]

ADDITIONAL STATISTICS IN EVIDENCE-BASED PHYSICAL THERAPY

In addition to the traditional statistics described here there are several other calculations used to evaluate the usefulness of diagnostic tests, prognostic indicators, interventions, and outcome measures. An ideal diagnostic test is one that always correctly identifies patients with the disorder ("true positives") as well as those individuals free of it ("true negatives").[10] The degree to which a diagnostic test can meet these expectations is established by the values calculated for a test's *sensitivity*, *specificity*, *positive predictive value*, and *negative predictive value*.[5,6] A diagnostic test's usefulness also depends upon the extent to which the result increases or decreases the probability of the presence of disease in individual patients, as indicated by its *positive* or *negative likelihood ratios*.[5,6] Details about these calculations and their interpretation are provided in Chapter 10. Prognostic indicators are useful when they can quantify via an *odds ratio* the odds that a patient/client will develop or avoid the disease or disorder of interest,[5] as described in Chapter 11. Interventions, on the other hand, are evaluated by the degree to which they reduce the risk of a bad outcome or increase the probability of a good outcome, as well as by the number of patients required for treatment (*number needed to treat*) before one good outcome occurs.[5,6] Details about these calculations and their interpretation are provided in Chapter 12. Finally, outcome measures such as the DASH[9] are most useful when they are responsive to change, as discussed in Chapter 13.

Investigators often use these calculations in combination with traditional statistical tests and provide the results for readers to consider. Physical

Table 9–6 Nonparametric statistical tests of differences.

Statistic	Purpose	Indications for Use	Method for Use	Information Provided	Limitations or Important Caveats
Mann–Whitney U	• To examine differences between 2 groups	• Comparisons of characteristics between groups at start of study • Comparison of outcomes due to risk factor or treatment	• Designed for use with nonparametric data or problematic parametric data (e.g., non-normally distributed)	• Ranks the data for each group • U-statistic • p-value	• Does not assume normal distribution of data • Can be used with small sample sizes
Wilcoxon Rank Sum	• To examine differences between 2 groups	• Comparisons of characteristics between groups at start of study • Comparison of outcomes due to risk factor or treatment	• Designed for use with nonparametric data or problematic parametric data (e.g., non-normally distributed)	• Rank sum of the data for each group • z-score • p-value	• Does not assume normal distribution of data • Can be used with small sample sizes
Wilcoxon Signed Rank Test	• To examine differences within the same group	• Pre-test/Post-test designs in which subjects act as their own controls	• Examines differences in the median values between the experimental condition and control condition • Designed for use with nonparametric data (ordinal, nominal)	• Ranks the difference between each pair of numbers • z-score • p-value	• None

Chi-Squared Goodness-of-Fit Test	• To examine differences between 2 groups	• To determine "goodness of fit" between data from sample and data estimated from population	• Compares actual to expected frequencies • Typically used with nominal data	• Chi-square statistic (χ^2) • p-value	• In goodness-of-fit tests it is preferable that the actual frequencies match the expected frequencies; this match will be indicated by a **nonsignificant** result
Kruskal-Wallis H	• To examine the difference between 3 or more groups (control group and experimental groups)	• Designs in which the independent variable (e.g., the treatment) has 3 or more levels • Used when there is only 1 dependent variable (outcome) • May be used with parametric data if it is not normally distributed	• Designed for use with nonparametric data (ordinal, nominal)	• Ranks • H-statistic • p-value	• Does not assume normal distribution of data • Can be used with small sample sizes • Will only tell you that a difference exists—will NOT tell you where the difference is (e.g., which groups are different) • Requires additional ("post hoc") statistical tests to determine which groups are different from one another

continues

Table 9–6 Nonparametric statistical tests of differences *(continued)*.

Statistic	Purpose	Indications for Use	Method for Use	Information Provided	Limitations or Important Caveats
Friedman's ANOVA	• To examine differences among repeated measures on subjects within the same group	• Repeated measures designs in which subjects act as their own controls • Used when there is only 1 dependent variable (outcome)	• Examines differences in rank sums among repeated measures • Designed for use with nonparametric data (ordinal, nominal)	• Rank sums • F-statistic, or Friedman's chi-square statistic • p-value	• Does not assume normal distribution of data • Can be used with small sample sizes • Will only indicate that a difference exists—will NOT indicate where the difference is (e.g., which groups are different) • Requires additional ("post hoc") statistical tests to determine which groups are different from one another

Table 9–7 Nonparametric statistical tests of relationships.

Statistical Test	Purpose	Indications for Use	Method for Use	Information Provided	Limitations or Important Caveats
Chi-Squared Test of Independence	• To answer the question "Is there a relationship between 2 variables?"	• Epidemiological studies (e.g., case-control designs)	• Compares actual to expected frequencies of the variables • Designed for use with nominal level data	• Chi-square (χ^2) statistic • p-value	• This procedure is designed to test whether two sets of data are independent of each other • a **significant** result indicates that the variables are not independent (therefore, they have an association)
Spearman Rank Correlation Coefficient	• To answer the question "Is there a relationship between 2 variables?"	• Designs used to assess the reliability of measures • Designs used to assess the association between 2 variables	• Designed for use with ordinal level data	• Correlation coefficient (ρ); indicates the strength of the association from -1 to $+1$ (negative to positive) • p-value	• Synonyms = correlation, association, relationship • Assumes the data are linearly related • Association does not equal causation

continues

Table 9–7 Nonparametric statistical tests of relationships *(continued)*.

Statistic Test	Purpose	Indications for Use	Method for Use	Information Provided	Limitations or Important Caveats
Kappa	• To answer the question "Is there a relationship among 3 or more variables?"	• Designs used to assess the reliability of repeated measures • Designs used to assess the association among 3 or more pairs of variables	• Designed for use with nominal level data	• Reliability coefficient (k); indicates the strength of the association from −1 to +1; • p-value	• Synonyms = correlation, association, relationship • Assumes the data are linearly related
Logistic Regression	• To answer the question "What is the probability of an event occurring based on the value of a known factor?"	• Prognosis studies	• Dependent variable (y) is nominal (dichotomous) level data • Predictor (x) [independent variable] may be nominal, interval, or ratio level data	• b = the amount of change in y per unit change in x • SE = standard error of the estimate • r = the strength of the relationship between x and y (−1 to +1) • r^2 = the percent of variance in y explained by x • F-statistic to determine if $r^2 > 0$ • p-value for r^2 • Confidence interval for the predicted value of y	• Works best when the independent variable is highly correlated with the dependent variable

Multiple Logistic Regression	• To answer the question "What is the probability of an event occurring based on the value of 2 or more known factors?"	• Prognosis studies • Independent variables may be entered into the regression equation in several ways: ◦ All together in a block ◦ One at a time (forward step-wise) ◦ All together with removal one at a time (backward step-wise)	• Predictions performed with 2 or more independent variables • Dependent variable (y) is nominal (dichotomous) • Predictor (x) [independent variable] may be nominal, interval, or ratio level data • Exp (β) = odds ratio • F- or t-statistic to determine if Exp (β) > 0 and/or $R^2 > 0$ • p-value for Exp (β) and R^2 • Confidence interval for the predicted value of y and Exp (β)	• b= the amount of change in y per unit change in x • SE = standard error of the estimate • R = the strength of the relationship between x's and y • R^2 = the percent of variance in y explained by x's	• Works best when the independent variable is highly correlated with the dependent variable • Assumes independent variables are not correlated with one another

therapists reviewing the evidence also may be able to calculate these values from data provided by authors who use traditional statistics alone. Straus *et al.* provide the necessary formulas to perform the calculations in their critical appraisal worksheets, a modified version of which is located in Appendix B.[6]

STATISTICAL IMPORTANCE

As noted at the outset of this chapter, the goal of statistical testing is to evaluate the data in an objective fashion. Two methods by which investigators assess the importance of their statistical results are the p-value and the confidence interval. In both instances, researchers must choose a threshold that indicates at what point they will consider the results to be significant, rather than a chance occurrence. A declaration of statistical significance is synonymous with rejection of the null hypothesis (i.e., "there is no difference [relationship]").

p-Values

The *p-value* is the probability that the study's findings occurred due to chance.[1] For example, a p-value equal to 0.10 is interpreted to mean that there is a 10 percent probability that a study's findings occurred due to chance. The statistics software program used to perform the test of differences or relationships also calculates this probability. Authors provide information about this "obtained" p-value with the rest of their results. The *alpha level* (α) or significance level, is the term used to indicate the threshold the investigators have selected to detect statistical significance, the traditional level of which is 0.05.[11] Obtained p-values lower than the 0.05 threshold indicate even lower probabilities of the role of chance. Authors identify an alpha level in the methods section of their study or they simply may indicate in their results that the p-values calculated as part of the statistical tests were lower than a critical value. In either case, investigators select alpha levels to reduce the opportunity of making a *Type I error*—when a difference or relationship is identified that really does not exist.[3] The lower the alpha level (and resulting obtained p-value), the lower the opportunity for such an error.

The limitation of a p-value is that it is a dichotomous—"yes/no"—answer to the question about significance. This approach leaves no room for finer interpretations based on an assessment that uses continuous level information. Sterne and Smith argue that this approach to determining the importance of a statistical test result is limited for two reasons:

1) A threshold value (e.g., 0.05) is arbitrary; and,
2) There are other means by which to evaluate the importance of a study's result using continuous values—specifically, the confidence interval.[11]

These authors contend that the context of the study, along with other available evidence, is as important as the p-value for determining whether the results are meaningful. Furthermore, p-values considerably lower than 0.05 (e.g., 0.001) are more convincing that the null hypothesis can be rejected.

Confidence Intervals

By comparison, the *confidence interval* is a range of scores within which the true score for a variable is estimated to lie.[3] Narrower intervals mean less variability in the data. The thresholds for confidence intervals are the probability levels within which they are calculated, the typical values of which are 90 percent, 95 percent and 99 percent. If investigators select a 95% confidence interval (95% CI)—the traditional value utilized—then they are indicating the range within which there is a 95 percent probability that the true value for the population is located. Sim and Reid point out that a confidence interval provides information about statistical significance, while also characterizing a statistical result's precision and accuracy.[12] An interval that includes the value "zero" indicates that the null hypothesis—"there is no difference (relationship)"—cannot be rejected. Furthermore, a narrow interval range (e.g., 95 percent) indicates that the result obtained is close to the true value (precision), while a wider interval range (e.g., 99 percent) increases the chance the population value will be included (accuracy). These confidence intervals are consistent with p-values of 0.05 and 0.01, respectively. In both instances, an evidence-based physical therapist can read the information provided and accept or reject the importance of the result based on its statistical significance; but the confidence interval provides the additional information about the range of possible population values.

The debate about the appropriateness of p-values likely will continue for the foreseeable future. An evidence-based physical therapist's job is to understand the information provided about p-values and/or confidence intervals because the relative objectivity of these values is an important counterbalance to the subjective human appraisal of the same results.

Power

Statistical significance is dependent in part upon a study's sample size. Investigators have a vested interest in determining the number of subjects that are required in order to detect a significant result. *Power* is the probability that a statistical test will detect, if present, a relationship between two or more variables or a difference between two or more groups.[1,3] Failure to achieve adequate power will result in a *Type II error*, a situation in which the null hypothesis is accepted incorrectly (a false negative). Fortunately, investigators can identify the minimum sample size required for their study by conducting a power analysis. This technique requires investigators to select their desired alpha level, effect size, and power. The threshold for power often is set at 0.80, which translates into a 20 percent chance of committing a Type II error.[2] Software programs designed to perform these analyses will calculate the number of subjects required to achieve these criteria. Essentially, the larger the sample size the greater the opportunity to detect a meaningful difference or relationship if it is present. p-Values will be lower and confidence intervals will be narrower when adequate sample sizes are obtained.

CLINICAL RELEVANCE

As noted, statistical tests along with their obtained p-values and confidence intervals help researchers and evidence-based physical therapists objectively evaluate the data collected from subjects. The next challenge is to determine whether the study's results are useful from a clinical perspective. As an example, imagine a study in which investigators examine the effectiveness of an aerobic exercise program on the functional exercise capacity of elderly subjects as measured using a graded treadmill test. One possible result of the study is that a statistically significant difference (e.g., $p < 0.05$) is found between subjects in the exercise group as compared to subjects in a "usual activity" group. If the change in performance in the exercise group amounts to five additional minutes on the treadmill, then most people would probably agree that a clinically meaningful improvement occurred. On the other hand, if the exercise group only gains one-and-a-half additional minutes on the treadmill, then this finding may not translate into an improvement in subjects' ability to perform daily tasks, despite the statistical significance of the finding. In other words, the results would not be clinically relevant.

An alternative scenario is that the study's results produce a p-value greater than the threshold for significance (e.g., $p > 0.05$). If the exercise group increased its treadmill time by five minutes, but the p-value equaled 0.08, evidence-based physical therapists might still be inclined to try the aerobic exercise program with their patients. In other words, therapists might be willing to accept an increased probability (8 percent versus 5 percent) that the study's results occurred due to chance because an additional five minutes of exercise capacity might translate into improved household mobility. Researchers sometimes acknowledge the potential for this type of scenario by using the phrase "a trend toward significance." As noted in the previous section, debate continues regarding which p-value represents the best threshold for statistical significance. A confidence interval may provide additional insights if the researchers provide this information; however, the statistical result is the same (e.g., 0.05 and 95% CI). Ultimately, evidence-based physical therapists will have to weigh all of the information in their own minds in order to make a decision about applying the evidence to patient/client management.

SUMMARY

Statistics are tools researchers use to understand and evaluate the data they collect from subjects. As is true for clinical tools, statistical tests have defined purposes, indications for their use, specified methods for their application, and limitations or caveats regarding their performance. They also provide information in a particular form. These tools are designed to describe, to answer questions about differences and relationships, and to provide insight into the usefulness of diagnostic tests, prognostic indicators, and outcomes measures. The importance of statistical results is evaluated through the use of probabilities and confidence intervals. Evidence-based physical therapists must use their clinical judgment and expertise to determine whether statistical findings will be relevant to clinical practice.

Exercises

Questions 1–3 pertain to the following scenario:

Study Hypothesis: "Calcium consumption is associated with osteoporosis in post-menopausal women."

Alpha Level: ≤ 0.05

Results: (n = 75 subjects)

Subject Age (years)

Mean	56.6
Median	61.2
Std. Deviation	8.43
Range	32–97
$\chi^2 = 5.46$	$p = 0.07$

	Osteoporosis (+)	Osteoporosis (−)
<1000 mg CA^{2+}	25	22
>1000 mg CA^{2+}	12	16

1) What type of statistical test is being used in this scenario?
   a) Chi-squared test
   b) Spearman rank correlation
   c) Two-way analysis of variance
   d) Wilcoxon rank sum test
2) Based on the results reported, you would expect the study's authors to:
   a) Accept the hypothesis
   b) Consider the hypothesis proven
   c) Reject the hypothesis
   d) None of the above
3) These results conflict with numerous other studies using larger sample sizes. What type of error most likely occurred to cause this discrepancy?
   a) Math error
   b) Test choice error
   c) Type I error
   d) Type II error

Questions 4–5 pertain to the following scenario:

Study Question: "Does patient gender predict the use of thrombolytic therapy ("clot busters") for patients presenting to the emergency room with signs of stroke?"

Variables and Measures: Gender = male or female   Age = years
Clot busters = yes or no

4) What kind of statistical analysis should be used to answer the actual question posed?
   a) Descriptive statistics
   b) Test of differences
   c) Test of relationships
   d) None of the above
5) Which statistical test would be most appropriate to analyze the question posed?
   a) Logistic regression
   b) Linear regression
   c) Pearson product moment correlation
   d) Spearman rank correlation coefficient

Questions 6–8 pertain to the following scenario:

Study Question: "Will weight decrease in mildly obese teenagers as a result of an 8-week high protein, low carbohydrate diet, plus exercise?"

Alpha level: ≤ 0.05

Results: (n = 10)   weight = pounds

Subject	Weight 1	Weight 2
1	211	194
2	173	169
3	186	170
4	165	172
.	.	.
.	.	.
.	.	.
10	201	195
	$\bar{x}_1 = 188.2$	$\bar{x}_2 = 180$

6) Which statistical test is most appropriate to analyze this data?
   a) Independent t-test
   b) One-way ANOVA test
   c) Paired t-test
   d) Two-way ANOVA test
7) The statistical test returns an obtained p-value of 0.243. Based on these results you would conclude:
   a) Diet plus exercise affects weight
   b) Diet plus exercise does not affect weight
   c) The findings are irrelevant
   d) The findings are not plausible
8) This study represents a:
   a) Between-groups analysis with dependent measures
   b) Between-groups analysis with independent measures
   c) Within-group analysis with dependent measures
   d) Within-group analysis with independent measures

Questions 9–11 pertain to the following scenario:

A sampling distribution of data indicates a mean = 63 and a 95 percent confidence interval of 32 to 100.

9) The 95 percent confidence interval indicates the probability that the obtained mean is:
   a) Between 32 and 100
   b) Less than 32
   c) More than 100
   d) Zero
10) The wide confidence interval suggests that the variability in the distribution is:
   a) Absent
   b) High

c) Irrelevant
d) Low

11) The standard deviation of the error terms in this sampling distribution is referred to as the:
    a) Power
    b) Range
    c) Standard error of the mean
    d) Standard error of the measure

Questions 12–13 pertain to the following scenario:

Study Question: "What is the effect of hours of daylight and depression on exercise frequency?"

Depression: Depressed or not depressed based on inventory score threshold
Hours of Daylight: 8 or 12
Exercise (F)requency: Times per week
Alpha Level: ≤ 0.01
Results: (n = 100)

	F	p- value
Daylight Hours	10.62	0.001
Depression	4.89	0.263
Hours x Depression	13.21	0.03

12) What type of statistical test is used in this study?
    a) One-way ANOVA test
    b) Two-way ANOVA test
    c) Three-way ANOVA test
    d) None of the above

13) How would you interpret the results presented above?
    a) Depression affects exercise frequency
    b) Hours of daylight affects exercise frequency
    c) There is no interaction effect
    d) b and c

Questions 14–16 pertain to the following scenario:

Study Question: "Can length of hospital stay following total hip replacement be predicted by patient demographic and clinical characteristics?"

- n = 200 total hip replacement cases from one Boston hospital
- Length of stay (LOS) = Number of days in the hospital

Alpha Level: ≤ 0.05

Patient Demographics	Patient Clinical Characteristics
Age (years)	Post-op hemoglobin (deciliters)

Gender (1 = female, 0 = other)
Race (1 = white, 0 = other)
Post-op white blood cell count (deciliters)
Nausea (1 = yes, 0 = no)

(β)		Std. Betas	p-value
0.417	AGE	0.251	0.020
−0.103	GENDER	0.102	0.171
0.893	RACE	0.015	0.082
−1.430	HEMOGLOBIN	0.269	0.050
2.590	WHITE BLOOD CELLS	0.182	0.001
0.960	NAUSEA	0.003	0.040

Constant = 3.9

14) The statistical test used in this study is a:
   a) Multiple linear regression
   b) Multiple logistic regression
   c) Simple linear regression
   d) Simple logistic regression

15) The negative sign in front of the unstandardized beta for hemoglobin implies that:
   a) As hemoglobin goes down, length of stay goes down
   b) As hemoglobin goes up, length of stay goes down
   c) As hemoglobin goes up, length of stay goes up
   d) Hemoglobin does not influence length of stay

16) How would you interpret the standardized beta results and p-value for nausea?
   a) Not statistically significant but important
   b) Not statistically significant and unimportant
   c) Statistically significant with maximal influence on LOS
   d) Statistically significant with minimal influence on LOS

References

1. Portney LG, Watkins MP. *Foundations of Clinical Research: Applications to Practice.* 2d ed. Upper Saddle River, NJ: Prentice Hall Health; 2000.
2. Polit DF, Beck CT. *Nursing Research: Principles and Methods.* 7th ed. Philadelphia, PA: Lippincott Williams & Wilkins; 2003.
3. Domholdt E. *Rehabilitation Research: Principles and Applications.* 3d ed. St Louis, MO: Elsevier Saunders; 2005.
4. Munro BH. *Statistical Methods for Health Care Research.* 5th ed. Philadelphia, PA: Lippincott Williams and Wilkins; 2005.
5. Herbert R, Jamtvedt G, Mead J, Hagen KB. *Practical Evidence-Based Physical Therapy.* Edinburgh, Scotland: Elsevier Butterworth Heinemann; 2005.
6. Straus SE, Richardson WS, Glaziou P, Haynes RB. *Evidence-Based Medicine: How to Practice and Teach EBM.* 3d ed. Edinburgh, Scotland: Elsevier Churchill Livingstone; 2005.

7. Batavia M. *Clinical Research for Health Professionals: A User-Friendly Guide*. Boston, MA: Butterworth-Heinemann; 2001.
8. Mini Mental State Exam. Available at: http://www.hartfordign.org/publications/trythis/issue03.pdf. Accessed March 1, 2006.
9. Disability of the Arm, Shoulder & Hand (DASH). Available at: http://www.dash.iwh.on.ca/assets/images/pdfs/dash_quest.pdf. Accessed March 1, 2006.
10. Helewa A, Walker JM. *Critical Evaluation of Research in Physical Rehabilitation: Towards Evidence-Based Practice*. Philadelphia, PA: WB Saunders & Company; 2000.
11. Sterne JAC, Smith GD. Sifting the evidence—what's wrong with significance tests? *BMJ*. 2001; 322(7280):226–231.
12. Sim J, Reid N. Statistical inference by confidence intervals: Issues of interpretation and utilization. *Phys Ther*. 1999; 79(2):186–195.

Part III

Appraising the Evidence

Chapter 10

Appraising Evidence About Diagnostic Tests

One of the most widespread diseases is diagnosis.

—Karl Kraus

OBJECTIVES

Upon completion of this chapter the student/practitioner will be able to:

1. Discuss the purposes and processes of diagnosis and differential diagnosis in physical therapy.
2. Critically evaluate evidence about diagnostic tests including:
   a. Important questions to ask related to research validity; and
   b. Measurement properties of reliability and validity.
3. Interpret and apply information provided by the following calculations:
   a) Sensitivity;
   b) Specificity;
   c) Positive and negative predictive values;
   d) Positive and negative likelihood ratios;
   e) Pre- and posttest probabilities;
   f) Test threshold;
   g) Treatment threshold.
4. Evaluate p-values and confidence intervals to determine the potential importance of reported findings.
5. Discuss considerations related to the application of evidence about diagnostic tests to individual patients/clients.

Terms in This Chapter

Bias: Results or inferences that systematically deviate from the truth "or the processes leading to such deviation."[1(p. 251)]

Concurrent Validity: A method of criterion validation that reflects the relationship between a measure of interest and a criterion ("gold standard") measure, both of which have been applied within the same time frame.[2]

Confidence Interval: A range of scores within which the true score for a variable is estimated to lie within a specified probability (e.g., 90%, 95%, 99%).[2]

Criterion Validity: The degree to which a measure of interest relates to an external criterion measure.[3]

Diagnosis: "A process that integrates and evaluates data" obtained during a patient/client examination, often resulting in a classification that guides prognosis, the plan of care and subsequent interventions.[4(p. 45),5]

Differential Diagnosis: A process for distinguishing among "a set of diagnoses that can plausibly explain the patient/client's presentation."[6(p. 673)]

Face Validity: A subjective assessment of the degree to which an instrument appears to measure what it is designed to measure.[7]

Gold Standard (or Reference Standard): A diagnostic test or measure that provides a definitive diagnosis.[1]

Masked (Blinded): In diagnosis studies, the lack of knowledge of prior test results.

Measurement Reliability: The extent to which repeated measurements agree with one another. Also referred to as "stability," "consistency," and "reproducibility."[7]

Measurement Validity: The degree to which a measure captures what it is intended to measure.[7]

Negative Likelihood Ratio: The likelihood that a negative test result will be obtained in a patient/client with the condition of interest as compared to a patient/client without the condition of interest.[8]

Negative Predictive Value (NPV): The proportion of patients/clients with a negative test result who do not have the condition of interest.[9]

Pretest Probability: The odds (probability) that a patient/client has a condition based on clinical presentation before a diagnostic test is conducted.[9]

Positive Likelihood Ratio: The likelihood that a positive test result will be obtained in a patient/client with the condition of interest as compared to a patient/client without the condition of interest.[8]

Positive Predictive Value (PPV): The proportion of patients/clients with a positive test result who have the condition of interest.[9]

Posttest Probability: The odds (probability) that a patient/client has a condition based on the result of a diagnostic test.[9]

Prevalence: Proportion of individuals with a condition of interest at a given point in time.[6]

p-value: The probability that a statistical finding occurred due to chance.

Reference Standard: See "Gold Standard."

Sensitivity: The proportion of individuals with the condition of interest that have a positive test result. Also referred to as "true positives."[9]

Specificity: The proportion of individuals without the condition of interest who have a negative test result. Also referred to as "true negatives."[9]

Standard Error of Measurement (SEM): "The standard deviation of measurement errors" obtained from repeated measures.[2(p. 560)]

Test Threshold: The probability below which a physical therapist determines that a suspected condition is unlikely and forgoes diagnostic testing.[6]

Treatment Threshold: The probability above which a physical therapist determines that a diagnosis is likely and forgoes further testing in order to initiate treatment.[6]

INTRODUCTION

Diagnosis is a process in which patient data are collected and evaluated in order to classify a condition, determine prognosis, and identify possible interventions.[4,5] *Differential diagnosis* is the method by which doctors (of medicine, physical therapy, and so on) use information to make decisions between two or more alternatives to explain why their patient has a set of signs and symptoms.[6] In both cases, the conclusions reached are informed by results from the patient history, clinical examination, and associated diagnostic tests.

Diagnostic tests have three potential purposes in physical therapy 1) to help focus the examination in a particular body region or system; 2) to identify potential problems that require physician referral; and, 3) to assist in the classification process.[10] The decision to perform a diagnostic test rests on a clinician's estimation of the probability that a patient has the condition that is suspected based on clinical examination findings and relevant subjective history. In Figure 10-1, Guyatt and Rennie describe a continuum of probabilities from 0 to 100 percent along which are two decision points: the "test threshold" and the "treatment threshold."[6]

The *test threshold* is the probability below which a diagnostic test will not be ordered because the possibility of the particular diagnosis is so remote. The *treatment threshold* is the probability above which a test will not be ordered because the possibility of the particular diagnosis is so great that immediate treatment is indicated. Fritz and Wainner refer to this decision

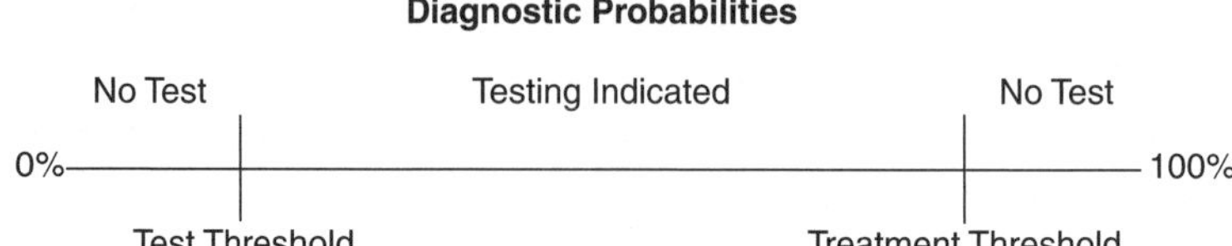

Figure 10–1 Diagnostic test and treatment thresholds.

Reprinted from *Users' Guides to the Medical Literature*, Gordan Guyatt and Drummon Rennie, Chapter 1C, Copyright (2002), with permission from the American Medical Association.

point as the "action threshold."[10] In between these two decision points are the probabilities for which administering a test or tests is indicated in order to rule in or rule out the suspected diagnosis.

Successful diagnosis and differential diagnosis depend, in part, on the availability and use of tests that are reliable and valid. A test that has demonstrated *measurement reliability* produces stable results over time, while a test that has demonstrated *measurement validity* is said to capture correctly what it is supposed to be measuring.[7] Physical therapists primarily use clinical tests to examine their patients/clients, although the latitude to order imaging studies and other diagnostic tests is granted to those in military practice. Civilian therapists also may have opportunities to recommend diagnostic tests during consultations. In either case, a physical therapist should consider the evidence about tests in order to improve the quality, safety, and efficiency of care and to support the patient/client's values and preferences.

STUDY CREDIBILITY

Evidence pertaining to tests physical therapists use first should be evaluated with an assessment of its research validity. Higher research validity provides greater confidence that a study's findings are believable. Appraisal of evidence about tests starts with the questions itemized in Table 10–1. These questions are adapted from the critical appraisal worksheets developed by the Oxford Center for Evidence-Based Medicine.[11] Their purpose is to help physical therapists determine whether there are problems with a study's design that may have biased the results.[9]

1. **Did the investigators compare results from the test of interest to results from a gold (or reference) standard test?**

   This question addresses the need to confirm a diagnosis via a gold standard test, such as a radiographic image, laboratory result, or surgical or autopsy finding.[1] A *gold standard* (or *reference standard*) test

Table 10–1 Questions to assess the validity of evidence about diagnostic tests and measures.

1. Did the investigators compare results from the test of interest to results from a gold (or reference) standard test?
2. Were the individuals performing and interpreting each test's results unaware (i.e., masked, or blinded) of the other test's results?
3. Did the investigators include subjects with all levels or stages of the condition being evaluated by the diagnostic test of interest?
4. Did all subjects undergo the gold standard diagnostic test?
5. Did the investigators repeat the study with a new set of subjects?

should have superior capability because of its technological features and/or its own track record of reliability and validity. In addition, the purpose and potential outcomes of the gold standard test should be consistent with the purpose and outcomes of the diagnostic test of interest.[10] Performing an x-ray to assess the usefulness of a functional balance scale would not be a meaningful comparison despite the technological superiority of radiography. Comparison to an appropriate gold standard test allows researchers to verify the measurement validity of the diagnostic test of interest. Readers should be aware, however, that the true usefulness of the gold standard itself often cannot be verified because a reference against which to compare it does not exist. At a minimum, face validity of the gold standard test is essential in these cases. The possibility that the gold standard will be replaced over time as technology evolves also should be acknowledged.[8]

2. **Were the individuals performing and interpreting each test's results unaware (i.e., masked, or blinded) of the other test's results?**

   Ideally, the diagnostic test of interest and the gold standard test will be applied to subjects by examiners who are *masked* (or *blinded*). Masking the individuals responsible for administering the different tests further enhances validity by minimizing tester *bias*. In other words, the possibility is reduced that a positive or negative finding will occur on one test as a result of knowledge of another test's result.

3. **Did the investigators include subjects with all levels or stages of the condition being evaluated by the diagnostic test of interest?**

   This question focuses on the utility of the test in various clinical scenarios. For example, different levels of severity may characterize the condition of interest such that the identification of each level is essential to guide prognosis and treatment. An example relevant to physical therapy is the use of grades to rank the severity of ligament damage that has occurred during a lateral ankle sprain. Grade I represents minimal tearing with maintenance of full function and strength. Grade II reflects a partial ligament tear with mild joint laxity and functional loss. Grade III indicates a full thickness ligament tear with complete joint laxity and functional loss.[12] Each of these levels requires a progressively greater treatment intensity and recovery time; therefore, it is preferable that a diagnostic test be evaluated for its ability to differentiate among these grades. The ability of the test to distinguish between those who have been treated for the ankle sprain and those who have not also is helpful to assess the patient's progress. Finally, a test that can discriminate among other similar conditions (e.g., fracture, tendonopathy) will be useful in the differential diagnostic process.[1,10]

4. **Did all subjects undergo the gold standard diagnostic test?**
   This question clarifies the degree to which the investigators may have introduced bias into the study by administering the gold standard test to a select group of subjects previously evaluated by the test of interest. This selective evaluation may occur in situations in which the gold standard is expensive and/or when subjects are judged to have a low probability of having the condition of interest.[10] The ability of a test to identify correctly someone with (or without) the condition will be misleading if only those subjects who tested positive are followed up with the gold standard. Specifically, the diagnostic accuracy of the test of interest may be overestimated in these situations.
5. **Did investigators repeat the study with a new set of subjects?**
   This question alludes to the possibility that the research findings regarding a diagnostic test occurred due to chance. Repeating the study on a second group of subjects who match the inclusion and exclusion criteria outlined for the first group provides an opportunity to evaluate the consistency (or lack thereof) of the test's performance. Often this step is not included in a single research report due to insufficient numbers of subjects and/or lack of funds. As a result, evidence-based physical therapists must read several pieces of evidence about the same diagnostic test if they wish to verify its usefulness to a greater degree.

Additional Considerations

Additional concerns pertaining to research design in evidence about diagnostic tests include the presence or absence of a detailed description of the:

1. Setting in which the research was conducted;
2. Inclusion and exclusion criteria used to select subjects; and,
3. Protocol for the test(s) used, including scoring methods.

This information allows evidence-based physical therapists to determine if the clinical test of interest is applicable and feasible in their environment (1, 3) and if the subjects included resemble the patient/client about whom there is a question (2).

Most of these questions serve as an initial screening of the evidence to determine its potential usefulness—that is, its research validity. Readers should note that these same screening questions may be asked about methodologic studies of measures physical therapists use to quantify impairments and functional limitations. Herbert *et al.* suggest that research articles that fail to meet many of the criteria indicated by these questions should be set aside and a new evidence search initiated when possible.[8] In the absence of this opportunity, the evidence should be considered carefully in light of its limitations, especially when a test or measure of interest is associated with a significant degree of risk to the patient/client.

STUDY RESULTS

Reliability

Evidence-based practice relies on tests of relationships to determine reliability of tests and measures. Verification of reliability is an acknowledgement that all measures are scores that are composed of the "true value" and error. Error may be the result of the subject, the observer, the instrument itself, and/or the environment in which the test or measure was performed.[2,7] A correct diagnosis depends in part on the ability to minimize error during the testing process to avoid a false positive or false negative result. Investigators also use tests of relationships to demonstrate the intra- or interrater reliability of their test administrators. The need to demonstrate that those collecting the data can do so in a reproducible manner over many subjects is driven by the threat to research validity known as "instrumentation" (Chapter 8).

Examples of statistics commonly used in physical therapy research about tests and measures include the *standard error of measurement (SEM)*, the Pearson's Product Moment Correlation (r), the Intraclass Correlation Coefficient (ICC), Spearman's rho (ρ), and Kappa (κ). As noted in Chapter 9, all of these tests assess the strength of the association between measures collected on patients or research subjects. The first two tests are designed for use with interval or ratio level data, while the second two are designed for use with ordinal and nominal data, respectively. Pearson's r and Spearman's rho compare only two measures, while the ICC and Kappa can be used to compare multiple pairs of measures simultaneously. Portney and Watkins offer the following criteria by which to judge the strength of the correlation coefficient:[7(p. 494)]

- 0.00–0.25 little or no relationship
- 0.26–0.50 fair degree of relationship
- 0.51–0.75 moderate to good relationship
- 0.76–1.00 good to excellent relationship

A p-value or confidence interval also may be used to assess the statistical significance and clinical usefulness of the relationship tested.

Validity

The validity of diagnostic tests or measures may be evaluated from several perspectives. The first approach is to consider the *face validity* of the instrument or technique. A test evaluating lower extremity muscle performance would not have face validity for assessing ligament integrity. The second approach is to assess statistically the relationship between results from the test or measure of interest and the results from the gold standard test or measure. The statistical tests described in the previous section also apply here. Higher correlation coefficients indicate greater correspondence between the results of the different tests. In other words, the test of interest provides the same information as the gold standard. This statistical approach is used to verify *criterion validity* or *concurrent validity*, or both.[2,3]

Finally, measurement validity may be evaluated through mathematical calculations based on a two-by-two (2 × 2) table (Figure 10–2). A 2 × 2 table is

	+ Lung Cancer	– Lung Cancer
+ Smoking	A	B
– Smoking	C	D

Figure 10–2 A 2 × 2 table used for epidemiological research on smoking and lung cancer.

the basis for the Chi-square test of association and is a commonly used method of classifying nominal data in epidemiological studies that are evaluating the association between a risk factor and disease. The classic example of this scenario is the association between cigarette smoking and lung cancer.

Figure 10–2 should be interpreted in the following manner:

- Cell (a) represents the individuals who smoked and who developed lung cancer;
- Cell (b) represents individuals who smoked and did not develop lung cancer;
- Cell (c) represents people who did not smoke and who developed lung cancer; and,
- Cell (d) represents people who did not smoke and who did not develop lung cancer.

The 2 × 2 table is easily adapted for evaluation of diagnostic tests by changing the labels for the rows to reflect a positive diagnostic test result and a negative diagnostic test result, respectively.

A valid diagnostic test will consistently produce true positives or true negatives, or both.[1] In addition, the test will produce information that allows the physical therapist to adjust his or her estimate of the probability that a patient has the condition of interest. The following mathematical calculations based on the 2 × 2 table in Figure 10–3 are used to determine whether a diagnostic test meets these standards.

Sensitivity

A diagnostic test is said to be *sensitive* when it is capable of correctly classifying individuals with the condition of interest (true positives).[9] This information allows evidence-based physical therapists to determine which test may be most appropriate to use when a particular condition is sus-

	+ Disorder	− Disorder
+ Test Result	True Positives (a)	False Positives (b)
− Test Result	False Negatives (c)	True Negatives (d)

Figure 10–3 A 2 × 2 table used for the evaluation of diagnostic tests.

pected. Most authors provide the value for sensitivity (0–100%) of the test they evaluated; however, the sensitivity also can be calculated using the following formula:

$$\text{Sensitivity} = \frac{\text{Patients with the condition who test positive (a)}}{\text{All patients with condition (a+c)}}$$

There is an important caveat for tests that are highly sensitive (good at detecting people with a condition): when a negative result is obtained using a highly sensitive test, then a clinician can say with confidence that the condition can be ruled out. In other words, false positives are so unlikely that the test will catch most, if not all, of those individuals with the condition. Therefore, a negative test result for a highly sensitive test indicates the person is condition-free. Sackett *et al.* developed the mnemonic **SnNout** (Sn = sensitive test, N = negative result, out = rule out disorder) to help remember this caveat.[13]

Specificity

A diagnostic test is said to be *specific* when it is capable of correctly classifying individuals without the condition of interest (true negatives).[9] Like sensitivity, specificity indicates which test may be appropriate to use for a suspected condition. Most authors provide the value for specificity (0–100%) of the test they evaluated; however, the specificity also can be calculated from the 2 × 2 table:

$$\text{Specificity} = \frac{\text{Patients without the condition who test negative (d)}}{\text{All patients without the condition (b+d)}}$$

There is an important caveat for tests that are highly specific (good at detecting people without the condition): when a positive result is obtained using this test then a clinician can say with confidence that the condition can be ruled in. In other words, false negatives are so unlikely that the test will catch most, if not all, of those individuals without the condition. Therefore, a positive test result for a highly specific test indicates a person has the condition. The mnemonic **SpPin** (Sp = specific test, P = positive test result, in = rule in disorder) is the reminder about this situation.[13]

Receiver Operating Characteristic (ROC) Curves

Unfortunately, sensitivity and specificity have limited usefulness for two reasons 1) they indicate a test's performance in individuals whose status is known (e.g., they have or do not have the condition); and, 2) they reduce the information about the test to a choice of two options based on the threshold, or cut point, according to which a result is classified as positive or negative. Different test cut points require recalculation of sensitivity and specificity, a situation that is inefficient when a range of test scores may indicate a range of severity of a condition.[1]

One way to improve the usefulness of sensitivity and specificity calculations is the creation of a ROC curve. An ROC curve is a graphical way to evaluate different test scores with respect to the number of true positive and false positive results obtained at each threshold or cut point. In effect, the curve allows an investigator to identify the signal to noise ratio of any score the diagnostic test can produce.[7] This is a much more efficient approach than creating a 2 × 2 table for each possible diagnostic test value.

An ROC curve is plotted in a box, the y-axis of which represents the test's sensitivity or true positive rate and the x-axis of which represents 1 − specificity or the false positive rate. A perfect test will only have true positive results, so it will not matter what test score is selected as a threshold to determine the presence of a condition. When that happens, the ROC curve essentially stays along the y-axis (Figure 10–4).

Diagnostic tests are rarely perfect—an ROC curve typically starts along the y-axis, but eventually bends away from it and trails out along the x-axis. In these cases, a curve that reflects more true positives than false positives or greater signal to noise will fill the box (Figure 10–5).

If the curve is a perfect diagonal line, then the diagnostic test produces the same number of true positive and false positive results for any score and the determination of a diagnosis is reduced to a coin flip (Figure 10–6).

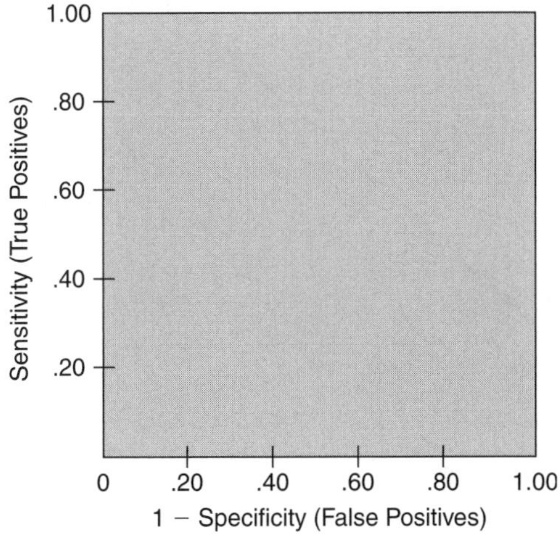

Figure 10–4 A Receiver Operating Characteristic (ROC) curve for a perfect test.

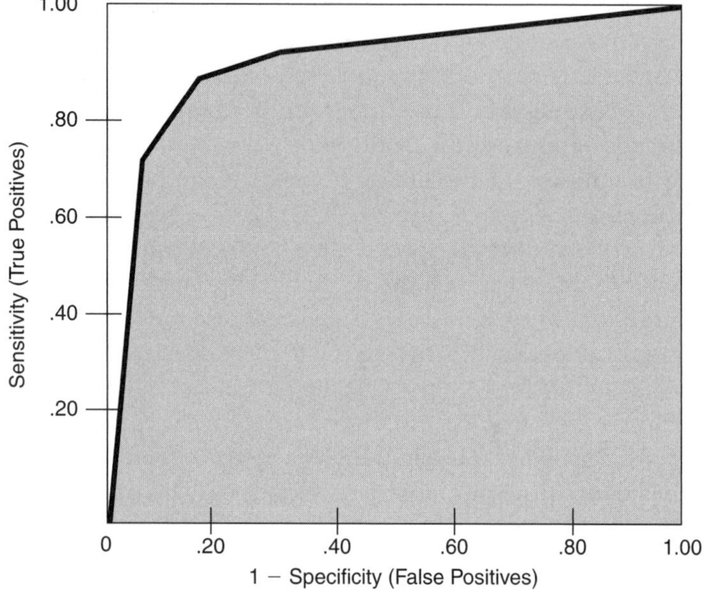

Figure 10–5 A Receiver Operating Characteristic (ROC) curve for an imperfect but useful test.

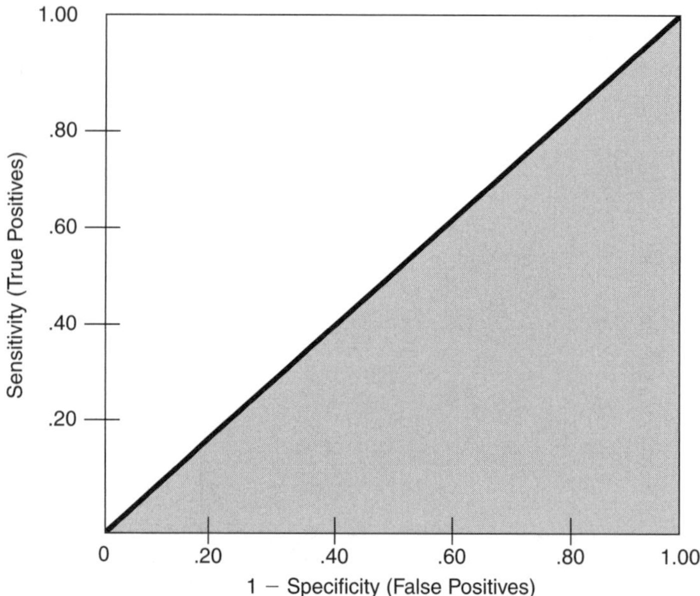

Figure 10–6 A Receiver Operating Characteristic (ROC) curve for a test with results equal to chance.

Investigators examine the curve to determine its area and to identify the most useful cut point or points among the available diagnostic test scores. The area under the curve simply represents the true and false positives for each and every score obtained on the diagnostic test or for specific cut points that the investigators wish to evaluate. A higher true positive rate results in a bigger area under the curve. Assuming an imperfect test, the threshold score is the point at which the curve starts to bend away from the y-axis because that is the point when the false positive rate starts to increase. In other words, that is the point at which the diagnostic test provides the most information about people who have the problem and people who do not.

Positive Predictive Value

The *positive predictive value* (PPV) describes the ability of a diagnostic test to correctly determine the proportion of patients with the disease from all of the patients with positive test results.[9] This value is consistent with clinical decision making in which a test result is used to judge whether or not a patient has the condition of interest.[10] Most authors provide the PPV (0–100 percent) of the test they evaluated; however, the PPV also can be calculated from the 2 × 2 table:

$$\text{Positive Predictive Value} = \frac{\text{Patients with the condition who test positive (a)}}{\text{All patients with positive test results (a+b)}}$$

Negative Predictive Value

The *negative predictive value* (NPV) describes the ability of a diagnostic test to correctly determine the proportion of patients without the disease from all of the patients with negative test results.[9] This value also is consistent with the clinical decision-making process. Most authors provide the NPV (0–100 percent) of the test they evaluated; however, the NPV also can be calculated from the 2 × 2 table:

$$\text{Negative Predictive Value} = \frac{\text{Patients without the condition who test negative (d)}}{\text{All patients with negative test results (c+d)}}$$

There is an important caveat regarding the positive and negative predictive values of diagnostic tests—these values will change based on the overall prevalence of the condition. In other words, the PPV and NPV reported in a study will apply only to scenarios in which the proportion of individuals with the condition is the same as that used in the study. *Prevalence* may change over time as preventive measures or better treatments are implemented. For these reasons, the PPV and NPV generally are not as useful as other measures of diagnostic validity.[14]

Likelihood Ratios

Likelihood ratios are another method by which to establish the validity of a diagnostic test. There are three advantages to using likelihood ratios. First, the ratios can be calculated for all levels of test results (not just positive and negative). Second, they are not dependent on the prevalence of the condition in the population.[9] Third, the ratios can be applied to individual patients/clients, whereas sensitivity, specificity, and positive and negative predictive values, refer to groups.

A *positive likelihood ratio* (LR+) indicates the likelihood that a positive test result was obtained in a person with the condition as compared to a person without the condition. A *negative likelihood ratio* (LR−) indicates the likelihood that a negative test result was observed in a person with the condition as compared to a person without the condition.[8] Likelihood ratios have values greater than or equal to zero. An LR+ will have values greater than one. An LR− will have values less than one. A test with a likelihood ratio equal to one is said to produce a result that is no better than chance (e.g., a coin flip) in terms of identifying whether a person is likely to have, or not have the condition.[14]

Most authors provide the likelihood ratio of the test they evaluated; however, the ratio also can be calculated from the 2 × 2 table or when authors provide sensitivity and specificity information:

$$\text{LR+} = \frac{\text{Sensitivity}}{1 - \text{Specificity}} \text{ or } \frac{(a/a+c)}{[1-(d/b+d)]}$$

$$\text{LR−} = \frac{1 - \text{Sensitivity}}{\text{Specificity}} \text{ or } \frac{[1-(a/a+c)]}{(d/b+d)}$$

Using Likelihood Ratios in Practice

A test's likelihood ratio can be applied in clinical practice with the use of a nomogram as depicted in Figure 10-7.[15]

The nomogram helps a clinician determine whether performing the test will provide enough additional information to be worth the risk and expense of conducting the procedure on a specific patient/client. Use of a nomogram requires the following steps:

- *Determine the patient/client's pretest probability of the condition*

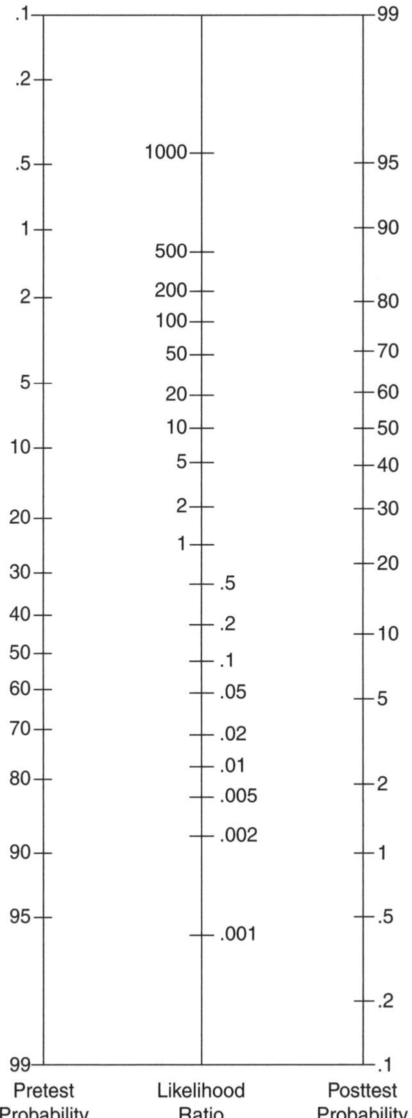

Figure 10–7 A nomogram.

Source: Fagan TJ. Nomogram for Bayes's theorem. *N Engl J Med.* 1975; 293:257.

This step requires physical therapists to estimate the proportion of individuals who have the condition they suspect based on the data gathered during the patient/client history and initial examination. This estimate is a percentage value and can be determined by:

1. The known prevalence of the condition in the population (per epidemiological studies);
2. The known prevalence of the condition in patients/clients referred to the therapist's clinic; or,
3. Gut instinct about the probability this patient/client has the problem.

The proportion should be identified on the line on the left hand side of the nomogram labeled *pretest probability*.

- *Identify the likelihood ratio for the test*

The likelihood ratio is identified from the best available evidence and should be identified on the middle line of the nomogram.

- *Connect the dots*

A straight edge should be used to draw a line from the pretest probability through the likelihood ratio for the test to the line on the right of the nomogram entitled *posttest probability*. This value also is expressed as a percentage and indicates the probability that the patient/client has the condition of interest now that a test result has been obtained.

Guyatt and Rennie provide the following guidelines for interpreting likelihood ratios:[6(pp. 128–129)]

- LR+ > 10 or LR− < 0.10 = large and conclusive change from pre- to posttest probability;
- LR+ = 5–10 or LR− = 0.10–0.20 = moderate change from pre- to posttest probability;
- LR+ = 2–5 or LR− = 0.20–0.50 = small, but sometimes important change from pre- to posttest probability;
- LR+ = 1–2 or LR− = 0.50–1.0 = negligible change in pretest probability.

Evaluating a Diagnostic Test—Calculations Based on Study Results

The following is an illustration of the use of a 2 × 2 table and nomogram with results from an actual study about a diagnostic test. Van Dijk *et al.* examined the usefulness of delayed physical examination for the diagnosis of ankle sprains resulting in ligament rupture.[16] Confirmation of the diagnosis was obtained through arthrography. One of the clinical procedures performed to assess the integrity of the anterior talofibular ligament was the anterior drawer test. Figure 10-8 is a 2 × 2 table with results from the anterior drawer test and the arthrography.

	+ Ligature Rupture	− Ligature Rupture
+ Anterior Drawer	90	9
− Anterior Drawer	27	28

Figure 10–8 Anterior drawer test and arthrography results from van Dijk *et al.*[13]

Calculations using these data produce the following values for sensitivity, specificity, positive and negative predictive values, and likelihood ratios.

Sensitivity	90/117	= 0.77
Specificity	28/37	= 0.76
Positive Predictive Value	90/99	= 0.91
Negative Predictive Value	28/55	= 0.51
+ Likelihood Ratio	.0.77/1-0.76	= 3.21
− Likelihood Ratio	0.23/0.76	= 0.31

The authors concluded that, based on these results and data from other examination procedures, a delayed physical examination was sufficient to diagnose an ankle ligament rupture and was less invasive (and presumably less costly) than arthrography.

Figure 10–9 illustrates an application of the likelihood ratios using a nomogram. The prevalence of ligament rupture in the study was 76 percent; therefore, this value serves as the pretest probability in this example. The light gray line indicates that a positive likelihood ratio of 3.2 increases the probability that an individual has a ligament tear to approximately 92 percent, while the dark gray line indicates that a negative likelihood ratio of 0.30 decreases the probability that an individual has a ligament tear to approximately 38 percent. Assuming this study's research validity is sound, these changes in the pretest probability are large enough to suggest that the anterior drawer test is a worthwhile procedure to perform when a lateral ankle sprain is suspected.

Practical Use of Likelihood Ratios

Using a nomogram may be helpful in medical practice because the diagnostic tests physicians order often are expensive, invasive, and/or potentially risky to the patient. Deciding whether there is value added to clinical deci-

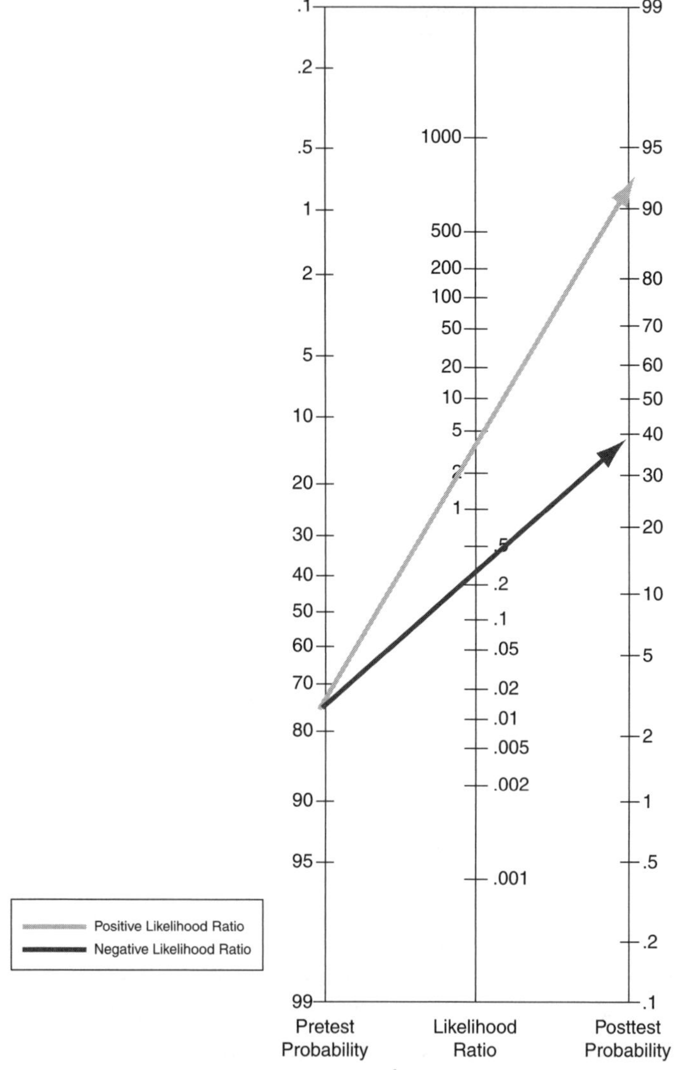

Figure 10–9 Likelihood ratios for the anterior drawer test for ankle ligament rupture from van Dijk *et al.*[13]

sion making by conducting another test makes sense under these circumstances. Civilian physical therapy practice often does not have to confront concerns about cost and invasiveness of diagnostic tests because therapists usually are prohibited from ordering and/or performing these procedures. However, clinical examination techniques often cause pain and, in some circumstances, have a high enough level of risk associated with them that their added value also should be considered. In addition, the contribution of a diagnostic test to accurate classification of the patient's condition should be acknowledged in an effort to direct treatment. Under these circumstances, a nomogram may be useful as illustrated by the anterior drawer test example. Physical therapists with diagnostic test ordering privileges, as well as those who perform diagnostic electrophysiological examinations, will have even greater opportunities to put this simple tool to use.

Evidence-based physical therapists also may determine the shift from pretest to posttest probabilities via calculations provided by Sackett *et al.*[13] The procedure requires conversion of probabilities to odds and back again using the following steps (as illustrated with the use of the data from the ankle study):

$$\textbf{(1) Pretest odds} = \frac{\textbf{Pre-test probability}}{\textbf{1} - \textbf{pretest probability}} = \textbf{0.76/0.24} = \textbf{3.16}$$

$$\textbf{(2) Posttest odds} = \textbf{Pretest odds} \times \textbf{Likelihood ratio} = \textbf{3.16} \times \textbf{3.2} = \textbf{10.13}$$

$$\textbf{(3) Posttest probability} = \frac{\textbf{Posttest odds}}{\textbf{Posttest odds} + \textbf{1}} = \textbf{10.13/11.13} = \textbf{91\%}$$

Whether using the nomogram or doing the math, therapists should evaluate the final posttest probability against the identified treatment threshold to determine if intervention, or further diagnostic testing, is warranted.[10]

THE MEANING OF STUDY RESULTS

In addition to the correlation coefficients, sensitivity, specificity, predictive values, and likelihood ratios reported in studies, investigators also provide information to determine the "meaningfulness"—or potential importance—of their results. The two primary ways to convey potential importance are the p-value and the confidence interval. A *p-value* indicates the probability that the result obtained occurred due to chance. The smaller the p-value (e.g., < 0.05), the more important the result is statistically because the role of chance is so diminished, although not eliminated.

A *confidence interval* represents a range of scores within which the true score for a variable is estimated to lie within a specified probability (e.g., 90%, 95%, 99%).[2] A likelihood ratio is meaningful if it lies within the confidence interval; however, a narrow range or interval is preferred for the purposes of validity. In other words, a narrow confidence interval suggests that the likelihood ratio in the study is close to the "true" likelihood ratio within the identified probability (e.g., 95%). Unfortunately there are no criteria by which to judge whether a confidence interval is "too wide." Remember that if a confidence interval around a likelihood ratio contains the value "one," then the true value includes chance (a coin flip), a finding that invalidates the result obtained by the researchers.[13] Authors may acknowledge this situation by stating that their result was not statistically significant.

Remember also that authors choose what their threshold values for statistical significance will be. In the case of p-values, the traditional threshold is alpha (α) ≤ 0.05. In the case of confidence intervals, the traditional probability is 95 percent. Ultimately, these are arbitrary choices, which means that evidence-based physical therapists must use their clinical judgment and expertise to determine the clinical meaningfulness or importance of a study's findings. This challenge will be apparent when results just miss significance (i.e., $p = 0.07$) or when confidence intervals are wide. Nevertheless, a study that minimizes bias and that demonstrates strong statistical significance with narrow confidence intervals should be taken seriously in terms of the information it provides.

EVIDENCE AND THE PATIENT/CLIENT

Once the validity of a study about a diagnostic test or measure is established and the importance of its results confirmed, the final step is to determine whether the evidence is appropriate for use with an individual patient/client. This is the point in the process during which the physical therapist must add his or her clinical expertise and judgment, along with the patient/client's preferences and values, to the information gleaned from the research.

There are several practical considerations before putting the evidence into practice. First, the test of interest should be available, practical, and safe in the setting in which the physical therapist practices. A test that requires an immobile piece of expensive equipment, such as a Biodex System 3[17], likely will be more appropriate for use in an outpatient clinic than in a skilled nursing facility. Second, the test should have demonstrated performance on patients/clients that resemble the individual with whom the physical therapist is working. These commonalities may include age, gender, signs, symptoms, previous activity or functional levels, comorbidities, and so on. Important differences may indicate a need to discard the test in favor of another option. Third, the therapist must consider whether he or she can estimate pretest probabilities for his or her patient/client. Rarely encountered diagnoses may make this step difficult both in terms of the therapist's experience and available epidemiologic data. A reasonable pretest probability is essential to determining whether the test's results will add information by revising the probability of a diagnosis upward or downward. Evidence that provides ambiguous answers to these considerations will demand more of the physical therapist in terms of his or her clinical judgment about the usefulness and safety of a diagnostic test.

In addition to addressing these practical issues, the physical therapist also must take into account his or her patient/client's preferences and values with respect to their health status and its management. Exploration of these issues occurs during the initial interview and continues throughout the episode of care. Areas of interest or concern for the patient/client may include, but are not limited to:[18,19]

a) The potential risk of injury or pain involved with the procedure;
b) Whether sufficient benefit will occur once the test results are known;
c) Cost– financial, as well as time away from work, school, or family;
d) Confidence in the test and/or the examiner; and,
e) Appreciation of and belief in the value of scientific evidence.

Individual cultural and social norms will shape the direction of these issues for the patient/client as well as for family members or other caregivers involved in the situation.

Ideally, both the physical therapist and the patient/client will agree upon the optimal course of action. However, the ethical principle of autonomy dictates that the patient/client must decide whether the diagnostic test or measure is worth the effort and risk to undergo the procedure. Reluctance may translate into suboptimal performance that further confounds results of the clinical examination, a situation that the physical therapist must take into account as he or she considers the data obtained.

FINAL THOUGHTS ABOUT DIAGNOSIS IN PHYSICAL THERAPY

The need for evidence about diagnostic tests is intuitive in military physical therapy practice where test-ordering privileges are granted and in civilian outpatient physical therapy practice in states with direct access to physical therapy services. Home health physical therapists also may find themselves using this type of information when they encounter a patient whose signs and symptoms differ from those exhibited at the last visit. Physical therapists working in inpatient settings, on the other hand, may wonder if the concept of diagnosis even applies to their practice. After all, the patient has been admitted with a diagnostic label such as "stroke," "myocardial infarction," or "hip fracture." Physical therapists do not need to decide which tests to perform to rule in or rule out these conditions. However, each of these patients requires physical therapy for a movement-related impairment, the classification of which must be determined from a variety of potential options. For example, exercise intolerance after myocardial infarction may be due to diminished aerobic capacity and/or due to peripheral muscle weakness. Physical therapists must perform clinical examination procedures to determine which of these problems underlies the poor exercise response in order to design and execute the most effective plan of care;[10] therefore, they must decide which procedures are the most useful to obtain the necessary information. In that sense, evaluation of evidence about diagnostic tests is relevant to physical therapists in all practice settings.

Table 10–2 provides a checklist to guide the evaluation of evidence about diagnostic tests for use in any practice setting.[11,20] Alternatively, readers might consider use of the worksheet adapted from the Oxford Center for Evidence-Based Medicine located in Appendix B. A strategy worth considering is the creation of reference notebooks that contain completed checklists or worksheets along with their associated research articles. These compendia could facilitate the use of evidence regarding diagnostic tests for all physical therapists in a particular setting.

Table 10–2 Evidence about diagnostics tests—quality appraisal checklist.

Research Validity of the Study	
Did the investigators compare results from the test of interest to results from a gold (or reference) standard test?	___ Yes ___ No
Were the individuals performing and interpreting each test's results unaware (i.e., masked, or blinded) of the other test's results?	___ Yes ___ No
Did the investigators include subjects with all levels or stages of the condition being evaluated by the diagnostic test of interest?	___ Yes ___ No
Did all subjects undergo the gold standard diagnostic test?	___ Yes ___ No
Did the investigators repeat the study with a new set of subjects?	___ Yes ___ No
Do you have enough confidence in the research validity of this paper to consider using this evidence with your patient/client?	___ Yes ___ Undecided ___ No
What results do the authors report related to your clinical question?	
Sensitivity ______________________	
Specificity ______________________	
Positive Predictive Value(s) ______________________	
Negative Predictive Value(s) ______________________	
+ Likelihood Ratio(s) ______________________	
− Likelihood Ratio(s) ______________________	

Correlation Coefficient(s) ______________________________

Other ______________________________

How important are the results?

Obtained p-values for each statistic reported by the authors:

Obtained confidence intervals for each statistic reported by the authors:

Is this test reliable and valid? If yes, continue below.	___ Yes ___ No
What is the pretest probability that your patient/client has the condition of interest?	________%
What is the posttest probability that your patient/client has the condition of interest if you apply this test?	________%
Do the subjects in the study resemble your patient/client?	___ Yes ___ No
Can you perform this test safely and appropriately in your clinical setting given your current knowledge and skill level and your current resources?	___ Yes ___ No
Does the test fit within the patient/client's expressed values and preferences?	___ Yes ___ No
Will you use this diagnostic test for this patient/client?	___ Yes ___ No

SAMPLE CALCULATIONS

		Target Disorder (Biceps Pathology & SLAP Lesion)		
From Holtby and Razmjou[20]		Present	Absent	**Totals**
Diagnostic Test Result (Yergason's)	Positive (Pain in bicipital groove or GH joint)	**a** 9	**b** 6	**a+b** 15
	Negative (No pain in bicipital groove or GH joint)	**c** 12	**d** 22	**c+d** 34
Totals		**a+c** 21	**b+d** 28	**a+b+c+d** 49

Sensitivity = a/(a+c) = 9/21 = 43% (0.43)
Specificity = d/(b+d) = 22/28 = 79% (0.79)
Likelihood ratio for a positive test result = LR+ = sens/(1−spec) = 0.43/0.21 = 2.05
Likelihood ratio for a negative test result = LR− = (1−sens)/spec = 0.57/0.79 = 0.72
Positive Predictive Value = a/(a+b) = 9/15 = 60%
Negative Predictive Value = d/(c+d) = 22/34 = 65%
Pretest probability (prevalence) = (a+c)/(a+b+c+d) = 21/49 = 43% (0.43)
Pretest odds = prevalence/(1−prevalence) = 0.43/0.57 = 0.75
Posttest odds = pretest odds × LR = 0.75 × 2.05 = 1.54
Posttest probability = posttest odds/(posttest odds +1) = 1.54/2.54 = 61%

YOUR CALCULATIONS

		Target Disorder		
From Holtby and Razmjou[20]		Present	Absent	**Totals**
Diagnostic Test Result	Positive	a	b	a+b
	Negative	c	d	c+d
Totals		a+c	b+d	a+b+c+d

Source: Based upon material developed by the Oxford Center for Evidence-Based Medicine (2006) (www.cebm.net); used with permission.

SUMMARY

Diagnostic tests are an essential component of physical therapy practice in any setting. The most useful tests are those that have demonstrated reliability and validity with patients/clients similar to the individual with whom the physical therapist is working. Reliability is demonstrated through statistical tests of relationships among repeated testing. Validity is demonstrated through statistical and mathematical comparisons to a gold standard test, the application of which will provide a definitive diagnosis. A receiver operating characteristic (ROC) curve may be used to identify important thresholds or cut points in a diagnostic test's scoring system. The likelihood ratio is the most flexible measurement property for clinical use because it can be calculated for a spectrum of test results. Evidence about diagnostic tests should be evaluated to verify research validity and to determine if the results are useful and important for application with patients/clients in the physical therapist's practice. The final decision should reflect both the therapist's clinical judgment and the patient/client's preferences and values.

Exercises

1. Differentiate between a test threshold and a treatment threshold.
2. Differentiate between reliability and validity of a diagnostic test.
3. Explain why a masked comparison to a gold standard is a necessary step in establishing the validity of a diagnostic test of interest.
4. Differentiate between the sensitivity and specificity of a diagnostic test. What does it mean when sensitivity is low, but specificity is high? What does it mean when sensitivity is high and specificity is low?
5. Explain why positive and negative predictive values for diagnostic tests are limited in their usefulness.
6. Differentiate between a positive and negative likelihood ratio. What does it mean when a likelihood ratio equals one?
7. Differentiate between pretest and posttest probabilities. How does a likelihood ratio interact with these two values?
8. Use the following 2 × 2 table to calculate the sensitivity, specificity, positive and negative predictive values, and positive and negative likelihood ratios for a hypothetical diagnostic test:

	+ Condition	− Condition
+ Test	138	108
− Test	35	238

   Interpret the results for each of the calculations.

9. Assume that a patient has a pretest probability of 30 percent for the diagnosis of interest in Question # 8. Use the nomogram in Figure 10–8 and determine the posttest probabilities for the positive and negative likelihood ratios obtained in question #8.
10. A study regarding the diagnostic test in Question #8 provides the following confidence intervals for the positive and negative likelihood ratios:

    + LR 95% CI (0.87, 6.8)

    − LR 95% CI (0.20, 0.74)

    What do these confidence intervals indicate about the usefulness of each likelihood ratio?

References

1. Helewa A, Walker JM. *Critical Evaluation of Research in Physical Rehabilitation: Towards Evidence-Based Practice.* Philadelphia, PA: W.B. Saunders Company; 2000.

2. Domholdt E. *Rehabilitation Research: Principles and Applications.* 3d ed. St. Louis, MO: Elsevier Saunders; 2005.
3. Polit DF, Beck CT. *Nursing Research: Principles and Methods.* 7th ed. Philadelphia, PA: Lippincott Williams & Wilkins; 2003.
4. American Physical Therapy Association. Guide to Physical Therapist Practice. 2d ed. *Phys Ther.* 2001; 81(1):9–744.
5. Higgs J, Jones M. *Clinical Reasoning in the Health Professions.* 2d ed. Oxford, England: Butterworth-Heinemann; 2000.
6. Guyatt G, Rennie D. *Users' Guides to the Medical Literature: A Manual for Evidence-Based Clinical Practice.* Chicago, IL: AMA Press; 2002.
7. Portney LG, Watkins MP. *Foundations of Clinical Research: Applications to Practice.* 2d ed. Upper Saddle River, NJ: Prentice Hall Health; 2000.
8. Herbert R, Jamtvedt G, Mead J, Hagen KB. *Practical Evidence-Based Physical Therapy.* Edinburgh, Scotland: Elsevier Butterworth-Heinemann; 2005.
9. Straus SE, Richardson WS, Glaziou P, Haynes RB. *Evidence-Based Medicine: How to Practice and Teach EBM.* 3d ed. Edinburgh, Scotland: Elsevier Churchill Livingstone; 2005.
10. Fritz JM, Wainner RS. Examining diagnostic tests: an evidence-based perspective. *Phys Ther.* 2001; 81(9):1546–1564.
11. Critically Appraising the Evidence. Worksheets for Diagnosis. Oxford Center for Evidence-Based Medicine Web site. Available at: www.cebm.net. Accessed July 15, 2005.
12. Safran MR, Benedetti RS, Bartolozzi AR III, Mandelbaum BR. Lateral ankle sprains: a comprehensive review Part I: etiology, pathoanatomy, histopathogenesis, and diagnosis. *Med Sci Sports Exerc.* 1999; 31(7):S429–S437.
13. Sackett DL, Straus SE, Richardson WS, Rosenberg W, Haynes RB. *Evidence-Based Medicine: How to Practice and Teach EBM.* 2d ed. Edinburgh, Scotland: Churchill Livingstone; 2000.
14. Davidson M. The interpretation of diagnostic tests: A primer for physiotherapists. *Aust J Physiother.* 2002; 48(3):227–233.
15. Fagan TJ. Nomogram for Bayes's theorem. *N Engl J Med.* 1975; 293(5):257.
16. van Dijk CN, Lim LSL, Bossuyt PMM, Marti RK. Physical examination is sufficient for the diagnosis of sprained ankles. *J Bone Joint Surg.* 1996; 78(6):958–962.
17. Biodex System 3. Biodex Medical Systems Web site. Available at: http://www.biodex.com/rehab/system3/system3_feat.htm. Accessed November 1, 2005.
18. King M, Nazareth I, Lampe F, Power B, Chandler M *et al.* Conceptual framework and systematic review of the effects of participants' and professionals' preferences in randomized controlled trials. *Health Technol Assess.* 2005; 9(35):1–191.
19. Davey HM, Lim J, Butow PN, Barratt AL, Houssami N, *et al.* Consumer information materials for diagnostic breast tests: Women's views on information and their understanding of test results. *Health Expectations.* 2003; 6(4):298–311.
20. Holtby R, Razmjou H. Accuracy of the Speed's and Yergason's tests in detecting biceps pathology and SLAP lesions: Comparison with arthroscopic findings. *Arthroscopy.* 2004; 20(3):231–236.

Chapter 11

Appraising Evidence About Prognoses

Prediction is very difficult, especially about the future.

—Niels Bohr

Objectives

Upon completion of this chapter the student/practitioner will be able to:

1. Discuss the three uses of prognosis in physical therapy practice;
2. Critically evaluate evidence about prognoses including:
   a. Important questions to ask related to research validity; and,
   b. Statistical approaches for identification of prognostic indicators.
3. Interpret and apply information provided by:
   a. Survival curves;
   b. Odds ratios;
   c. Relative risks;
   d. Hazard ratios.
4. Evaluate p-values and confidence intervals to determine the potential importance of reported findings.
5. Discuss considerations related to the application of evidence about prognosis to individual patients/clients.

Terms in This Chapter

Bias: Results or inferences that systematically deviate from the truth "or the processes leading to such deviation."[1(p. 251)]

Case-Control Design: A retrospective epidemiological research design used to evaluate the relationship between a potential exposure (e.g., risk factor) and an outcome (e.g., disease or disorder); two groups of subjects—one of which has the outcome (the case) and one which does not (the control)—are compared to determine which group has a greater proportion of individuals with the exposure.[2]

Cohort Design: A prospective epidemiological research design used to evaluate the relationship between a potential exposure (e.g., risk factor) and an outcome (e.g., disease or disorder); two groups of subjects—one of which has the exposure and one of which does not—are monitored over time to determine who develops the outcome and who does not.[2]

Confidence Interval: A range of scores within which the true score for a variable is estimated to lie within a specified probability (e.g., 90%, 95%, 99%).[3]

Hazard Ratio: An estimate of the relative risk of developing the problem of interest over the course of the study, weighted by the number of subjects available.[2]

Inception Cohort: A group of subjects that are followed over time starting early in the course of their disease or disorder.[4]

Masked (also referred to as "Blinded"): In prognosis studies, the lack of knowledge of risk or of prognostic factors.

Odds Ratio: The odds that an individual with a prognostic (risk) factor had an outcome of interest as compared to the odds for an individual without the prognostic (risk) factor.[2,4]

Prognosis: A prediction about the future status of a patient/client with respect to either disease or disorder development, disease or disorder outcome, and/or response to physical therapy intervention.[5]

Prognostic Factor: A demographic, diagnostic, or comorbid characteristic of a patient/client that confers increased or decreased chances of positive or adverse outcomes from a disease/disorder or from interventions.[2,4]

p-value: The probability that a statistical finding occurred due to chance.

Relative Risk: The ratio of the risk of developing a disorder in patients with a prognostic (risk) factor compared to the risk in patients without the prognostic (risk) factor.[2,4]

Risk Factor: A demographic, diagnostic, or comorbid characteristic of a patient/client that confers increased or decreased chances of development of a disease or disorder.[2,4]

Survival Curve: A graphic representation of the frequency of an outcome of interest over time created by plotting the percentage of individuals who are free of the outcome at successive points in time.[2,4]

INTRODUCTION

Prognosis is the process of predicting the future about a patient/client's condition. Physical therapists develop prognoses about 1) the risk of developing a future problem 2) the ultimate outcome of an impairment or functional limitation, and 3) the results of physical therapy interventions.[5,6] Prognostic estimates are formulated in response to questions posed by patients/clients and their families, as well as to indicate the purpose of the therapist's plan of care. In both instances the predicted outcome includes a time frame for its development,[5] again to satisfy patient/client expectations, but also to address payer interests with respect to the duration and intensity of the physical therapy episode of care. This chapter focuses on the evaluation of evidence that informs physical therapists' prognoses for their patients/clients.

Risk of a Future Adverse Event

Physical therapists' concerns about the risk for developing future problems generally are focused on patients for whom a primary medical diagnosis or impairment already is established. Risk mitigation is employed as part of secondary and tertiary prevention strategies in these situations.[5] Common examples of potential problems patients may develop include:

- Skin breakdown as a result of sensation loss (as in diabetes and stroke) or immobility (as in spinal cord injury and casting);
- Reinjury with return to work or athletic activities following joint sprain or muscle strain; and,
- Falls as a result of neurologic insult (as in stroke or brain injury).

As physical therapists have moved into primary health promotion and wellness, their focus has broadened to include primary prevention efforts with clients, such as addressing the risk for development of cardiovascular disease, osteoporosis, or arthritis as a result of inactivity. The goal in all of these examples is to prevent adverse events that may occur years in the future.

Ultimate Outcomes

Physical therapists formulate prognoses related to the ultimate outcome of movement-related impairments. In addition, they are often asked what the ultimate outcome of a condition will be. Unlike the risk for future events, the ultimate outcome of a condition or impairment is easier to conceptualize in some respects because of the many clinical observations that have been catalogued about the natural course of various diagnoses.[6] Prognostic questions regarding ultimate outcomes that physical therapists may encounter (or have themselves) resemble these examples:

- Will I always need oxygen for activity?

- Will I walk without a walker again?
- Will my shoulder always be painful when I pitch?
- Will my child be able to attend school like other children?

These are the questions raised by patients and caregivers, as well as by students and professionals with limited experience with various patient problems. In addition, there are questions about the timeline for change that both patients and therapists wonder about, including:

- How long will it take for this patient's incision (bone, tendon, ligament) to heal?
- When will this patient regain sensation in his hand after carpal tunnel surgery?
- How long before this patient can resume driving?

and so on. Identifying the ultimate outcome of a condition or impairment in terms of progress, regression, death, or cure provides the context in which the plan of care is formulated and treatment-related prognostic estimates are determined.

Results from Physical Therapy Interventions

Predictions about the results produced by interventions are reflected in the goals physical therapists write for their patients/clients. Whether directed toward remediation of impairments, functional limitations, or disabilities, goals indicate what therapists expect in terms of responses to treatment.[5] In addition, this information is tied to a timeline such as the number of days, weeks, or visits anticipated to achieve the specified outcome(s). The therapist's challenge is to consider the likelihood of achievement, within the specified timeline, of the outcomes identified for a given patient/client. For example, a patient's ability to learn a home exercise program prior to hospital discharge following total knee arthroplasty may be dependent upon the individual's cognitive abilities and support from family or caregivers. The status of each of these factors may alter the therapist's estimate of the likelihood of goal attainment. As noted above, prognoses about treatment responses are subsets of the prediction of ultimate outcomes.

ELEMENTS OF PROGNOSIS

The examples above make the point that prognoses have three elements 1) the outcome (or outcomes) that are possible; 2) the likelihood that the outcome (or outcomes will) occur; and, 3) the time frame required for their achievement.[4] Identification of patient/client characteristics that may influence the outcomes identified are of particular interest. As noted in Chapter 3, relevant characteristics may be sociodemographic—such as age, gender, race/ethnicity, income, education, and social support—or clinical, such as disease stage, severity, time since onset, recurrence, and/or the presence of comorbid conditions. The general term that describes characteristics predictive of any type of future outcomes is *prognostic factors*. Predictors of future adverse events usually are referred to as *risk factors*.[2,4] In both cases, the challenge is to identify which of these many pieces of information available about a patient/client are most predictive of the potential outcomes.

Because making predictions is an integral part of physical therapy management, it is important for therapists to be familiar with evidence about prognoses for the patients/clients in their practice. This is especially true because daily practice often limits therapists' ability to follow up with patients/clients over a long enough period of time in order to determine if the outcomes they predicted really came true. In addition, they only see a limited, nonrepresentative set of individuals with a particular disorder which adds a great deal of bias to their prediction estimates.[6] Evaluation of the best available evidence can help physical therapists overcome these natural practice limitations and improve their prognostic abilities.

STUDY CREDIBILITY

Evidence pertaining to prognoses first should be evaluated with an assessment of its research validity. Higher research validity provides greater confidence that a study's findings are reasonably free from *bias*. In other words, the results are believable. Appraisal of evidence about prognoses starts with the questions itemized in Table 11–1. These questions are adapted from the critical appraisal worksheets developed by the Oxford Center for Evidence-Based Medicine.[7] Their purpose is to help physical therapists determine whether there are problems with a study's design that may have biased the results.[2,4]

1. **Did the investigators provide sufficient information to describe the sample in their study?**

   One of the first concerns investigators must address with respect to their sample is its definition. Clearly articulated inclusion and exclusion criteria should be used to ensure that subjects fit the definition of individuals who have, or who are at risk for, the outcome of interest. For example, a study examining risk factors for the development of "arthritis" should specify whether the origin of the disorder of interest is systemic (e.g., rheumatoid arthritis) or

Table 11-1 Questions to assess the validity of evidence about prognosis.

1. Did the investigators provide sufficient information to describe the sample in their study?
2. Are the subjects representative of the population from which they were drawn?
3. Did all subjects enter the study at the same (preferably early) stage of their condition?
4. Was the study time frame long enough to capture the outcome(s) of interest?
5. Did the investigators collect outcome data from all of the subjects enrolled in the study?
6. Were outcome criteria operationally defined?
7. Were the individuals collecting the outcome measures masked (or blinded) to the status of prognostic factors in each subject?
8. Does the sample include subgroups of patients for whom prognostic estimates will differ? If so, did the investigators conduct separate subgroup analyses or statistically adjust for these different prognostic factors?
9. Did investigators repeat the study with a new set of subjects?

biomechanical (e.g., osteoarthritis). The pathology associated with these two forms of joint disease are sufficiently different from one another that risk factors are likely to differ to some degree. An operational definition of the disorder and the criteria by which it will be recognized will improve the validity of any associated risk factors.

2. **Are the subjects representative of the population from which they were drawn?**

   The issue of representativeness pertains to the degree to which investigators were able to capture all eligible subjects during the time frame of the study. Enrolling some individuals and not others may indicate that there are systematic differences between participants and nonparticipants, the consequence of which is different prognostic estimates for each group.[6] Of course, investigators cannot force all eligible patients to participate; however, they can perform statistical comparisons between participants and nonparticipants to determine whether the sample is representative of the population of interest. Statistically significant differences between the groups suggest that biased prognostic estimates may have resulted.

3. **Did all subjects enter the study at the same (preferably early) stage of their condition?**

   This question is particularly salient for longitudinal *cohort design* designs. Investigators must determine at what point patients should be gathered for study. This decision is dependent in part upon the nature of the disease or disorder of interest and in part upon the research question. An acute problem, such as muscle soreness after initiation of a new exercise routine, would require study immediately at onset because the problem is self-limiting within a few days. On the other hand, a chronic disease such as osteoarthritis may be studied at several points along its evolution depending upon what the investigators want to know relative to prognosis from a given point in time. Understandably, patients too far along in the course of their disorder may achieve the outcome of interest early in the study and give a false sense of the time frame involved in the disorder's evolution.[4] The preferred starting point for prognosis studies is just after a disease or disorder becomes clinically apparent. Subjects assembled at this point are referred to as an an *inception cohort*.[4] Regardless of the starting point selected, the goal is to avoid a sample that is so heterogeneous that predicting future outcomes and their associated predictors and time frames becomes unworkable.

4. **Was the study time frame long enough to capture the outcome(s) of interest?**

   The length of follow-up time of a study will be dependent upon which outcomes or events are being anticipated. The time frame identified must be possible for the human body to achieve the outcome from a physiological or psychological standpoint. If the time is too short, then a possible outcome will be missed.[4] Studies of rare events usually use a retrospective *case-control design* because of the low likelihood of a patient developing the problem in a prospective fashion.

5. **Did the investigators collect outcome data from all of the subjects enrolled in the study?**

   The ability to capture the outcomes of all subjects is important because attrition for any reason may provide a skewed representation of which outcomes occurred and when. Ideally, investigators will be able to determine what happened to subjects who left the study in order to evaluate whether the outcomes were truly different than for those who remained. Differences between subjects who remained and subjects who dropped out indicate that bias likely has been introduced to the prognostic estimates. Straus *et al.* describe a "5 and 20 rule" in which the loss of 5 percent of subjects likely has little impact, whereas the loss of 20 percent (or more) of subjects will undermine study validity to a considerable extent. Investigators also may conduct sensitivity analyses in which they calculate "best case" and "worst case" scenarios to determine the degree to which outcomes are affected by attrition.[4] Evidence-based physical therapists may then make their own decisions about whether the worst case scenario reflects bias that undermines the study's value.

6. **Were outcome criteria operationally defined?**

   This question addresses the validity of the measures used to capture the outcome(s) of interest. A clear definition of the outcome(s) or event(s) is necessary to avoid misidentification. Investigators should articulate specific clinical and/or testing criteria prior to the start of data collection.

7. **Were the individuals collecting the outcome measures masked (or blinded) to the status of prognostic factors in each subject?**

   Ideally, those identifying the outcome(s) or event(s) will be *masked*, or ignorant of the subjects' prognostic or risk factors. Prior knowledge of subject status may introduce tester bias into the study because expectations about the outcomes may influence application and interpretation of the measures used to capture them.

8. **Does the sample include subgroups of patients for whom prognostic estimates will differ? If so, did the investigators conduct separate subgroup analyses or statistically adjust for these different prognostic factors?**

   A subgroup is a smaller group of subjects who have a characteristic that distinguishes them from the larger sample. This characteristic is anticipated to influence the outcome of interest such that a different prognostic estimate is likely to be identified. Consider a hypothetical study about risk factors for the development of knee pain in individuals who are at least 80 years old. Age, along with associated ailments such as arthritis, might be reasonable predictors of this outcome. However, if some of the subjects are also obese, then their development of knee pain may be influenced by their weight in addition to the other relevant characteristics. This difference in outcome development and expression for the subgroup of obese patients may confound the results for the total sample.

   Ideally, investigators will identify these additional prognostic factors and isolate them in some fashion. The simplest approach is to conduct separate analyses—in this case, for elderly subjects who are obese and for elderly subjects who are not. An alternative approach is to test a statistical model to predict the knee pain using the entire sample, while adjusting for body weight or body mass index.[8] In either case, an evidence-based physical therapist should consider what additional factors may predict or influence the outcome of interest and review the evidence to determine whether these factors were accounted for.

9. **Did investigators repeat the study with a new set of subjects?**
   This question alludes to the possibility that the research findings regarding prognostic or risk factors occurred due to chance. Repeating the study on a second group of subjects who match the inclusion and exclusion criteria outlined for the first group provides an opportunity to evaluate whether the same predictive factors are identified. One strategy is to assemble a group of subjects and randomly select half of them to create the prognostic model, which can then be retested on the remaining half. Often, this step is not included in a single research report due to insufficient numbers of subjects and/or lack of funds. As a result, evidence-based physical therapists must read several pieces of evidence about the same prognostic or risk factors if they wish to verify the factors' usefulness to a greater degree.

Additional Considerations

Additional concerns pertaining to research design in evidence about prognoses include the presence or absence of a detailed description of the:

1. Inclusion and exclusion criteria used to select subjects; and,
2. Operational definitions of the prognostic or risk factors.

This information allows evidence-based physical therapists to determine if the subjects included resemble the patient/client about whom there is a question (1) and if the predictive factors are identifiable and measurable (2).

STUDY RESULTS

Prognosis research uses both descriptive statistics, as well as tests of relationships to identify prognostic or risk factors. The descriptive statistics usually are reported as proportions, such as the percent of subjects with a particular risk factor who developed a pressure ulcer or the percent of subjects with a certain prognostic factor who returned to work. These values may be reported over time or at a certain point in time (commonly the median).[4] Another descriptive approach is the creation of a *survival curve* that plots the number of events or outcomes over time. Survival curves are calculated most commonly when investigators are evaluating the development of adverse events such as death, side effects from treatment, and loss of function. Any dichotomous outcome may be depicted in this fashion. Figure 11-1 illustrates a generic example in which an increasing proportion of subjects experience an adverse outcome of interest over ten years.

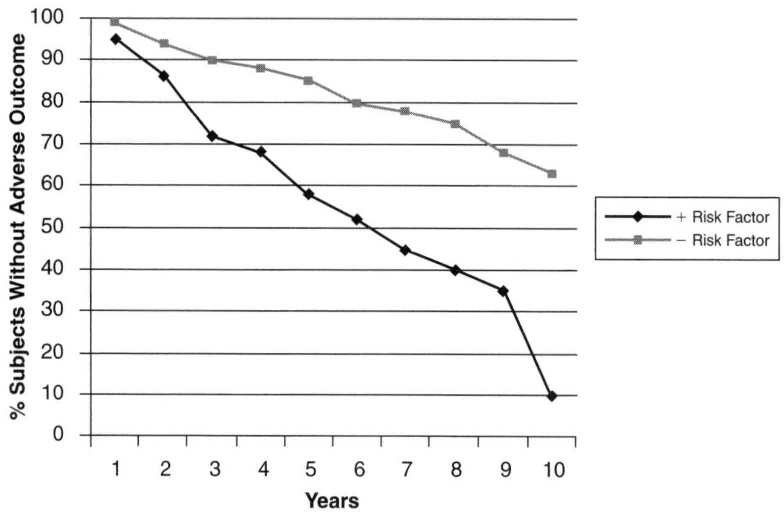

Figure 11-1 Survival curves illustrating a good and poor prognosis for development of an adverse outcome.

Subjects in the lower curve represent those who have a suspected risk factor, while subjects in the upper curve do not. The slope of these curves gives an immediate visual idea regarding how quickly (or slowly) the outcome of interest occurred.[4,9] Both the data points and the slope indicate a poorer prognosis for subjects represented by the lower curve as compared to those represented by the upper curve. By the ten year mark 90 percent of the subjects in the risk factor group experienced the adverse outcome compared to only 37 percent in the nonrisk factor group. Clearly, these dramatic numbers make a compelling case for identifying this hypothetical risk factor in future patients.

Statistical tests related to prognosis may take the form of simple associations or more sophisticated predictions via regression analyses. Association tests such as Pearson's r, Spearman's rho, and chi-square may be used in situations where a new relationship between a predictive factor and an outcome is being explored to determine whether further investigation is indicated. These tests provide the least amount of information because they evaluate an association between two variables, but do not provide a prediction about an outcome. Regression analyses, on the other hand, are used to predict the value of the outcome, as well as to determine the relative contribution of each prognostic or risk factor to this result. Both linear and logistic regression approaches may be used for evaluating predictors depending upon whether the outcome is continuous or dichotomous in nature.

Multiple logistic regression is implemented frequently because this technique produces odds ratios (OR) for each factor retained in the equation. *Odds ratios* reflect the odds that an individual with a prognostic (risk) factor had an outcome of interest, as compared to the odds for an individual without the prognostic (risk) factor.[2,4] The odds are derived in consideration of all of the other independent variables in the regression equation.[9] Odds ratios have the same values as likelihood ratios—that is, zero to infinity. Values less than one are recognized as decreased odds, while values greater than one are recognized as increased odds. A value equal to one is a coin flip; in other words, the odds of developing the outcome of interest are no better than chance.

Table 11-2 provides results of a logistic regression analysis from an hypothetical study about predictors of reinjury upon return to work. The odds ratio is indicated by the symbol "Exp (**B**)." Interpretation of odds ratios is similar to the interpretation of likelihood ratios. For example, the odds ratio for body mass index in Table 11-2 is 2.398. This result would be interpreted to mean that subjects with a higher body mass index had more than twice the odds of suffering reinjury compared to subjects with a lower body mass index. On the other hand, the odds ratio for job satisfaction—0.790—indicates decreased odds for reinjury. This result is consistent with the negative sign in front of the **B** coefficient which indicates that higher job satisfaction is inversely related to reinjury.

Odds ratios also can be calculated from a 2 × 2 table for an individual variable. Figure 11-2 represents data from a hypothetical study of fall risk in relation to the presence or absence of peripheral neuropathy. The equation for calculating odds ratios from the table is:

$$OR = [A/B] / [C/D] \text{ or } AD/BC$$

Table 11-2 Results from a hypothetical study examining predictors of reinjury following return to work.

Variable	Beta (B)	SE	p-value	Exp(B)-Odds Ratio	95% CI
Age (years)	0.181	0.049	0.102	1.198	0.98, 2.67
Body Mass Index (> 30 kg/m^2)	1.078	0.431	0.031	2.398	1.79, 3.56
Smoker (+)	0.389	0.084	0.070	1.475	0.93, 4.05
Prior Injury (+)	1.908	0.560	0.005	6.739	4.32, 7.23
Job Satisfaction (Visual analog scale)	−0.986	0.341	0.022	0.790	0.69, 0.98
Constant	6.327	2.45	0.000		

	+ Fall > 1 time	– Fall > 1 time
+ Neuropathy	**A** 43	**B** 20
– Neuropathy	**C** 25	**D** 38

Figure 11–2 A 2 × 2 table for calculating odds ratios from a hypothetical study about falls.

Using the data in the table produces an odds ratio of 3.27; in other words, the odds that a subject with peripheral neuropathy fell more than once are three times the odds for a subject without neuropathy. This approach is useful when only one indicator is being evaluated; more than one factor or predictor requires a regression approach to isolate the effects of each predictor in the presence of the others.

Finally, investigators may report relative risks (RR) and hazard ratios for risk factors for a particular outcome. *Relative risks* are the ratio of the risk of developing a disorder in patients with a prognostic (risk) factor compared to the risk in patients without the prognostic (risk) factor.[2,4] *Hazard ratios* commonly are reported in conjuction with survival curves. These values reflect relative risk for an outcome over time. As their names imply, these estimates are used in the context of adverse events. Conceptually, they are similar to odds ratios in that comparisons are made between the group that has the risk factor and the group that does not. Interpretation also is comparable: ratios greater than one indicate increased risk, ratios less than one indicate reduced risk, and ratios equal to one indicate that the risk of developing the outcome of interest is no better than chance.

Relative risks are different from odds ratios in that their calculation is based on the incidence of the outcome within the total group of subjects with (or without) the risk factor. This distinction is important because, by definition, relative risks are used in longitudinal studies in which the incidence of an outcome of interest can be determined for individuals with, and without, the risk factor. They cannot be calculated in case-control designs in which the investigators define the number of subjects with and without the outcome and then identify risk factor distribution retrospectively.[4] Relative risks can be calculated from 2 × 2 tables using the following equation:

$$RR = [A/A + B] / [C/C + D]$$

Using the data from Figure 11–1, the relative risk of falls is 1.72, which means that subjects with neuropathy have more than 1.5 times the risk for falling as compared to subjects without neuropathy. Relative risks generally have lower values than odds ratios because the former value is a ratio of rates of events rather than a ratio of actual events. When the event rates are low, the relative risk and odds ratio will approach each other. Readers must be cognizant of which estimate is used in order to interpret the study's results appropriately.

THE MEANING OF STUDY RESULTS

In addition to the correlation coefficients, odds ratios, relative risks, and hazard ratios reported in studies, investigators also provide information to determine the "meaningfulness"—or potential importance—of their results. The two primary ways to convey potential importance are via the p-value and the confidence interval. As noted in previous chapters, the smaller the *p-value* (e.g., < 0.05), the more important the result is statistically because the role of chance is so diminished, although not eliminated.

A *confidence interval* represents a range of scores within which the true score for a variable is estimated to lie within a specified probability (e.g., 90%, 95%, 99%).[3] An odds ratio, relative risk, or hazard ratio is meaningful if it lies within the confidence interval. As with any other estimate, a narrower confidence interval is preferred because it suggests that the ratio of interest is close to the "true" ratio according to the specified probability (i.e., 95%). Unfortunately, there are no criteria by which to judge whether a confidence interval is "too wide." Remember that if a confidence interval around an odds ratio, relative risk, or hazard ratio contains the value "one" then the odds, risks, or hazards are no better than chance and the predictor is not useful.[9] Such a result also will be reported as statistically nonsignificant. Table 11-2 illustrates this situation for the prognostic factor "age."

Usually authors report the relevant confidence interval; however, readers also may calculate the interval for different estimates when they are not reported. Appendix B provides equations for confidence intervals for outcomes and various ratios. Finally, as noted in previous chapters, authors choose what their threshold values will be for p-values and confidence intervals. In the former case, the traditional threshold is alpha $(\alpha) \leq 0.05$. In the latter case, the traditional probability is 95 percent. Ultimately, these are arbitrary choices which means that evidence-based physical therapists must use their clinical judgment and expertise to determine the clinical meaningfulness or importance of a study's findings.

EVIDENCE AND THE PATIENT/CLIENT

As with all evidence, a prognosis study must be examined to determine if the subjects included resemble closely enough the patient/client to whom the results may be applied. The unique twist to the use of prognosis evidence is the degree to which it will influence what therapists will tell their patients/clients about their future, as well as how treatment planning will be affected, if at all.[6] Predictions about the future can be complicated by expectations, fears, desires, and many other emotions that define the human experience. Although the evidence may be objective and unemotional, its implications may not be. This is where clinical judgment comes into play as therapists will have to decide whether their patients' potential to experience an outcome is unique to him or her or matches the tendency of the group in the study. That conclusion, as well as the patient/clients' values, will provide direction to therapists about how to use the information in the management process.

Table 11-3 provides a checklist to guide the evaluation of evidence about prognosis for use in any practice setting.[7]

Table 11-3 Evidence about prognoses—quality appraisal checklist.

Research Validity of the Study	
Did the investigators provide sufficient information to describe the sample in their study?	___ Yes ___ No
Are the subjects representative of the population from which they were drawn?	___ Yes ___ No
Did all subjects enter the study at the same (preferably early) stage of their condition?	___ Yes ___ No
Was the study time frame long enough to capture the outcome(s) of interest?	___ Yes ___ No
Did the investigators collect outcome data from all of the subjects enrolled in the study?	___ Yes ___ No
Were outcome criteria operationally defined?	___ Yes ___ No
Were the individuals collecting the outcome measures masked (or blinded) to the status of prognostic factors in each subject?	___ Yes ___ No
Does the sample include subgroups of patients for whom prognostic estimates will differ?	___ Yes ___ No
If so, did the investigators conduct separate subgroup analyses or statistically adjust for these different prognostic factors?	___ Yes ___ No
Did investigators repeat the study with a new set of subjects?	___ Yes ___ No
Do you have enough confidence in the research validity of this paper to consider using this evidence with your patient/client?	___ Yes ___ Undecided ___ No

What results do the authors report related to your clinical question?

Correlation Coefficient(s) ________________________________

Coefficients of Determination ________________________________

Odds Ratios ________________________________

Relative Risk ________________________________

Other ________________________________

____

How important are the results?

Obtained p-values for each statistic reported by the authors:

Obtained confidence intervals for each statistic reported by the authors:

How likely are the outcomes over time (based on your experience or on the proportion of subjects in the study who achieved the outcome)?

Do the subjects in the study resemble your patient/client? If no, how are they different? ___ Yes ___ No

Will sharing information from this study about prognostic indicators or risk factors help your patient/client given their expressed values and preferences? ___ Yes ___ No

How will you use this information with your patient/client?

Source: Based upon material developed by the Oxford Center for Evidence-Based Medicine (2006) (www.cebm.net); used with permission.[7]

SUMMARY

Prognosis is the process of predicting a future outcome for a patient/client. Developing prognostic estimates from clinical practice alone is difficult because of the limited exposure physical therapists have to a representative group of individuals at risk for, or known to have, a particular problem. Evidence about prognosis for physical therapy-related problems is limited, but should be evaluated when possible to improve the prognostic estimation process. Verification of the validity, importance, and relevance of the evidence about prognosis is central to the ability to use the information with patients/clients. Sensitivity to patient/client values and preferences is equally important in light of the potential emotional impact of sharing information about unfavorable prognoses.

Exercises

1. Describe the three focus areas of prognosis in physical therapy patient/client management and give clinical examples of each.
2. Describe the three elements of a prognostic estimate and give a clinical example that includes all of the relevant information.
3. Explain why clinical practice is insufficient for establishing precise prognostic estimates.
4. Explain why the length of time and completeness of follow-up is essential to the validity of prognosis studies.
5. Explain why it is important for prognosis studies to include subjects with the spectrum of the disease or disorder of interest.
6. Explain why adjustment for other factors is important when subgroups of subjects have different prognostic estimates for an outcome.
7. Differentiate between odds ratios, relative risks, and hazard ratios. Provide interpretations for ratios that have values less than one, equal to one, and greater than one.
8. Explain the usefulness of an odds ratio, relative risk, or hazard ratio when its associated confidence interval includes the value one.
9. Use the following 2 ×2 table to calculate the odds ratio and relative risk for the hypothetical outcome:

	+ Outcome	− Outcome
+ Prognostic Factor	97	68
− Prognostic Factor	38	130

   Interpret the results for each of the calculations. Why is the odds ratio different than the relative risk?

10. A study regarding the prognostic factor in Question #9 provides the following confidence interval for the odds ratio:

    OR 95% CI (2.05, 22.8)

    What does this confidence interval indicate about the usefulness of this odds ratio?

References

1. Helewa A, Walker JM. *Critical Evaluation of Research in Physical Rehabilitation: Towards Evidence-Based Practice*. Philadelphia, PA: W.B. Saunders Company; 2000.

2. Guyatt G, Rennie D. *Users' Guides to the Medical Literature: A Manual for Evidence-Based Clinical Practice*. Chicago, IL: AMA Press; 2002.
3. Domholdt E. *Rehabilitation Research: Principles and Applications*. 3d ed. St Louis, MO: Elsevier Saunders; 2005.
4. Straus SE, Richardson WS, Glaziou P, Haynes RB. *Evidence-Based Medicine: How to Practice and Teach EBM*. 3d ed. Edinburgh, Scotland: Elsevier Churchill Livingstone; 2005.
5. American Physical Therapists Association. Guide to Physical Therapist Practice. 2d ed. *Phys Ther*. 2001; 81(1):9–744.
6. Herbert R, Jamtvedt G, Mead J, Hagen KB. *Practical Evidence-Based Physical Therapy*. Edinburgh, Scotland: Elsevier Butterworth-Heinemann; 2005.
7. Critically Appraising the Evidence. Worksheets for Prognosis. Oxford Center for Evidence-Based Medicine Web site. Available at: www.cebm.net. Accessed March 1, 2006.
8. Altman DG. Systematic reviews of evaluations of prognostic variables. *BMJ*. 2001; 323(7306):224–228.
9. Portney LG, Watkins MP. *Foundations of Clinical Research: Applications to Practice*. 2d ed. Upper Saddle River, NJ: Prentice Hall Health; 2000.

Chapter 12

Appraising Evidence About Interventions

To do nothing is sometimes a good remedy.

—Hippocrates

OBJECTIVES

Upon completion of this chapter the student/practitioner will be able to:

1. Discuss the contribution of evidence to the decision making about interventions for patients/clients.
2. Critically evaluate evidence about interventions including the:
   a. Important questions to ask related to research validity; and,
   b. Relative merits of experimental, quasi-experimental and nonexperimental designs.
3. Interpret and apply information provided by the following calculations:
   a. Absolute benefit increase;
   b. Absolute risk reduction;
   c. Effect size;
   d. Intention to treat;
   e. Number needed to treat;
   f. Relative benefit increase;
   g. Relative risk reduction.
4. Evaluate p-values and confidence intervals to determine the potential importance of reported findings.
5. Discuss the role of the minimal clinically important difference in determining the potential usefulness of an experimental intervention.
6. Discuss considerations related to the application of evidence about interventions to individual patients/clients.

Terms in This Chapter

Absolute Benefit Increase (ABI): The absolute value of the difference in rates of positive outcomes between the intervention group and the control group (expressed as a percentage).[1]

Absolute Risk Reduction (ARR): The absolute value of the difference in rates of adverse outcomes between the intervention group and the control group (expressed as a percentage).[1]

Attrition: Loss of subjects in a study for reasons such as death, hospitalization, illness, decision to withdraw, or loss of contact.

Bias: Results or inferences that systematically deviate from the truth "or the processes leading to such deviation."[2(p.251)]

Concealment: The methods by which investigators hide information about group assignment from individuals responsible for enrolling subjects.[3]

Confidence Interval: A range of scores within which the true score for a variable is estimated within a specified probability (e.g., 90%, 95%, 99%) to lie.[4]

Control Group Event Rate (CER): The percentage of subjects who improved in the control group.

Effectiveness: The extent to which an intervention produces a desired outcome under usual clinical conditions.[2]

Effect Size: The magnitude of the difference between two mean values; may be standardized by dividing this difference by the pooled standard deviation in order to compare effects measured by different scales.[5]

Efficacy: The extent to which an intervention produces a desired outcome under ideal conditions.[2]

Experimental Design: A research design in which the behavior of randomly assigned groups of subjects is measured following the purposeful manipulation of an independent variable(s) in at least one of the groups; used to examine cause-and-effect relationships between an independent variable(s) and an outcome(s).[4,6]

Experimental Group Event Rate (EER): The percentage of subjects who improved in the experimental group.

Imputation: A term referring to a collection of statistical methods used to estimate missing data.[7]

Intention-to-Treat Analysis: Statistical analysis of data from subjects according to the group to which they were assigned despite noncompliance with the study protocol.[3]

Intervention: The purposeful use of various physical therapy procedures and techniques, in collaboration with the patient/client and, when appropriate, caregivers, in order to effect a change in the patient/client's condition.[8]

Masked (Blinded): In intervention papers, the lack of knowledge about to which group a subject has been assigned.

Minimal Clinically Important Difference (MCID): "The smallest treatment effect that would result in a change in patient management, given its side effects, costs, and inconveniences."[9(p. 1197)]

Nonexperimental Design (also referred to as an Observational Study): A study in which controlled manipulation of the subjects is lacking;[4] in addition, if groups are present, assignment is predetermined based upon naturally occurring subject characteristics or activities.[1]

Number Needed to Treat (NNT): The number of subjects treated with an experimental intervention over the course of a study required to achieve one good outcome or prevent one bad outcome.[10]

Placebo: "An intervention without biologically active ingredients."[3(p. 682)]

Quasi-Experimental Design: A research design in which there is only one subject group or in which randomization to more than one subject group is lacking; controlled manipulation of the subjects is preserved.[11]

Randomized Clinical Trial (also referred to as a Randomized Controlled Trial and a Randomized Controlled Clinical Trial)[RCT]: A clinical study that uses a randomization process to assign subjects to either an experimental group(s) or a control (or comparison) group. Subjects in the experimental group receive the intervention or preventive measure of interest and then are compared to the subjects in the control (or comparison) group who did not receive the experimental manipulation.[4]

Relative Benefit Increase (RBI): The absolute value of the rate of increase in positive outcomes for the intervention group relative to the control group (expressed as a percentage).[1]

Relative Risk Reduction (RRR): The absolute value of the rate of decrease in adverse outcomes for the intervention group relative to the control group (expressed as a percentage).[1]

INTRODUCTION

At the conclusion of the examination and evaluation process, physical therapists identify the *interventions* that are available to address identified patient/client needs. A number of factors may influence decisions about which treatments to choose that are derived from both the therapist and the patient/client. For example, the physical therapist will a) determine whether the signs and symptoms fit an established classification scheme; b) consider the complexity of the case; c) prioritize the problem list; d) determine what resources are required, as well as their availability; e) identify the patient/client's educational needs; and, f) make a judgment about enablers and barriers to patient/client adherence to the treatment plan. These issues will be evaluated in the context of past experiences with similar patients/clients, as well as within the ethical, legal, and socioeconomic parameters that inform practice.[8] On the other hand, the patient/client will offer his or her perspective on priorities, resources, educational needs, and adherence challenges in a manner that reflects his or her preferences and values about the usefulness of physical therapy, the effort required to recover or adapt function, and the opportunities lost as a result of spending time and money on rehabilitation, rather than on other activities or material pursuits.

As physical therapists and patients/clients review various treatment options they also consider the tradeoffs between the benefits and risks for each intervention. This deliberation may be illustrated by the following questions:

a) If this intervention (versus another) is applied, will the condition improve, regress, remain unchanged, or will a new problem develop?
b) If this intervention (versus another) is not applied, will the condition improve, regress, remain unchanged, or will a new problem develop?

Ideally, the answer to these questions will include details about the different responses possible, as well as estimations about the likelihood of their occurrence. Physical therapists may use previous experience with similar patients/clients, as well as theoretical premises based in biological plausibility, to answer these questions. As noted in Chapter 1, however, past experience is subject to bias and biological plausibility may be refuted in unexpected ways. The incorporation of the best available evidence about the efficacy or effectiveness of different therapeutic approaches adds to this deliberative process by helping physical therapists and patients/clients consider their options from an objectively tested point of view.

STUDY CREDIBILITY

Evidence pertaining to interventions physical therapists use first should be evaluated with the questions itemized in Table 12–1. These questions are adapted from the critical appraisal worksheets developed by the Oxford Center for Evidence-Based Medicine.[12] Their purpose is to help physical therapists determine whether there are problems with a study's design that may have biased the results.[1]

1. **Did the investigators randomly assign (or allocate) subjects to groups?**

   This question represents a minimum threshold in the evidence selection process. Randomization of subjects to groups is the as-

Table 12–1 Questions to determine the validity of evidence about interventions

1. Did the investigators randomly assign (or allocate) subjects to groups?
2. Was each subject's group assignment concealed from the people enrolling individuals in the study?
3. Did the groups have similar sociodemographic, clinical, and prognostic characteristics at the start of the study?
4. Were subjects, clinicians, and outcome assessors masked (or blinded) to the subjects' group assignment?
5. Did the investigators manage all of the groups in the same way except for the experimental intervention(s)?
6. Did subject attrition (e.g., withdrawal, loss to follow-up) occur over the course of the study?
7. Did the investigators collect follow-up data on all subjects over a time frame long enough for the outcomes of interest to occur?
8. Were subjects analyzed in the groups to which they were assigned?

signment method most likely to reduce *bias* by creating groups with equally distributed characteristics (see Chapter 6). Groups that are equivalent at the start of the study are necessary in order to isolate the impact, if any, of the experimental intervention. Investigators who used a randomized allocation process usually announce that fact in the title or abstract of the paper, making it easy for a reader to identify such studies. The importance of this research design feature is emphasized by proponents of evidence-based practice who propose that research papers that do not include randomized subject assignment should be set aside in favor of a new literature search.[1,3,13] Unfortunately, many questions of interest to physical therapists are addressed by quasi-experimental and nonexperimental studies without randomized group assignment. The potential role of these designs is discussed later in this section.

2. **Was each subject's group assignment concealed from the people enrolling individuals in the study?**

   The issue of *concealment* alludes to the possibility that study personnel may interfere with the randomization process such that bias is introduced into the study. This interference may be well intended. For example, investigators may feel compelled to respond to logistical challenges that make study participation difficult for the subjects, the research personnel, or the facilities. Prior knowledge of subject assignment during the enrollment period would allow the investigators to reassign subjects to resolve these problems.[3] In so doing, however, equal distribution of characteristics is undermined, resulting in the introduction of an alternative explanation for the study's results. Unfortunately, the concealment of group assignment during the enrollment period often is not addressed one way or the other in physical therapy research. Readers should not assume concealment was performed unless explicitly stated.

3. **Did the groups have similar sociodemographic, clinical, and prognostic characteristics at the start of the study?**

   Although randomized assignment methods are likely to result in equal groups at the start of the study, this result is not guaranteed. This question acknowledges this fact by asking whether the investigators confirmed group equality through statistical analysis of the relevant sociodemographic, clinical, and prognostic characteristics. This information may be found in tables and text reported in the section describing subjects or in the results section of the paper, depending upon journal formatting demands. Ideally, investigators will adjust for the imbalances in these factors in their statistical analyses. However, readers should note any statistically significant differences among the groups and consider whether, and in what ways, those differences may have played a role in the study's results.

4. **Were subjects, clinicians, and outcome assessors *masked* (or *blinded*) to the subjects' group assignment?**

   This question explores the possibility that subject, study personnel, or clinician behavior may have changed during the study as a result of knowledge about the group to which a subject was assigned. As discussed in Chapter 8, subjects may increase their efforts in the hopes of achieving the anticipated outcomes or decrease their efforts as a result of frustration that they are not in the experimental treatment group. In addition, clinicians responsible for training subjects in the study may provide added encouragement to compensate for allocation to the control group. Finally, outcomes assessors may unconsciously introduce bias into the measurement process because of expectations about how subjects in each group will respond over the course of the study.

   As Herbert *et al.* note, it often is impractical to mask group assignment from the subjects in physical therapy research.[13] The one exception is the modification of electrotherapeutic modalities, such as ultrasound, to give the appearance of normal function without providing actual therapeutic effects. Creation of sham interventions for exercise and mobilization techniques often is not possible. As a result, physical therapists are likely to find research papers in which only the outcomes assessors are masked to group assignment. The potential for changes in subject behavior as a result of knowledge of their group assignment should be considered when evaluating the study's results.

5. **Did the investigators manage all of the groups in the same way except for the experimental intervention(s)?**

   This question clarifies the degree to which group equality was maintained when study personnel and/or clinicians interacted with subjects over the course of the project. Ideally, the only difference between or among the study groups will be the application of the experimental intervention. Other factors such as a) the timing of treatment applications and outcomes measurement, b) the environmental conditions in which these activities are performed, and c) the methods for provision of instructions and application of treatments or measures should be comparable across groups so that the effect, if any, of the experimental intervention may be isolated. The reader should note any differences in group management and consider whether, and in what ways, these differences may have influenced the study's results.

6. **Did subject attrition (e.g., withdrawal, loss to follow-up) occur over the course of the study?**

   Readers must determine whether all of the subjects who were enrolled at the start of the study remained at the end of the study. The loss of subjects, or *attrition*, may unbalance the groups such that inequalities in group characteristics influence the study's results. For example, groups that were previously equal in the proportion of male and female subjects now may be unequal in gender distribution. If there is an expectation that gender may influence the outcome of the study independent of the experimental intervention, then this imbalance is problematic. In addition, statistical power may be undermined due to the decrease in sample size.

   Attrition may occur for numerous reasons including death, illness, loss of interest by the subjects, or new circumstances making participation difficult. In addition, subjects may be dropped from the analyses when individual data points are missing from their cases. A variety of statistical methods are available for estimating data in order to avoid this reduction in sample size.[7] Details about these *imputation* methods are beyond the scope of this textbook. Readers should understand, however, that these methods provide estimates of the missing information that may introduce error to various degrees depending upon the approach selected.[13,14] When imputation is not performed, then the reader must make a qualitative decision about whether bias likely has been introduced because of attrition. Several authors recommend that a loss of five percent or less probably is inconsequential, whereas losses of 15–20 percent or more probably have undermined the internal validity of the study.[1,13] Investigators may explicitly discuss the loss of subjects in the text of the paper or they may indicate attrition by noting the number (via the symbol "n") of subjects included in each of the analyses summarized in tables or figures.[13]

7. **Did the investigators collect follow-up data on all subjects over a time frame long enough for the outcomes of interest to occur?**

   The issue regarding subject follow-up involves the time frame over which the study is conducted. Readers must determine whether the time allotted for the study was long enough for the outcomes of interest to occur. For example, a hypothetical study about an experimental strength training technique should be conducted over at least several weeks in order for changes in muscle fiber size and performance to develop.[15] Depending upon the research question, data may be collected beyond the immediate conclusion of the intervention phase in order to determine over what length of time any treatment effects remain. In this scenario, the time frame(s) selected for follow-up are at the discretion of the investigators; however, they should be consistent with the actual purpose of the study. Understandably, the longer the study is conducted the greater the chance for attrition to occur.

8. **Were subjects analyzed in the groups to which they were assigned?**

   The final question used to assess an intervention study's validity pertains to situations in which some of the subjects are not compliant with the protocol for their assigned group. Noncompliance may occur because of factors outside of the subjects' control, such as illness, or because of purposeful decisions by the subjects not to participate according to plan. As noted above, the latter situation is likely to occur when subjects determine to which group they have been assigned and change their behavior as a result of this knowledge. If noncompliant subjects are still available for collection of follow-up data, then investigators may implement an *intention-to-treat analysis* in which the outcome data are analyzed according to group assignment.[14,16] In other words, statistical comparisons between the intervention and control groups are made as if every subject complied with the protocol for their group. The results likely will reflect a reduction in the effect size of the treatment; however, Herbert *et al.* point out that this reduction is what one should expect if subjects (or patients) are not compliant with the treatment.[13] An intention-to-treat analysis is valued primarily because it preserves the randomized allocation process and, therefore, the baseline equality of group characteristics. In addition, sample size is maintained. There is some debate regarding the appropriateness of using imputed data from subjects lost to follow-up in these analyses because of the potential for error in the estimates. Sensitivity analyses provide an alternative approach to determine the impact on effect size of "best case" and "worst case" scenarios in which outcomes for missing subjects are assumed to be all favorable or all unfavorable, respectively. Authors should state clearly which, if any, analytic technique was used.

ADDITIONAL CONSIDERATIONS

In addition to the eight questions itemized above, concerns pertaining to research design in evidence about interventions include the presence or absence of a detailed description of the:

1. Setting in which the research was conducted;
2. Inclusion and exclusion criteria used to select subjects; and,
3. Protocol for the intervention(s) used.

This information allows evidence-based physical therapists to determine if the intervention of interest is applicable and feasible in their environment (1, 3) and if the subjects included resemble the patient/client about whom there is a question (2).

Issues Related to Study Design

Affirmative answers to most of the questions above are possible only in randomized controlled trials; however, the question of the validity of intervention papers is complicated by an ongoing debate regarding the relative merits of *experimental, quasi-experimental, and nonexperimental (or observational) research designs.* The evidence hierarchies promulgated by evidence-based practice sources consistently place experimental studies (e.g., randomized clinical trials) higher in ranking than the other two study types.[1,3,13] The rationale underlying this order is the ability of experimental designs to minimize bias by virtue of numerous controls directing subject assignment and management, study procedures, and study personnel knowledge and behavior. Evidence suggesting that lower forms of evidence tend to overestimate treatment effects due to bias reinforce the value of experimental designs.[17,18] Unfortunately, randomized clinical trials are complex and expensive endeavors that may be logistically difficult to produce depending upon the intervention in question. In addition, randomization to groups may be unethical if the necessary comparison is "no care" or a treatment alternative associated with high risk. Finally, experimental designs do not, by defintion, resemble everyday clinical practice in which any number of factors may influence both therapist and patient/client behavior, as well as outcomes from interventions. This latter point challenges the external validity of results from *randomized clinical trials.*

Britton *et al.* conducted a systematic review in response to this debate over study design.[17] These authors found that experimental designs are not inevitably better than quasi-experimental designs. For example, randomized clinical trials may produce a smaller effect size if they over-select subjects whose conditions are less severe, resulting in a smaller capacity to benefit from the experimental treatment. Such a scenario is reasonable to expect given the stringent exclusion criteria often used in experimental research designs. On the other hand, a treatment effect may be overestimated due to the potential influence of subject preferences in unmasked randomized trials. The authors also reported that quasi-experimental studies may produce comparable results to randomized clinical trials, provided that adjustment for group differences in important baseline prognostic factors is performed and that the same subject exclusion criteria are used. A subsequent systematic review drew similar conclusions comparing effects reported in randomized clinical trials to those reported in quasi-experimental and nonexperimental (observational) studies.[18] These reviews do not provide a definitive resolution to this debate. Both noted difficulties making direct comparisons among different studies of the same intervention because of small, but important, differences in inclusion and exclusion criteria and intervention protocols. In addition, they indicated that a consistent level of detail regarding study procedures for quasi-experimental and nonexperimental designs is lacking, making a thorough assessment of potential sources of bias a challenge.

In spite of the emphasis on experimental designs, Straus *et al.* and Guyatt and Rennie do acknowledge that quasi-experimental and nonexperimental designs may be appropriate for determining the potential ineffectiveness or harm from an intervention of interest.[1,3] On a more practical level, physical therapists may find that the only research available to them to answer a question about interventions is not in the form of a randomized controlled trial. Rejecting this evidence because it is lower on the hierarchy would leave therapists without options beyond practice as it is currently conducted. Ultimately, evidence-based physical therapists will be required to use their clinical expertise and judgment regarding the potential usefulness of a quasi-experimental or nonexperimental study, keeping in mind that these research designs always are more vulnerable to bias.

STUDY RESULTS

Studies about interventions may use descriptive statistics to elaborate on subject characteristics and to summarize baseline measures of performance. Whether or not an experimental treatment had an effect, as compared to an alternative or control, may be determined by "tests of differences"—those statistical tests that compare groups based on means, ranks, or frequencies. Recall that these tests come in parametric (e.g., *t*-test, ANOVA) and nonparametric (e.g., Kruskal-Wallis, chi-squared) forms depending on whether the outcome measure is ratio, interval, ordinal, or nominal. In addition, which test is used depends upon whether the investigator is comparing only two groups or more than two groups. Finally, researchers need to decide if they are going to adjust for covariates (e.g., ANCOVA) and whether they are looking at only one outcome or multiple outcomes (e.g., MANOVA). While these statistical tests indicate if a difference resulted from the experimental treatment, they do not provide information about the size of the treatment effect. This piece of information is vital in order to know if the resulting outcome may be clinically meaningful for the physical therapist and the patient/client.

Treatment Magnitude—Continuous Data

One method for determining the magnitude of treatment impact is to calculate an *effect size*. This approach is appropriate for intervention studies in which the outcomes are continuous measures. An effect size identifies the extent of the difference between two group means.[5] In its simplest form, the effect size is calculated by subtracting the mean outcome value for the control group from the mean outcome value for the experimental group at the conclusion of the study. In studies in which the comparison group is an alternative intervention rather than a true control (no intervention or *placebo*), then the "experimental group" may represent the larger mean score of the two groups. For example, imagine a hypothetical study in which a customized ankle-foot orthosis (AFO) is compared to a molded arch support to determine if increased support of the foot and ankle improves the ambulatory ability of children with spastic hemiplegia. If the average walking distance in the AFO group was 250 feet further than in the arch support group at the conclusion of the study, then the effect size produced by the customized AFO is 250 feet.

A standardized version of the effect size is created when the variation in scores is included in the calculation (Figure 12–1). This approach evaluates the extent of overlap, if any, in the distribution of scores for each group (Figure 12–2). Standardized effect sizes often are utilized when investigators want to compare the magnitude of impact from the same intervention across different outcome measures within a study[19,20] or across numerous studies evaluated in a systematic review (Chapter 14). As noted in Chapter 6, standardized effect sizes also are used in power calculations to determine the minimum sample size needed to detect a statistically significant difference or relationship, if it is present.

Standardized effect sizes often have a value between zero and one although they may be less than zero or greater than one. The following guidelines have been recommended by some authors for interpreting standardized effect sizes:[4,5]

- 0.20 minimal effect size
- 0.50 moderate effect size
- 0.80 large effect size

However, an argument can be made that this scale has the potential to diminish the clinical relevance of smaller treatment effects when compared to other available alternatives.[21] In other words, interventions with small effect sizes may still be clinically meaningful to a physical therapist or a patient/client.

Treatment Magnitude—Dichotomous Data

An alternative method by which to demonstrate the magnitude of treatment impact is to calculate the change in the rate (expressed as a percentage) of developing the outcome of interest. This approach is useful when the outcome is captured using a dichotomous measure—either the outcome

$$\frac{\text{Mean Score of Group 1} - \text{Mean Score of Group 2}}{\text{Pooled Standard Deviation}}$$

$$\text{Pooled Standard Deviation} = \sqrt{\frac{(N_{exp} - 1)SD^2_{exp} + (N_{control} - 1)SD^2_{control}}{N_{exp} + (N_{control} - 2)}}$$

Figure 12–1 Calculation of standardized effect size.

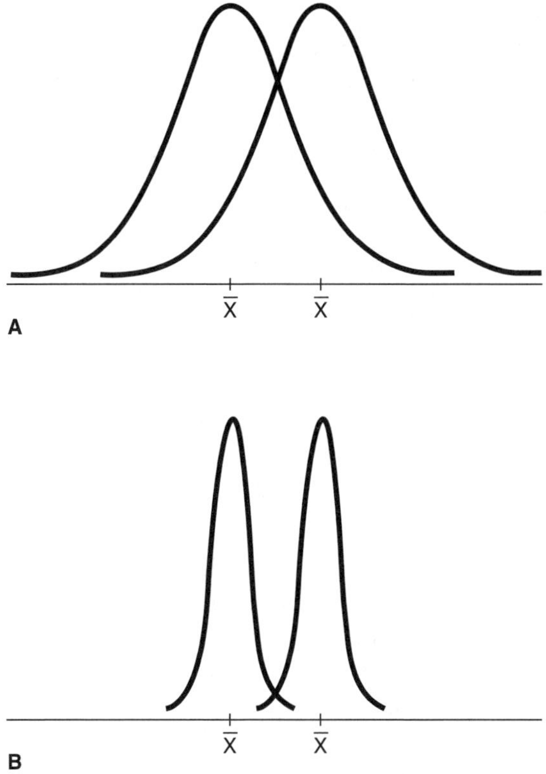

Effect of within-group variability on the overlap of sampling distributions.
A, High variability leads to overlap of sampling distributions.
B, Low variability leads to minimal overlap of sampling distributions.
$\bar{X}$ = mean.

Figure 12–2 Illustration of the influence of group variability on effect size.
Source: Reprinted from *Rehabilitation Research: Principles and Applications*, 3d edition, Elizabeth Domholdt, page 294, Copyright (2005), with permission from Elsevier.

happened or it did not. The first step in this process is to determine whether the outcome of interest is beneficial or harmful to the subjects. Santos *et al.* considered a beneficial outcome when they investigated potential improvements in submaximal exercise capacity following an aerobic training program for overweight pregnant women.[22] On the other hand, Emery *et al.* considered a harmful outcome when they studied whether a home balance training program prevented sports-related injuries in adolescent high school students.[23]

Changes in the rates of beneficial outcomes may be reflected by calculations of the increase in benefit achieved due to application of the experimental intervention. In the exercise study, the investigators wanted to know the extent to which aerobic training made a difference in submaximal cadiorespiratory capacity. Investigators can capture the impact of aerobic training by determining the absolute benefit increase and relative benefit increase. The *absolute benefit increase (ABI)* is calculated as follows:

ABI = | Experimental group event rate (EER) − Control group event rate (CER)[1] |

These rates are the percentage of subjects who improved submaximal functional capacity in the exercise group and control group, respectively. Santos *et al.* reported an EER of 26 percent and a CER of 5 percent;[22] therefore, the ABI achieved through aerobic exercise training was 21 percent. The ABI is useful for discriminating between large and small treatment effects.[1]

Alternatively, the *relative benefit increase* (*RBI*) is calculated as follows:

$$\text{RBI} = \frac{|\ \text{Experimental group event rate (EER)} - \text{Control group event rate (CER)}^1\ |}{\text{Control group event rate (CER)}}$$

Using the same numbers from the prior calculation, the RBI in the exercise training study was 4.2 which should be interpreted to mean that aerobic exercise training increased submaximal functional capacity in the experimental group by 420 percent as compared to those who did not participate in the exercise program. Unlike the ABI, the RBI is insensitive to differences in magnitude of the treatment effect. For example, if 2.5 percent of the experimental group improved submaximal functional capacity versus 0.5 percent of the control group, the RBI would still be 420 percent. Yet, the actual difference between the two groups is only 2.0 percent which may have no clinical relevance depending on what other treatment techniques are available.

Changes in rates of adverse outcomes may be reflected by calculations of the reduction in risk achieved as a result of the experimental intervention. Risk reduction will be familiar to those with a background in public health epidemiology, as prevention of adverse events is a central theme in this service area. In the balance training study, the risk pertains to the development of sports-related injury as a result of presumed proprioceptive deficiencies. An appropriate exercise program may reduce this risk by improving static and dynamic balance through proprioceptive training. Investigators can capture the impact of the balance training program by determining the absolute risk reduction and the relative risk reduction. The *absolute risk reduction (ARR)* is calculated as follows:

ARR = | Control group event rate (CER) − Experimental group event rate (EER)[1] |

These rates are the percentage of subjects who developed a sports-related injury in the control group and experimental group, respectively. Emery *et al.*

reported a CER of 17 percent and an EER of 3 percent;[23] therefore, the ARR achieved by use of the balance training program was 14 percent. As with the ARI, the ARR is useful in distinguishing between small and large treatment effects.

Alternatively, the *relative risk reduction (RRR)* is calculated as follows:

$$\text{RBI} = \frac{|\text{ Control group event rate (CER)} - \text{Experimental group event rate (EER)}^1 \text{ }|}{\text{Control group event rate (CER)}}$$

Using the same numbers from the prior caculation, the RRR in the balance training study was 0.82. In other words, participation in the balance training program reduced the risk of developing a sports-related injury by 82 percent as compared to subjects who did not participate in the program. The RRR is limited in the same fashion as the RBI in that it is insensitive to small treatment effects.

Readers should note that the absolute and relative benefit and risk calculations can be derived from 2 × 2 tables if authors provide the data in their results. Tables 12–2 and 12–3 illustrate this approach for both the Santos *et al.* and Emery *et al.* studies. However, results from hand calculations may vary slightly from those reported depending upon whether the authors round values with decimal points up or down.

Table 12–2 Results from a study of aerobic exercise training in overweight pregnant women.[22]

	+ Improved VO_2	− Improved VO_2
+ Aerobic Exercise Program	a 10	b 28
− Aerobic Exercise Program	c 2	d 36

VO_2 = Oxygen consumption at anaerobic threshold in exercise test

$$\text{ABI} = a/(a+b) - c/(c+d) = 10/38 - 2/38 = 0.21 \times 100\% = 21\%$$

$$\text{RBI} = \frac{a/(a+b) - c/(c+d)}{c/(c+d)} = \frac{10/38 - 2/38}{2/38} = 4.2 \times 100\% = 420\%$$

Table 12–3 Results from a study of balance training for reducing sports-related injuries.[23]

	+ Sports Injury	− Sports Injury
+ Balance Program	a 2	b 58
− Balance Program	c 10	d 50

$$\text{ARR} = c/(c+d) - a/(a+b) = 10/60 - 2/60 = 0.14 \times 100\% = 14\%$$

$$\text{RRR} = \frac{c/(c+d) - a/(a+b)}{c/(c+d)} = \frac{10/60 - 2/60}{10/60} = 0.80 \times 100\% = 80\%$$

THE MEANING OF STUDY RESULTS

As is the case for evidence about diagnostic tests and prognostic indicators, p-values and confidence intervals may be employed in evidence about interventions to help determine the statistical importance of a study's results. Recall that a p-value indicates the probability that the result obtained occurred due to chance. The smaller the p-value (e.g., < 0.05) the more convincing the results become because the role of chance is so diminished, although not eliminated. P-values usually are reported in conjunction with statistical tests of differences to determine whether an experimental intervention was more effective than a control or comparison intervention. As noted above, it is helpful to know that a difference in outcome occurred, but it is more helpful to know the magnitude of that difference. For this reason, a p-value usually is not sufficient by itself to help determine the potential importance of findings in an intervention study.

Confidence intervals are more helpful in determining the potential meaningfulness of study findings because they establish the precision (or lack thereof) of effect sizes, as well as of absolute and relative benefit and risk calculations. Recall that a *confidence interval* represents a range of scores within which the true score for a variable is estimated within a specified probability (e.g., 90%, 95%, 99%) to lie.[4] There is an important difference, however, between confidence intervals calculated around values for treatment magnitude and confidence intervals calculated around the likelihood and odds ratios discussed in previous chapters. Specifically, the lower bound of confidence intervals for these ratios is zero, whereas it is possible for the lower bound of confidence intervals for treatment effects to be a negative number.

This difference is understandable if one considers what is being measured. Likelihood and odds ratios represent predictions about the probability of a specific outcome. As such, these ratios cannot have negative values in the mathematical sense. Put in practical terms, the statement "There is a −50% probability that a patient will have 'X' diagnosis or outcome" makes no sense. Either there is a probability of the diagnosis or outcome (however small or large) or there is not (the value zero). On the other hand, the evaluation of an experimental intervention in comparison to an alternative may produce one of three actual outcomes:

- Subjects who receive the experimental intervention improve (or reduce their risk) as compared to those who did not receive the intervention;
- Subjects who receive the experimental intervention remain unchanged as compared to those who did not receive the intervention; or,
- Subjects who receive the experimental intervention are worse off than those who did not receive the intervention.

As a result, it is possible to have negative values for both the measures of treatment magnitude (expressed as an effect size, ABI, ARR, RBI, or RRR), as well as for their confidence intervals.

Remember that authors choose what their threshold values will be for p-values and confidence intervals. In the case of p-values, the traditional threshold is an alpha (α) ≤ 0.05. In the case of confidence intervals, the traditional parameter choice is 95 percent certainty. Ultimately, these are arbitrary choices which means that evidence-based physical therapists must use their clinical judgment and expertise to determine the clinical meaningfulness of a study's findings.

EVIDENCE AND THE PATIENT/CLIENT

Once the validity of a study about an intervention is established and the statistical importance of its results confirmed, the final step is to determine whether the evidence is appropriate for use with an individual patient/client. This is the point in the process during which physical therapists must add their clinical expertise and judgment, along with the patient/client's preferences and values, to the information gleaned from the research. Whether to use an intervention with a patient/client depends in part upon the extent to which a study's results are clinically meaningful. As noted in Chapter 9, statistical significance does not equal clinical significance. However, physical therapists have tools with which to assess the relationship between these two judgments: the minimal clinically important difference and the number needed to treat.

Minimal Clinically Important Difference

The *minimal clinically important difference (MCID)* is defined as "the smallest treatment effect that would result in a change in patient management, given its side effects, costs, and inconveniences."[9(p. 1197)] In other words, the MCID reflects the minimal level of change required in response to an intervention before the outcome would be considered worthwhile in terms of a patient/client's function or quality of life. An intervention that produces a statistically significant change in study subjects that does not cross this change threshold is likely to be disregarded as unimportant from a clinical standpoint. Ideally, investigators will evaluate their own findings in light of a predetermined MCID. This value often is stated as part of a power calculation to determine an appropriate sample size. However, Chan *et al.* reported that authors of randomized clinical trials inconsistently evaluate clinical importance.[9] As a result, evidence-based physical therapists must make their own determination based on their knowledge of other evidence and their clinical experience, as well as on input from the patient/client for whom the intervention is being considered.[13]

Number Needed to Treat (NNT)

Interventions with large effects may still have limited usefulness if the associated outcomes are rare. Alternatively, interventions with modest effects may be more meaningful if the outcomes occur frequently. Investigators may estimate the number of subjects that must receive the intervention in order for one subject to increase his or her benefit (or reduce his or her risk).[10] This calculation is referred to as the *number needed to treat (NNT)* and is determined using one of the following equations:

$$NNT = 1/ABI \text{ or } NNT = 1/ARR$$

In the aerobic training study, the NNT is 1/0.21 or 5. In the balance training study, the NNT is 1/0.14 or 7. In other words, investigators need to treat five overweight pregnant women or seven adolescent high school students in order to improve submaximal functional capacity in one woman or prevent one sports-related injury in one student, respectively. These values do not indicate which women or students will benefit—only that one of them is likely to do so within the parameters of this study.[10] The NNT also should be interpreted within the timelines (12 weeks and six months) of their respective studies. Understandably, a smaller NNT along with a shorter timeline implies greater potential usefulness of the intervention. Physical therapists also may evaluate the precision of an NNT through the use of confidence intervals reported or calculated for these values.

Readers may calculate the NNT if authors provide the necessary information about event rates in their results. However, hand-calculated results may vary from those reported depending on how values with decimals are handled. The tendency is to be conservative in estimating the NNT, as is illustrated in the study by Emery *et al.*[23] Although they rounded the event rates for calculation of the absolute risk reduction, they left these values intact for calculation of the NNT, thereby producing NNT = 8, rather than the 7 calculated above.

The NNT calculated from a study refers to the group of subjects, not to the individuals, within it. In order to apply this value to an individual patient/client, physical therapists must consider the extent to which that person's probability of achieving the outcome of interest matches the probability of subjects in the study.[1] This determination is reached by considering the likelihood of achieving the desired outcome if the patient/client does not receive the intervention. As a result, the reference point used from the evidence is the probability for the control group (e.g., the control group event rate [CER]). Emery *et al.* reported a CER of 16.6 percent;[23] therefore, a therapist working with a high school athlete should consider whether that individual's risk is higher or lower than 16.6 percent given the degree to which this person's characteristics match those of the control group. This information may be used in combination with the relative risk reduction from the study to determine a number needed to treat for the individual athlete.

Fortunately, mathematical equations are not required for this purpose as a nomogram has been created to facilitate this evaluation of treatment effect for an individual patient/client (Figure 12–3).[24] The nomogram works in a similar fashion to that created for use with likelihood ratios. The individual patient/client's risk for the outcome of interest is identified on the line to the far left. A straightedge is applied from this point through the relative risk reduction from the study located on the center line to determine the NNT on the line to the far right. For example, the gray line on the figure indicates that, for an athlete with a risk of injury of less than the control group (10 percent), and a relative risk reduction from Emery *et al.* of 80 percent,[23] the NNT is approximately fifteen. Under these circumstances, the therapist might consider other interventions especially in light of the compliance issues reported in the study. On the other hand, if the athlete's risk is estimated to be 35 percent (dark gray line) then the NNT is reduced to approximately three. Under these circumstances, a physical

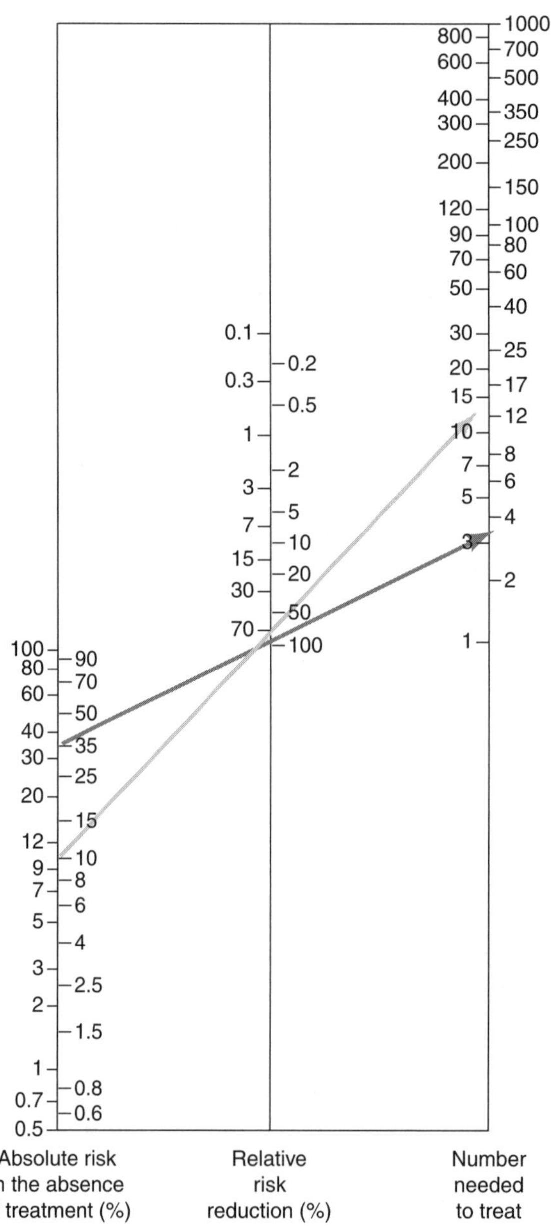

Figure 12–3 Nomogram for determining numbers needed to treat for individual patient/clients.

Source: Reprinted from The Number Needed to Treat: A Clinically Useful Nomogram in its Proper Context, Gilles Chatellier, Eric Zapletal, David Lemaitre, *et al.*, *British Medical Journal*, Volume 312, Copyright 1996, adapted with permission from BMJ Publishing Group, Ltd.

therapist and the high school athlete may decide to implement the balance training program.

Practical Considerations

In addition to the MCID and NNT, there are several practical considerations before putting the evidence about an intervention into practice. First, the intervention should be available, practical, and safe in the setting in which the physical therapist practices. Second, the intervention should have demonstrated performance on patients/clients that resemble the individual with whom the physical therapist is working. These commonalities may include age, gender, signs, symptoms, previous activity or functional levels, comorbidities and so on. Important differences may indicate a need to discard the intervention in favor of another option. Alternatively, therapists may decide to adapt the intervention to accommodate to a patient/client's limitations. For example, a joint mobilization technique performed in supine in a study may be modified by having the patient sit in a semirecumbent position to reduce the work of breathing associated with compromised cardiopulmonary function.

Physical therapists also must take into account their patient/client's preferences and values with respect to their health status and its management. Areas of interest or concern for the patient/client may include, but are not limited to:[25]

a) The potential risk of injury or pain involved with the intervention;
b) Whether sufficient benefit will occur to outweigh the risks;
c) Cost–including financial, as well as time away from work, school, or family;
d) Confidence in the physical therapist; and,
e) Appreciation of, and belief in the value of scientific evidence.

Individual cultural and social norms will shape the direction of these issues for the patient/client, as well as for family members or other caregivers involved in the situation.

Ideally, both the physical therapist and the patient/client will agree upon the optimal course of action. However, the ethical principle of autonomy dictates that the patient/client must decide whether the intervention is worth the effort and risk to undergo the procedure. The potential influence of patient/client preferences is addressed in more detail in Chapter 15.

Table 12-4 provides a checklist to guide the evaluation of evidence about interventions for use in any practice setting.[12] Answers to these questions should be considered in the context of the debate about the relative merits of experimental, quasi-experimental, and nonexperimental studies.

Table 12-4 Evidence about interventions—quality appraisal checklist.

Research Validity of the Study	
Did the investigators randomly assign (or allocate) subjects to groups?	___ Yes ___ No
Was each subject's group assignment concealed from the people enrolling individuals in the study?	___ Yes ___ No
Did the groups have similar sociodemographic, clinical, and prognostic characteristics at the start of the study?	___ Yes ___ No
Were subjects, clinicians, and outcome assessors masked (or blinded) to the subjects' group assignment?	___ Yes ___ No
Did the investigators manage all of the groups in the same way except for the experimental intervention(s)?	___ Yes ___ No
Did subject attrition (e.g., withdrawal, loss to follow-up) occur over the course of the study?	___ Yes ___ No
Were subjects analyzed in the groups to which they were assigned?	___ Yes ___ No
Did the investigators collect follow-up data on all subjects over a time frame long enough for the outcomes of interest to occur?	___ Yes ___ No
Did investigators repeat the study with a new set of subjects?	___ Yes ___ No
Do you have enough confidence in the research validity of this paper to consider using this evidence with your patient/client?	___ Yes ___ Undecided ___ No

What results do the authors report related to your clincical question?

Tests of Differences ______________________________

Effect Sizes______________________________

Absolute Benefit Increases ______________________________

Relative Benefit Increases ______________________________

Absolute Risk Reductions______________________________

Relative Risk Reductions ______________________________

Number Needed to Treat (Harm) ______________________________

Other ______________________________

How important are the results?

Obtained p-values for each statistic reported by the authors:

Obtained confidence intervals for each statistic reported by the authors:

Do these findings exceed a minimal clinically important difference?	___ Yes ___ No
Do the subjects in the study resemble your patient/client?	___ Yes ___ No
Can you perform this intervention safely and appropriately in your clinical setting given your current knowledge and skill level and your current resources?	___ Yes ___ No
Does the intervention fit within the patient/client's expressed values and preferences?	___ Yes ___ No
Do the potential benefits outweigh the potential risks of using this intervention with your patient/client?	___ Yes ___ No
Will you use this intervention for this patient/client?	___ Yes ___ No

SAMPLE CALCULATIONS—BENEFIT INCREASE

	+ Outcome	− Outcome
+ Intervention	a 72	b 55
− Intervention	c 40	d 78

CER = Control group event rate = c / (c+d) = 0.25 = 34%

EER = Experimental group event rate = a / (a+b) = 0.57 = 57%

		Relative Benefit Increase (RBI)	**Absolute Benefit Increase (ABI)**	**Number Needed to Treat (NNT)**
EER	CER	$\frac{EER - CER}{CER}$	EER − CER	1/ABI
57%	34%	56%	23%	4
		***95% CI**	10.9%–35.1%	3–9

*95% confidence interval (CI) on an NNT = 1/(limits on the CI of its ABI) =

$$\pm 1.96\sqrt{\left[\frac{CER \times (1-CER)}{\#\ \text{Control Pts}}\right] + \left[\frac{EER \times (1-EER)}{\#\ \text{Exper Pts}}\right]} =$$

$$\pm 1.96\sqrt{\left[\frac{0.34 \times 0.66}{118}\right] + \left[\frac{0.57 \times 0.43}{127}\right]} = \pm 12.1\%$$

SAMPLE CALCULATIONS—RISK REDUCTION

	+ Outcome	− Outcome
+ Intervention	a 10	b 50
− Intervention	c 26	d 34

CER = Control group event rate = c/(c+d) = 0.43 = 43%

EER = Experimental group event rate = a/(a+b) = 0.17 = 17%

		Relative Risk Reduction (RRR)	Absolute Risk Reduction (ARR)	Number Needed to Treat (NNT)
CER	EER	$\frac{CER - EER}{CER}$	CER − EER	1/ARR
43%	17%	60%	26%	4
		*95% CI	10.3%−41.7%	2−10

*95% confidence interval (CI) on an NNT = 1/(limits on the CI of its ARR) =

$$\pm 1.96\sqrt{\left[\frac{CER \times (1 - CER)}{\#\ Control\ Pts}\right] + \left[\frac{EER \times (1 - EER)}{\#\ Exper\ Pts}\right]} =$$

$$\pm 1.96\sqrt{\left[\frac{0.17 \times 0.83}{60}\right] + \left[\frac{0.43 \times 0.57}{60}\right]} = \pm 15.7\%$$

YOUR CALCULATIONS

	+ Outcome	− Outcome
+ Intervention	a	b
− Intervention	c	d

CER = Control group event rate = c/(c+d) =

EER = Experimental group event rate = a/(a+b) =

		Relative Benefit Increase (RBI)	Absolute Benefit Increase (ABI)	Number Needed to Treat (NNT)
EER	CER	(EER − CER)/CER	EER − CER	1/ABI
		***95% CI**		

*95% confidence interval (CI) on an NNT = 1/(limits on the CI of its ABI) =

		Relative Risk Reduction (RRR)	Absolute Risk Reduction (ARR)	Number Needed to Treat (NNT)
CER	EER	(CER − EER)/CER	CER − EER	1/ARR
		***95% CI**		

*95% confidence interval (CI) on an NNT = 1/(limits on the CI of its ARR) =

Source: Based upon material developed by the Oxford Center for Evidence-Based Medicine (2006) (www.cebm.net), with permission.[23]

SUMMARY

Physical therapists and patients/clients select interventions in consideration of a variety of objective and subjective factors. Evidence about interventions may inform the selection process if its design minimizes bias. The experimental research design has the greatest opportunity for control of bias; however, critics point out that the inherent restrictions in the design may limit the relevance of the evidence to "real-world" practice. Some published reports indicate that quasi-experimental and nonexperimental studies may provide acceptable results if adjustment for important prognostic factors is performed. Ultimately, evidence-based physical therapists must evaluate the evidence on its merits and use their clinical judgment to determine the strength of the research design. In addition to design issues, therapists also should evaluate the magnitude of reported treatment effects and consider whether the response to the experimental intervention is clinically worthwhile. This determination may be made when findings are compared to the minimal clinically important difference identified by researchers, therapists, and/or patients/clients.

Exercises

1. Discuss three factors that may influence the intervention selection process for physical therapists and for patients/clients.
2. Discuss the different perspectives in the debate regarding the relative usefulness of experimental, quasi-experimental, and nonexperimental designs.
3. Explain why it is important to mask those responsible for allocating subjects to groups.
4. Discuss the potential consequences of subject attrition. What are the advantages and disadvantages of estimating the lost data?
5. Explain the concept of an intention-to-treat analysis, including its purpose and benefits.
6. Explain why the magnitude of treatment effect provides more useful information than the results of a statistical test of differences.
7. Discuss the concept of effect size in both of its forms.
8. Use the following 2 × 2 table to calculate the experimental group and control group event rates, the absolute and relative risk reductions, and the number-needed-to-treat in this hypothetical study about an intervention to prevent pressure ulcers:

	+ Pressure Ulcer	− Pressure Ulcer
+ Intervention	6	38
− Intervention	17	32

Interpret the results for each of the calculations.

9. Discuss the concept of the minimal clinically important difference and its contribution to determining the potential usefulness of an experimental intervention.
10. The authors of the hypothetical study in Question #8 report a 95 percent confidence interval around the absolute risk reduction (ARR) is (14, 28). The minimal clinically important difference for the study is an ARR = 25 percent. Using this information, make an argument:
    a) In favor of using this intervention.
    b) Against using this intervention.

References

1. Straus SE, Richardson WS, Glaziou P, Haynes RB. *Evidence-Based Medicine: How to Practice and Teach EBM*. 3d ed. Edinburgh, Scotland: Elsevier Churchill Livingstone; 2005.
2. Helewa A, Walker JM. *Critical Evaluation of Research in Physical Rehabilitation: Towards Evidence-Based Practice*. Philadelphia, PA: W.B. Saunders Company; 2000.
3. Guyatt G, Rennie D. *Users' Guides to the Medical Literature: A Manual for Evidence-Based Clinical Practice*. Chicago, IL: AMA Press; 2002.
4. Domholdt E. *Rehabilitation Research: Principles and Applications*. 3d ed. St Louis, MO: Elsevier Saunders; 2005.
5. Batavia M. *Clinical Research for Health Professionals: A User-Friendly Guide*. Boston, MA: Butterworth-Heinemann; 2001.
6. Campbell DT, Stanley JC. *Experimental and Quasi-Experimental Designs for Research.* Boston, MA: Houghton Mifflin Company; 1963.
7. Tabachnik BG, Fidell LS. *Using Multivariate Statistics*. 4th ed. Boston, MA: Allyn & Bacon; 2006.
8. Guide to Physical Therapist Practice. 2d ed. *Phys Ther.* 2001; 81(1):7–944.
9. Chan KBY, Man-Son-Hing M, Molnar FJ, Laupacis A. How well is the clinical importance of study results reported? An assessment of randomized controlled trials. *CMAJ*. 2001; 165(9):1197–1202.
10. Dalton GW, Keating JL. Number needed to treat: A statistic relevant to physical therapists. *Phys Ther*. 2000; 80(12):1214–1219.
11. Cook TD, Campbell DT. *Quasi-Experimentation: Design and Analysis Issues for Field Settings*. Boston, MA: Houghton Mifflin Company; 1979.
12. Critically Appraising the Evidence. Worksheets for Therapy. Oxford Center for Evidence-Based Medicine Web site. Available at: www.cebm.net. Accessed March 15, 2006.
13. Herbert R, Jamtvedt G, Mead J, Hagen KB. *Practical Evidence-Based Physical Therapy*. Edinburgh, Scotland: Elsevier Butterworth-Heinemann; 2005.
14. Hollis S, Campbell F. What is meant by intention to treat analysis? Survey of published randomized controlled trials. *BMJ*. 1999; 319(7211):670–674.
15. Staron RS, Karapondo DL, Kraemer WJ, Fry AC, Gordon SE *et al.* Skeletal muscle adaptations during early phase of heavy-resistance training in men and women. *J Appl Physiol*. 1994; 76(3):1247–1255.

16. Montori VM, Guyatt GH. Intention-to-treat principle. *CMAJ*. 2001; 165(10):1339–1341.
17. Britton A, McKee M, Black N, McPherson K, Sanderson C *et al.* Choosing between randomized and non-randomised studies: A systematic review. *Health Technol Assess*. 1998; 2(13):i–iv, 1–124.
18. MacLehose RR, Reeves BC, Harvey IM, Sheldon TA, Russell IT, *et al.* A systematic review of comparisons of effect sizes derived from randomised and non-randomised studies. *Health Technol Assess*. 2000; 4(34):1–154.
19. Jette AM, Delitto A. Physical therapy treatment choices for musculoskeletal impairments. *Phys Ther.* 1997; 77(2):145–154.
20. Jette DU, Jette AM. Physical therapy and health outcomes for patients with spinal impairments. *Phys Ther.* 1997; 76(9):930–945.
21. "What is an Effect Size: A Guide for Users." Curriculum, Evaluation and Management Center Web site. Available at: http://www.cemcentre.org/ebeuk/research/effectsize/interpret.htm. Accessed February 14, 2006.
22. Santos IA, Stein R, Fuchs SC, Duncan BB, Ribeiro JP *et al.* Aerobic exercise and submaximal functional capacity in overweight pregnant women. *Obstet Gynecol.* 2005; 106(2):243–249.
23. Emery CA, Cassidy JD, Klassen TP, Rosychuk RJ, Rowe BH. Effectiveness of a home-based balance-training program in reducing sports-related injuries among healthy adolescents: A cluster randomized controlled trial. *CMAJ*. 2005; 172(6):749–754.
24. Chatellier G, Zapletal E, Lemaitre D, Menard J, Degoulet P. The number needed to treat: A clinically useful nomogram in its proper context. *BMJ*. 1996; 312(7028):426–429.
25. King M, Nazareth I, Lampe F, Power B, Chandler M *et al.* Conceptual framework and systematic review of the effects of participants' and professionals' preferences in randomized controlled trials. *Health Technol Assess*. 2005; 9(35):1–191.

Chapter 13

Appraising Evidence About Outcomes

Results are what you expect, and consequences are what you get.

—Ladies Home Journal

OBJECTIVES

Upon completion of this chapter the student/practitioner will be able to:

1. Discuss the purposes and potential benefits of evidence about outcomes and outcomes measures.
2. Critically evaluate evidence about outcomes including the:
    a. Important questions to ask related to validity; and
    b. Statistical approaches used.
3. Critically appraise evidence about the development and measurement properties of outcomes instruments.
4. Interpret and apply information provided by the following calculations:
    a. Cronbach's alpha;
    b. Effect size;
    c. Factor analysis;
    d. Floor and ceiling effects;
    e. Intraclass correlation coefficient;
    f. Kappa;
    g. Minimal detectable change;
    h. Minimal clinically important difference;
    i. Standardized response mean.
5. Evaluate p-values and confidence intervals to determine the potential importance of reported findings.
6. Discuss considerations related to the application of evidence about outcomes and outcomes measures to individual patients/clients.

Terms in This Chapter

Bias: Results or inferences that systematically deviate from the truth "or the processes leading to such deviation."[1(p.251)]

Case-Control Design: A retrospective epidemiological research design used to evaluate the relationship between a potential exposure (e.g., risk factor) and an outcome (e.g., disease or disorder); two groups of subjects—one of which has the outcome (the *case*) and one which does not (the *control*)—are compared to determine which group has a greater proportion of individuals with the exposure.[2]

Ceiling Effects: Failure of survey instruments to register higher scores for respondents whose health status has improved.[3]

Clinimetric Properties: The measurement properties of surveys or other indices used in clinical practice to obtain patients' perspectives about an aspect (or aspects) of their condition or situation.

Cohort Design: A prospective epidemiological research design used to evaluate the relationship between a potential exposure (e.g., risk factor) and an outcome (e.g., disease or disorder); two groups of subjects—one of which has the exposure and one of which does not—are monitored over time to determine who develops the outcome and who does not.[2]

Confidence Interval: A range of scores within which the true score for a variable is estimated within a specified probability (e.g., 90%, 95%, 99%) to lie.[3]

Construct Validity: The degree to which a measure matches the operational definition of the concept or construct it is said to represent.[4]

Content Validity: The degree to which items in an instrument represent all of the facets of the variable being measured.[3]

Criterion Validity: The degree to which a measure of interest relates to an external criterion measure.[5]

Cross-Sectional Study: A study that collects data about a phenomenon during a single point in time or once within a defined time interval.[6]

Effect Size: The magnitude of the difference between two mean values; may be standardized by dividing this difference by the pooled standard deviation in order to compare effects measured by different scales.[7]

Effectiveness: The extent to which an intervention or service produces a desired outcome under usual clinical conditions.[1]

Efficacy: The extent to which an intervention or service produces a desired outcome under ideal conditions.[1]

Factor Analysis: A statistical method used to identify a concise set of variables, or factors, from a large volume of data.[3]

Floor Effects: Failure of survey instruments to register lower scores for respondents whose status has declined.[3]

Imputation: A term referring to a collection of statistical methods used to estimate missing data.[8]

Internal Consistency: The degree to which subsections of an instrument measure the same concept or construct.[5]

Longitudinal Study: A study that looks at a phenomenon occurring over time.

Measurement Reliability: The extent to which repeated measurements agree with one another. Also referred to as "stability," "consistency," and "reproducibility."[4]

Measurement Validity: The ability of a test or measure to capture the phenomenon it is designed to capture.[4]

Minimal Clinically Important Difference (MCID): "The smallest treatment effect that would result in a change in patient management, given its side effects, costs, and inconveniences."[9(p.1197)]

Number Needed to Treat (NNT): The number of subjects treated with an experimental intervention over the course of a study required to achieve one good outcome or prevent one bad outcome.[6]

Observational Study (also referred to as a Nonexperimental Design): A study in which controlled manipulation of the subjects is lacking;[3] in addition, if groups are present, assignment is predetermined based upon naturally occurring subject characteristics or activities.[6]

Outcome: "The end result of patient/client management, which include the impact of physical therapy interventions;" may be measured by the physical therapist or determined by self-report from the patient/client.[10(p.43)]

Outcomes Research: The study of the impact of clinical practice as it occurs in the real world.[3,11]

Patient-Centered Care: Health care that "customizes treatment recommendations and decision-making in response to patients' preferences and beliefs. . . . This partnership also is characterized by informed, shared decision-making, development of patient knowledge, skills needed for self-management of illness, and preventive behaviors."[12(p.3)]

p-value: The probability that a statistical finding occurred due to chance.

Responsiveness: The ability of a measure to detect change in the phenomenon of interest.[13]

Standard Error of Measurement: The extent to which observed scores are disbursed around the true score; "the standard deviation of measurement errors" obtained from repeated measures.[3(p.560)]

Standardized Response Mean: An indicator of responsiveness based upon the difference between two scores (or the "change score") on an outcomes instrument.

Test-Retest Reliability: The stability of a measure as it is repeated over time;[3] also referred to as reproducibility.

INTRODUCTION

The *Guide to Physical Therapist Practice*, 2d edition describes *outcomes* as the "result of patient/client management, which include the impact of physical therapy interventions."[10(p.43)] Outcomes may be defined in terms of successful prevention of, remediation of, or adaptation to, impairments, functional limitations, or disabilities. The emphasis on *patient-centered care* and the processes of disablement has focused the discussion about outcomes on the latter two person-level concerns.[3,10,12] Physical therapists anticipate outcomes when they develop treatment goals with their patients/clients. They monitor progress toward these targets and adjust their plans of care in response to examination findings and to patient/client self-reports. Finally, they document the extent to which patients/clients achieve the desired outcomes during, and at the conclusion of, the episode of care. Essential to these processes are adequate methods for outcomes measurement, including the selection and application of instruments and procedures with established reliability and validity. This challenge is the same demand researchers face when determining the best way to measure the variables in their studies.

As with other elements of the patient/client management model, evidence may inform physical therapists about which person-level outcomes to expect at the conclusion of the episode of care. The available evidence, however, uses nonexperimental research designs that generally are considered suspect because of their greater potential for *bias*.[1,2,6,14] This concern is fueled by research that indicates that quasi-experimental and observational studies tend to overestimate treatment effects.[15,16] Evidence also may be used to assist decision making regarding the selection of outcome measures for practice. The purpose of this chapter is to provide information about the potential usefulness of observational studies about outcomes. In addition, considerations for the evaluation of evidence about outcomes and outcome measures are discussed.

OUTCOMES RESEARCH

Outcomes research is the study of the impact of clinical practice as it occurs in the "real world."[3,11] By definition, these studies focus on the *effectiveness*, rather than the *efficacy*, of therapeutic interventions across a wide variety of outcomes.[17] The research designs used in outcomes studies are nonexperimental (or *observational*); therefore, investigators collect information about the phenomenon of interest without purposefully manipulating subjects.[3] These designs are comparable to those used in studies of prognostic and risk factors.

Prospective outcome studies may be *cross-sectional* or *longitudinal* in nature. In the latter case, one or more groups, or cohorts, may be followed to determine what outcomes occur and who develops them. Their appeal is the ability to establish a temporal sequence in which an intervention clearly precedes an outcome, an essential contribution to causal inference. In addition, investigators are able to define the variables to be measured and to standardize data collection processes. Both design elements enhance the ability to answer the research question in a credible and useful manner. On the other hand, prospective studies may be logistically challenging in terms of subject identification and enrollment. Investigators must wait until potential subjects reveal themselves by virtue of admission to the clinical facility or service. Depending upon referral or procedure volume, the timeline for obtaining an adequate sample may be protracted considerably.

Retrospective outcomes studies also may be cross-sectional or longitudinal in nature; the latter is preferred as it is the only opportunity to establish a temporal sequence of interventions and outcomes. These designs commonly are used to take advantage of a wealth of secondary data available in institutional, commercial, and government healthcare-related databases.[3,18] Institutional databases refer to those created by hospitals, clinics, and health systems for internal use. Commercial databases refer to those developed for use by paying clients—such as Focus on Therapeutic Outcomes (FOTO), Inc.[19] and the Uniform Data System for Medical Rehabilitation—Functional Independence Measure (UDS-FIM)[20] —or to insurance company claims databases. Finally, government sources may be federal- or state-level and include databases maintained by the National Center for Health Statistics, the Agency for Healthcare Research and Quality, and the Centers for Medicare and Medicaid Services.[21]

The primary advantage of using data from these sources is the large sample size that can be generated in comparison to prospective studies. Large sample sizes enhance the ability of statistical tests to detect a difference if one exists. In addition, estimates of treatment effect are more precise.[3] Depending upon the database, it may be possible to make population-level estimates from the data it contains. A secondary benefit to using these databases is the variety of potential variables that may be accessed, including subject demographic characteristics, health service utilization and costs, and some clinical details. A third benefit is the opportunity to track subjects longitudinally, which may allow for causal inferences about the relationship between an intervention and an outcome.[18,21]

Retrospective outcomes research also may be conducted using medical records or abstracts of them produced for reimbursement purposes. The actual medical records are preferred because of the clinical data they provide, including details about 1) medical or surgical management and physical therapy interventions; 2) patient characteristics such as demographics, comorbidities, and functional status; and 3) outcomes of care. Gathering data can be time consuming, however, depending upon how large a sample the researcher hopes to obtain. In addition, the lack of standardization in terms of what and how clinicians document care may make it difficult for researchers to obtain consistent information within one record or across multiple records. Abstracts are more consistent in terms of the information they contain and require less time to review, but are considerably distilled versions of the medical record. As a result, they contain much less detail about the clinical status of patients and often do not have outcomes measures other than mortality or discharge destination.[3]

Regardless of the approach used, outcomes research should be evaluated in the same manner as evidence about diagnostic tests, prognostic factors, and interventions. Specifically, physical therapists should consider features of the design that may increase or reduce bias, the nature of the results provided, and their importance in statistical and clinical terms. Finally, findings from outcomes studies must be considered in light of patient/client preferences and values.

STUDY CREDIBILITY

Evidence pertaining to outcomes first should be evaluated with the questions itemized in Table 13-1. These questions focus on the design elements that may enhance the validity of observational studies.[22] Their purpose is to help physical therapists determine the extent to which the study's design may have produced biased results.

Table 13-1 Questions to determine the validity of evidence about outcomes.

1. Was this a study with more than one group?
2. Were the groups comparable at the start of the study?
3. If groups were not equal at the start of the study, was risk adjustment performed?
4. Were variables operationally defined and adequately measured by the data used for the study?
5. Was a standardized person-level outcomes instrument used?
6. Were standardized data collection methods implemented?
7. Did the intervention precede the outcome?
8. Were other potentially confounding variables accounted for in the analysis?
9. Were missing data dealt with in an appropriate manner?

1. **Was this a study with more than one group?**
   Outcomes studies will provide the most information if they include at least two groups: one that received the intervention of interest and one that did not. These designs are analogous to *case-control* and *cohort designs* used in evidence about prognostic factors. Group comparisions may allow investigators to evaluate the impact of different therapeutic approaches. Subjects are not randomly assigned to these groups, however; rather, their involvement is predetermined by the approach to their clinical management that is out of the investigator's control.[6] Group comparisons in observational studies cannot eliminate bias as there may be inherent subject characteristics that influence the selection of the clinical management approach. Nevertheless, these study designs are preferable to single group designs when available.
2. **Were the groups comparable at the start of the study?**
   As with study designs for interventions, a primary concern is the equality of groups at the start of an outcomes study. Baseline equality enhances the researcher's ability to isolate the effects, if any, of the intervention of interest. Unfortunately, the absence of random assignment may limit the degree to which subject characteristics may be distributed evenly between groups in an observational study.[22] Investigators can develop and implement specific inclusion and exclusion criteria that may achieve some level of group equality; however, these criteria generally are less stringent than those imposed during randomized controlled trials. At a minimum, investigators should perform statistical comparisons to evaluate which, if any, characteristics were different and what these differences mean for their analytic approach and their results.
3. **If groups were not equal at the start of the study, was risk adjustment performed?**
   Risk adjustment is the process by which patient/client outcomes are modified to reflect differences in important subject characteristics. Factors of interest often include, but are not limited to: patient/client age, gender, race/ethnicity, baseline functional or health status, presence of comorbidities, and severity or acuity of the condition of interest. In addition, social and environmental factors, such as family support, household income, and accessible living arrangements, may be used.[23] The ability to adequately risk adjust is dependent upon the availability of data about patient/client characteristics considered relevant to the outcome of interest. Secondary databases may provide challenges in this regard, particlarly due to their lack of

detailed clinical and physiological measures. A variety of methods for risk adjustment are available to outcomes researchers, the details of which are beyond the scope of this textbook. Readers who wish to learn more about these approaches are referred to *Risk Adjustment for Measuring Healthcare Outcomes*, 3d edition by Lisa Iezonni.[24]

4. **Were variables operationally defined and adequately measured by the data used for the study?**

The validity of any study is enhanced by the appropriate definition of and adequate measurement of its variables. Variables may be concrete observable phenomena such as height, weight, blood pressure, and heart rate. Each of these physiological parameters has one definition, although there may be multiple ways to measure them. Often, variables are more abstract concepts or constructs, however, such as strength, endurance, level of dependence, or health status. Each of these terms has more than one interpretation; therefore, investigators have an obligation to provide their own operational definitions to avoid confusion regarding measurement and the interpretation of subsequent results.

The ability to adequately measure variables in a study depends in part upon the *construct validity* of the measurement. This issue is particularly relevant for outcomes studies that use secondary data for their analyses. These data have been collected for purposes other than health care research. As a result, they may contain measures that are irrelevant or that are inadequately defined for the purposes of a particular study. Under these circumstances "proxy measures" may be required as substitutes for preferred measures of the variables of interest.[18] A common example is the use of the billing procedure code "therapeutic exercise" as a measure for a physical therapy intervention variable. This code does not provide details pertaining to exercise mode, intensity, or frequency, making it a blunt instrument at best for discerning treatment effectiveness. Secondary data also may be incomplete and/or inaccurate.[25] Accuracy problems often occur when conditions are labeled using diagnostic codes, in part because the codes are designed to support payment for services. The temptation to "up-code"—or assign diagnostic codes to enhance reimbursement—makes it difficult to know whether these indicators of clinical status are valid.[23]

A related issue is the relative availability of clinical data meaningful to physical therapists. Commercial databases such as FOTO[19] and UDS-FIM[20] are designed to measure patient-level functional performance, such as the ability to transfer, ambulate, and climb stairs. The

FIM instrument also provides information about the level of patient effort required to accomplish each functional task.[20] Institutional databases also may be customized to include more detailed clinical measures that are relevant to their practices and market demands. Government and insurance databases, on the other hand, often limit clinical detail to diagnostic and procedure codes or to mortality. These are undiscriminating measures that provide limited inferences about the impact of physical therapy on patient outcomes.[18,21,25]

Although the concerns discussed relate to secondary data, this question also should be addressed in prospective designs in which the investigators were able to define their variables and the methods with which they were measured. Important features include: clearly articulated operational definitions, rationales for the measures collected, verification of the reliability of data recorders or those collecting measures, and data audits to ensure accuracy and completeness. Inadequacies here decrease the credibility of the evidence and should be noted.

5. **Was a standardized person-level outcomes instrument used?**

   One way investigators can enhance the validity of an observational design is to select a standardized outcome instrument with established measurement properties. Specifically, instruments that are reliable, valid, and responsive to change are preferred in order to have confidence that the outcome of interest is being captured consistently and appropriately. An unstable instrument will make it difficult to determine whether change occurred in response to physical therapy interventions or because of problems with measurement variability. The issue of person-level measures pertains to the focus of outcomes research on functional limitations, disabilities, quality of life, and so on. The nature of these instruments and the methods for determining their performance are discussed later in this chapter.

6. **Were standardized data collection methods implemented?**

   Standardized data collection is another method by which investigators may impose some level of control in observational studies. The most control is achieved in prospective designs because investigators can design and implement their own procedures and forms for real-time data collection. They also may audit these processes to ensure their consistency and integrity. Problems with completeness or accuracy may be corrected as they occur. On the other hand, retrospective designs are limited to standardized data abstraction and maintenance procedures. The opportunity to influence the original data recording is, by definition, nonexistent in these studies. As a result, researchers using retrospective designs may find greater challenges with missing or inaccurate data elements.

7. **Did the intervention precede the outcome?**

   This question reflects an interest in potential causal connections between interventions and outcomes. Randomized clinical trials clearly are best suited to establishing cause and effect relationships because of the purposeful manipulation of the experimental intervention and because of the degree to which potential competing explanations may be managed. By definition, observational studies do not have these features. However, results from prospective and retrospective longitudinal designs may support causal inferences if the sequence of intervention and outcome can be established.[22] An investigator's ability to determine this temporal order is dependent upon the nature and integrity of the data being used, as well as the nature of the phenomenon being studied. For example, a study of the effectiveness of physical therapy for the management of acute ankle sprains likely will be able to demonstrate that the injury preceded the intervention based on the dates on which the diagnosis was established and physical therapy was initiated, respectively. On the other hand, chronic conditions, the symptoms of which ebb and flow in their own rhythm, may prove more challenging relative to determining whether the intervention was effective or the subjects experienced natural recovery.

8. **Were other potentially confounding variables accounted for in the analysis?**

   "Confounding" (or extraneous) variables are factors that are related both to the intervention and to the outcome. By defintion, subject characteristics may be confounding variables; however, if risk adjustment has been performed, then these factors have been accounted for. A key exception to this statement is the underlying motivation patients/clients may have for selecting a particular course of treatment. Time also may influence outcomes due to the potential for natural recovery.

   Other possible confounders in outcomes studies include characteristics of the healthcare providers and/or clinical facilities in which service occurs. For example, physical therapists may have varying professional degrees, specializations, amounts of experience, and so forth. If the study is large enough that the intervention of interest is provided by different therapists, then these factors may be important because they may influence how treatment is delivered. Similarly, clinical facilities may have different staff-to-patient ratios, skill mixes, payer mixes, and so on. Studies that use data from multiple sites also may require consideration of these factors, as they may influence decision making regarding the frequency of service delivery and the time spent with the patient/client.

Investigators conducting outcomes research should identify these potential confounding influences and account for them in their statistical analyses. This may be accomplished by stratifying the analysis according to subgroups (e.g., different levels of therapist experience or different clinical sites) or by adding these factors as control variables in a multivariate model.[22]

9. **Were missing data dealt with in an appropriate manner?**

   As noted above, missing data is a common challenge with secondary databases. Investigators have several options for dealing with missing data. First, they may exclude cases with incomplete information from the analysis. This strategy is perhaps the most forthright, but it may introduce bias by creating a sample that is predisposed to a particular outcome. Second, they may estimate missing values through statistical methods referred to as *imputation*.[8] These techniques may be as simple as averaging surrounding values and as complex as regression modeling. Error may be introduced in this process, but investigators may accept this consequence in order to preserve sample size and composition. At a minimum, researchers should report how much of the data were missing so that readers can make their own qualitative judgments about the nature and extent of potential bias introduced.

STUDY RESULTS

Outcomes studies may use the variety of statistical analyses included in evidence about diagnostic tests, prognostic factors, or interventions. These techniques include tests of differences and tests of relationships, as well as calcuations of likelihood ratios, odds ratios, and risk ratios. Tests of differences are appropriate for both between-group and within-group (e.g., single group) designs. Tests of relationships usually are regression analyses used to predict the level of an outcome given the presence of an intervention or interventions. A common approach is to use multivariate models in order to control for possible confounding variables.[22] Statistical test results that indicate a dose-response relationship are of particular interest. The presence of this association provides added support for a causal link between the intervention and the outcome.[22] Finally, calculation of ratios provides information about the magnitude of the effect or relationship. Interpretation of these different analyses is detailed in Chapters 9, 10, 11, and 12.

THE MEANING OF STUDY RESULTS

As with the other types of evidence discussed, evaluation of the statistical importance or meaningfulness of the results from outcomes studies depends upon the obtained p-values and confidence intervals. Investigators will indicate their threshold for statistical signficance; however, physical therapists should determine whether a *p-value* is of sufficient magnitude to be convincing. *Confidence intervals* provide the information necessary to determine the precision of the result within the specified probability.[3] Readers are reminded that interpretation of confidence intervals for ratios is different than for measures of *effect size*. In the former case, an interval that includes the value one indicates that the result may be due to chance. In the latter case, an interval that includes the value zero indicates that the true effect may be no change at all.

In addition to the statistical importance of the results, proponents of evidence-based medicine and practice acknowledge that "large" effects or "strong" relationships reported in observational studies should not be ignored, especially in cases where harmful outcomes are demonstrated.[6,14] There is no consensus about the minimum thresholds for "large" or "strong," so a common-sense judgment about the magnitude of the value in question is needed.

EVIDENCE AND THE PATIENT/CLIENT

As always, the decision to use evidence during clinical decision making for an individual depends upon the following factors:

1) The extent to which the patients/clients resemble the subjects in the study;
2) The extent to which the interventions of interest are feasible in the physical therapist's setting; and,
3) The concordance between the options outlined in the study and the patient/client's preferences and values.

Outcomes research may have an edge over other forms of evidence with respect to the first item, as inclusion and exclusion criteria tend to be less stringent than those used in randomized controlled trials.[14,15,26] As a result, samples tend to be more representative of populations typically served in clinical settings. With respect to preferences and values, physical therapists may find it helpful to discuss a *minimal clinically important difference* (MCID) threshold with the patient/client in order to determine the acceptable amount of change. If risk ratios are reported in the study, then it also may be possible to calculate the *number needed to treat* (NNT) to help make a determination about how much effort may be required to achieve the desired effect. Both of these approaches are detailed in Chapter 12.

Ultimately, using evidence about outcomes requires physical therapists to integrate their critical appraisal skills with their clinical judgment, perhaps more than would be the case when the evidence is a randomized clinical trial. Observational research designs are full of potential for bias that should not be ignored or overlooked. Nevertheless, the premise of this textbook is that these studies constitute evidence that may be more relevant to the circumstances in which patient/client management occurs. Careful evaluation of these studies' merits and thoughtful deliberation about their findings are reasonable and appropriate strategies given that outcomes research is nonexperimental in form. Physical therapists should inform their patients/clients about the relative limitations of these studies so that truly informed decisions may occur.

Table 13-2 provides a checklist to guide the evaluation of evidence about outcomes. Answers to these questions should be considered in the context of the debate about the relative merits of experimental, quasi-experimental and nonexperimental studies.

EVIDENCE ABOUT OUTCOME MEASURES

Outcomes may be captured through a physical therapist's objective examination or through the patient/client's perceptions about his or her status, or both. The patient/client's perspective usually is obtained through self-report survey instruments. Studies pertaining to the development of these measures are categorized as "methodological research." These studies, the designs of which are discussed in Chapter 5, also are nonexperimental. Their goal is to document how the instrument was developed and to establish its *clinimetric* (or measurement) *properties* with subjects representing the population of patients/clients for whom it is intended. All measures have some degree of error with which they are associated (e.g., the *standard error of measurement*). If that error is not understood, then interpretation of the results is problematic because it is not possible to know if what is being measured is the "true" score. An instrument that has demonstrated reliability, validity, and responsiveness is useful to investigators and to clinicians because measurement error is defined and can be accounted for.

Chapter 7 details the various forms of *measurement reliability, validity*, and responsiveness that may be evaluated for all measures physical therapists use. The application of these concepts to self-report measures used to capture person-level outcomes is described here. The goal is to help physical therapists evaluate evidence about the development and implementation of

Table 13–2 Evidence about outcomes—Quality Appraisal Checklist.

Research Validity of the Study	
Was this a study with more than one group?	___ Yes ___ No
Were the groups comparable at the start of the study?	___ Yes ___ No
If groups were not equal at the start of the study, was risk adjustment performed?	___ Yes ___ No
Were variables operationally defined and adequately measured by the data used for the study?	___ Yes ___ No
Was a standardized person–level outcomes instrument used?	___ Yes ___ No
Were standardized data collection methods implemented?	___ Yes ___ No
Did the intervention precede the outcome?	___ Yes ___ No
Were other potentially confounding variables accounted for in the analysis?	___ Yes ___ No
Were missing data dealt with in an appropriate manner?	___ Yes ___ No
Did investigators repeat the study with a new set of subjects?	___ Yes ___ No
Do you have enough confidence in the research validity of this paper to consider using this evidence with your patient/client?	___ Yes ___ Undecided ___ No

What results do the authors report related to your clinical question?

Tests of Differences ____________________

Effect Sizes ____________________

Absolute Benefit Increases ____________________

Relative Benefit Increases ____________________

Absolute Risk Reductions ____________________

Relative Risk Reductions ____________________

Number Needed to Treat (Harm) ____________________

Other ____________________

How important are the results?

Obtained p-values for each statistic reported by the authors:

Obtained confidence intervals for each statistic reported by the authors:

Do these findings exceed a minimal clinically important difference?	___ Yes ___ No
Do the subjects in the study resemble your patient/client?	___ Yes ___ No
Can you perform this intervention safely and appropriately in your clinical setting, given your current knowledge and skill level and your current resources?	___ Yes ___ No
Does the intervention fit within the patient/client's expressed values and preferences?	___ Yes ___ No
Do the outcomes fit within your patient/client's expressed values and preferences?	___ Yes ___ No
Do the potential benefits outweigh the potential risks of using this intervention with your patient/client?	___ Yes ___ No
Will you use this intervention for this patient/client?	___ Yes ___ No

Additional notes:

Source: Based upon material developed by the Oxford Center for Evidence-Based Medicine (2006) (www.cebm.net), with permission.

these instruments so that they may make informed decisions about which measures to use with their patients/clients.

IMPORTANT CLINIMETRIC PROPERTIES

The evaluative criteria used in this textbook are those recommended by the Scientific Advisory Committee of the Medical Outcomes Trust in 2003 (Table 13–3).[27] The authors make clear that these guidelines require further discussion and evaluation to determine their utility. Although they remain to be tested, these recommendations provide a reasonable basis for the appraisal of evidence about self-report outcome measures.

1. **Is there an adequate description of the survey development process, including identification of participants and methods for item development and testing?**

Evidence about the development of a new self-report instrument should include a description of the phenomenon to be captured. Disability, health status, and health-related quality of life are the person-level outcomes of interest most commonly addressed. These abstractions require operational definitions if they are to be successfully measured. The instrument's scope also should be described. Surveys may be written generically so that they can be used for patients/clients with a variety of conditions. Alternatively, they may be designed to focus on a specific condition or body region.

Once these features have been determined, then investigators will start the item development process. The use of focus groups is a common strategy to generate survey questions. This qualitative approach may be supplemented by the use of statistical methods, such as factor analysis, to organize items into common themes. Investigators should describe both of these processes including the characteristics of participants and criteria used to determine whether to keep or eliminate items. Additional features of the instrument, such as the ease with which subjects can read and understand the questions, also should be reported. Finally, investigators should make clear in which direction scores move as subjects improve or decline. A 0–100 scale in one instrument may have the anchors "0 = maximum disability," and "100 = no disability," respectively. Another instrument with the same numerical scale may be anchored in the opposite direction or "0 = no disability" and "100 = maximum disability." Readers should carefully note this information so as to avoid confusion when interpreting results of a study or a patient/client's own self-report.

Table 13–3 Questions to important clinimetric properties of self-report outcome measures.

1. Is there an adequate description of the survey development process, including identification of participants and methods for item development and testing?
2. Is the instrument reliable?
3. Is the instrument valid?
4. Is the instrument responsive?
5. Can the survey scores be interpreted in a meaningful way?
6. Is the instrument easy to administer?
7. If there is more than one method for administering this instrument, did the authors reexamine its measurement properties (Questions 2–6) for each mode?
8. If the instrument is being designed for use in other cultures or languages, did the authors reexamine its measurement properties (Questions 2–6) under these new conditions?

2. **Is the instrument reliable?**

   The reliability of a self-report instrument usually is established by testing for internal consistency and reproducibility. *Internal consistency* reflects the degree to which subsections of a survey measure the same concept or construct.[5] In other words, items within each dimension (e.g., physical function, emotional function, social function, etc.) should be highly correlated with one another. Reproducibility—also referred to as *test-retest reliability*—reflects the stability of repeated scores from respondents presumed to be unchanged over time. Demonstrating this form of reliability requires at least two administrations of the survey. Ideally, investigators will provide a detailed description of the methods used to establish reliability, as well as the characteristics of the subjects used and the conditions under which they were tested.

3. **Is the instrument valid?**

   Validity usually is examined on three fronts: content, construct, and criterion. *Content validity* is the degree to which items in an instrument represent all of the facets of the variable being measured.[3] In other words, if the survey is intended to measure the health-related quality of life of individuals with Parkinson's disease, then items should be phrased to reflect the experiences of individuals with this condition (e.g., stiffness interfering with movement, balance, and so on). The primary way in which content validity is established is by inviting content experts to help develop and/or comment upon items the investigators hope to use. These experts may be clinicians, patients, caregivers, or some combination of members from these groups.

   Construct validity is the degree to which a measure matches the operational definition of the concept or construct it is said to represent.[3] This approach to validity is theory driven. For example, investigators may hypothesize that individuals with Parkinson's disease have restrictions in physical and social function due to the symptoms of their condition. If this is the case, then the survey should contain questions that capture the constructs "physical function" and "social function." Construct validity also may be demonstrated if individuals with higher severity levels consistently report lower functioning on these subscales, as compared to individuals with milder forms of the disease.

   Criterion validity reflects the degree to which a measure of interest relates to an external criterion measure.[5] This is the same form of validity that is examined when diagnostic tests are compared to "gold standard" tests. The challenge is to find a "gold standard" self-report instrument. The most commonly used criterion measure is the Medical Outcomes Study Short Form–36 because of its demonstrated reliability and validity in a variety of patient populations around the world. The survey also has been norm referenced on healthy subjects.[28]

As with reliability, investigators should describe the methods by which they examined instrument validity, including the characteristics of the subjects they used and the conditions under which they were tested.

4. **Is the instrument responsive?**

   Responsiveness is the ability of a measure to detect change in the phenomenon of interest. "Change" may be defined simply as the smallest amount of difference the instrument can detect.[13] A responsive instrument will register change beyond measurement error. In addition, the degree to which an instrument can be responsive is dependent in part upon the scale that is used to measure the phenomenon. *Floor* and *ceiling effects* occur when the scale of the measure does not register a further decrease or increase in scores for the lowest or highest scoring individuals, respectively. Investigators should report which survey questions demonstrated floor and ceiling effects, along with the criteria used to maintain or eliminate problematic items.

5. **Can the survey scores be interpreted in a meaningful way?**

   From a qualitative perspective, the interpretation of scores starts with an analysis of the data's distribution relative to various influences the subjects experience, such as the initiation of treatment, the exacerbation of symptoms, the start of a new activity, and so on. Comparisons also may be made across subgroups of condition severity level or functional status. In both cases, the scores should reflect the meaning of the event or influence.[27] In other words, health-related quality of life would be anticipated to improve if an intervention is effective and to worsen if symptoms flare up. Comparisons with results from other studies using similar subjects and circumstances also may aid in the interpretation process.

   From a quantitative perspective, investigators may identify the minimal amount of change in the measure that is required to be meaningful.[29] "Meaningfulness" may be defined in an objective or subjective way. For example, investigators (or physical therapists) may identify the minimal change in range of motion at the knee required for a patient to climb stairs after a total knee arthroplasty. On the other hand, patients/clients may value ambulation more than stair climbing, in which case the minimal amount of change in range of motion at the knee will be different. Investigators should report how this minimal threshold for change was determined and which meaning they are using.

6. **Is the instrument easy to administer?**

   Developers of self-report instruments must balance the need for adequate measurement of the phenomenon with the practical realities of the clinic. A survey with many questions may be a disincentive to both patients/clients and physical therapists because of the time required to complete it. Similarly, the comprehension level needed to understand the questions should be as accessible as possible to the widest range of individual cognitive abilities. An additional administrative challenge may be the resources required to score the survey. The need for a computer or complex mathematical transformations may dissuade clinicians from adopting an otherwise useful outcome measure. Investigators should provide information about all of these issues.

   Physical therapists understandably want to see the survey instrument while they are reading the evidence about it. If it is included, then clinicians have the opportunity to judge for themselves what administrative demands may be required. Unfortunately, ownership issues often preclude publication to avoid copyright infringement.

Other Circumstances

Questions #7 and #8 in Table 13-3 reflect the need to repeat assessments of clinimetric properties when the survey instrument will be used under conditions different from those under which it was originally developed. These new circumstances may include translation into a different language, administration in a different format (such as oral rather than written), or administration to a different patient/client population. All of the same evaluative criteria apply in these situations.

A related issue is whether investigators repeated their study with a new set of subjects. This question alludes to the possibility that the research findings regarding an outcome measure are reflective only of the subjects in the study. Repeating the study on a second group of subjects who match the inclusion and exclusion criteria outlined for the first group provides an opportunity to evaluate the consistency (or lack thereof) of the measure's performance. If the authors have a large enough sample, then they might split it into two groups, evaluate the outcome measure on one group, and then repeat the evaluation using the second group. If not, then evidence-based physical therapists must read several pieces of evidence about the same outcome measure if they wish to verify its usefulness to a greater degree.

STUDY RESULTS

Results of an evaluation of an outcome measure's clinimetric properties may be presented in both qualitative and quantitative form. In both cases, physical therapists will find it easier to draw their own conclusions if more detail, rather than less, is provided.

Initial Survey Development

The statistical approach commonly implemented in survey development is *factor analysis*. The goal of the process is to determine whether items on a survey group together to form independent subsets or factors.[8] These factors should be intuitively meaningful based upon the content of the questions with which they are associated. For example, questions that address walking, running, climbing, and performing physical activities in the home likely reflect a factor that could be defined as "physical functioning." On the other hand, questions that address mood and emotional state may cluster together to form a subset regarding "psychological functioning."

There are a variety of factor analytic methods available. Investigators using these techniques often report which items grouped together, as well the strength of the association between each item and the factor. This association is represented by a "factor loading score" which is interpreted in the same manner as a correlation coefficient. Scores close to one indicate a strong association between the item and the factor. Threshold values usually are established below which items may be eliminated from the survey, thereby providing empirical support for the contents of the final instrument.

Reliability

Internal consistency usually is determined using Cronbach's alpha (α). This statistic evaluates the correlation among items within each dimension of the survey.[3] The standard identified by the Medical Outcomes Trust Scientific Advisory Committee is a correlation coefficient between 0.70 and 0.90–0.95.[27] Similarly, the intraclass correlation coefficient (ICC) and the kappa are the statistics used for test-retest reliability. Portney and Watkins suggest the following score interpretations for ICC statistics:[4]

- > 0.90 = "excellent agreement"
- > 0.75 = "good agreement"
- < 0.75 = "poor to moderate agreement"

Recommended standards for kappa are:

- 0.81–1.0 = "almost perfect agreement"
- 0.61–0.80 = "substantial agreement"
- 0.41–0.60 = "moderate agreement"
- 0.21–0.40 = "fair agreement"
- 0.01–0.20 = "slight agreement"
- < 0.00 = "poor agreement"[30]

Details about these statistical tests are described in Chapter 9.

Validity

Content validity is not tested statistically. Instead, investigators may describe the degree of consensus among content experts who review the survey. Construct validity also may be described qualitatively or it may be assessed via testing of hypothesized relationships among items or scale dimensions. Criterion validity, on the other hand, may be evaluated based on the relationship between scores on the survey and scores on a "gold standard" instrument. A high correlation coefficient suggests that the survey measures a comparable phenomenon. The challenge for investigators is to find an appropriate criterion against which to judge their instrument. Shorter versions of previously established surveys may be compared to their "parent" instrument.

Responsiveness

Responsiveness may be demonstrated through the calculation of an effect size or a standardized response mean, or both. The effect size may be the simple difference between the scores on the first and second administration of the survey. Alternatively, the calculation may include the standard deviation of the initial survey scores in order to capture the variability within the effect. The following guidelines have been recommended for interpreting this standardized effect size:[4]

- 0.80 large effect size
- 0.50 moderate effect size
- 0.20 minimal effect size

The *standardized response mean (SRM)* is similar in concept to the standardized effect size; however, the variability included in the calculation is the standard deviation of the change scores rather than the standard deviation of the initial scores. An SRM > 1.0 is a commonly stated threshold criteria for establishing responsiveness. Figure 13–1 provides the calculations for these indicators of responsiveness.

The limitations to responsiveness reflected by floor and ceiling effects may be detected when most of the answers to the questions on the survey are scored at the low end or the high end of the scale, respectively. If items demonstrating these effects are maintained, then investigators should describe the characteristics of individuals for whom the survey is not responsive.

Interpretability

As noted above, the interpretation of the meaning of survey scores may be achieved descriptively by evaluating patterns of responses in subsets of respondents defined by different characteristics or different circumstances. On the other hand, the minimal change needed to make a meaningful impact may be identified via opinion gathering, estimates using the standard error of measurement, or predictive modeling using receiver operating characteristic (ROC) curves.[29] Fortunately, this minimal clinically important difference will be reported in the units of the survey instrument (e.g., 12 points).

THE MEANING OF STUDY RESULTS

The statistical importance of the quantitative assessments of clinimetric properties are determined with p-values and confidence intervals in the same manner described in previous chapters. It goes without saying that an instrument with clearly established reliability and validity is worth considering, particularly as a way to measure outcomes of physical therapy interventions from the patient/client's point of view.

Effect Size	$\text{Mean}_{test1} - \text{Mean}_{test2}$
Standardized Effect Size	$(\text{Mean}_{test1} - \text{Mean}_{test2})/\text{SD}_{test1}$
Standardized Response Mean	$(\text{Mean}_{test1} - \text{Mean}_{test2})/\text{SD}_{difference}$

Figure 13–1 Calculations for indicators of responsiveness.

EVIDENCE AND THE PATIENT/CLIENT

All self-report instruments are developed and tested with a group of individuals that may be defined by the nature of their condition, as well as other characteristics such as age, gender, race/ethnicity, cognitive status, native language, and so forth. If the individual patient/client for whom the instrument is being considered is described by these attributes, then the survey may be an appropriate selection. Readers are reminded that the measurement properties of an instrument designed for one purpose should not be assumed to hold true when the survey is used under different circumstances. Additional considerations include the extent of the administrative burden described above.

Evidence Appraisal Tools

The evaluative criteria included here are recommended guidelines still under consideration by those interested in the performance of self-report measures. At the time of this publication, a generally accepted worksheet for appraisal of evidence about outcome measures does not exist. However, Bot *et al.* created their own checklist (Figure 13-2) as part of their systematic review of shoulder disability questionnaires.[31] The contents of the checklist are consistent with the criteria proposed by the Medical Outcomes Trust Scientific Advisory Committee.[27] The authors make clear that they created this tool only to facilitate their review process; their intent was not to promote this tool as a "standardized checklist," given that consensus has not been reached regarding evaluative criteria. Nevertheless, it is reproduced here to provide readers with a concise rendition of the information included in this chapter.

SUMMARY

Outcomes are the end result of physical therapy patient/client management. The focus on patient-centered care and the disablement process reinforces the need to understand treatment effectiveness in terms that are meaningful to the patient/client. Evidence in the form of outcomes research is challenging to use because of the vulnerability to bias inherent in its nonexperimental designs. Nevertheless, these studies constitute evidence worth considering, given their reflection of "real-world" physical therapy practice. Similarly, physical therapists should incorporate evidence in their decision making regarding which self-report outcomes measures to use. Instruments with demonstrated reliability, validity, and responsiveness are preferred when available.

Appendix W1. Checklist for rating the clinimetric quality of self-assessment questionnaires

Clinimetric property	Definition	Criteria used to rate the clinimetric quality
Content validity	The extent to which the domain of interest is comprehensively sampled by the items in the questionnaire.	1) patients were involved during item selection and/or item reduction 2) patients were consulted for reading and comprehension. Rating: + patients and (investigator or expert) involved ± patients only - no patient involvement ? no information found on content validity
Readability & comprehension	The questionnaire is understandable for all patients	Rating: + readability tested; result was good - inadequate readability ? no information found on readability and comprehension
Internal consistency	The extent to which items in a (sub)scale are intercorrelated; a measure of the homogeneity of a (sub)scale	1) Factor analysis was applied in order to provide empirical support for the dimensionality of the questionnaire. 2) Cronbach's alpha between 0.70 and 0.90 for every dimension/subscale Rating: + adequate design & method; factor analysis; alpha 0.70-0.90 ± doubtful method used - inadequate internal consistency ? no information found on internal consistency
Construct validity	The extent to which scores on the questionnaire relate to other measures in a manner that is consistent with theoretically derived hypothesis concerning the domains that are measured.	1) hypotheses were formulated 2) results were acceptable in accordance with the hypotheses 3) an adequate measure was used Rating: + adequate design, method, and result ± doubtful method used - inadequate construct validity ? no information found on construct validity
Floor & ceiling effects	The questionnaire fails to demonstrate a worse score in patients clinically deteriorated and an improved score in patients who clinically improved	1) descriptive statistics of the distribution of scores were presented 2) 15% of respondents achieved the highest or lowest possible score Rating: + no floor / ceiling effects - more than 15% in extremities ? no information found on floor and ceiling effects
Test-retest reliability	The extent to which the same results are obtained on repeated administrations of the same questionnaire when no change in physical functioning has occurred	1) calculation of an intraclass correlation coefficient (ICC); ICC > 0.70 2) time interval and confidence intervals were presented Rating: + adequate design, method, and ICC > 0.70 ± doubtful method was used - inadequate reliability ? no information found on test-retest reliability

Agreement	the ability to produce exactly the same scores with repeated measurements	1) for evaluative questionnaires reliability agreement should be assessed 2) limits of agreement, Kappa, or standard error of measurement (SEM) was presented Rating: + adequate design, method and result ± doubtful method used - inadequate agreement ? no information found on agreement
Responsiveness	The ability to detect important change over time in the concept being measured	1) for evaluative questionnaires responsiveness should be assessed 2) hypotheses were formulated and results were in agreement 3) an adequate measure was used (ES, SRM, comparison with external standard) Rating: + adequate design, method and result ± doubtful method used - inadequate responsiveness ? no information found on responsiveness
Interpretability	The degree to which one can assign qualitative meaning to quantitative scores	Authors provided information on the interpretation of scores: 1. presentation of means and SD of scores before and after treatment 2. comparative data on the distribution of scores in relevant subgroups 3. information on the relationship of scores to well-known functional measures or clinical diagnosis 4. information on the association between changes in score and patients' global ratings of the magnitude of change they have experienced Rating: + 2 or more of the above types of information was presented ± doubtful method used or doubtful description ? no information found on interpretation
Minimal clinically important difference (MCID)	The smallest difference in score in the domain of interest which patients perceive as beneficial and would mandate a change in patient's management	Information is provided about what (difference in) score would be clinically meaningful. Rating: + MCID presented - no MCID presented
Time to administer	Time needed to complete the questionnaire	Rating: + less than 10 minutes - more than 10 minutes ? no information found on time to complete the questionnaire
Administration burden	Ease of the method used to calculate the questionnaire's score	Rating: + easy: summing up of the items ± moderate: visual analogue scale (VAS) or simple formula - difficult: VAS in combination with formula, or complex formula ? no information found on rating method

Figure 13–2 Checklist for rating the clinimetric quality of self-assessment questionnaires.

Source: Reprinted from Clinimetric evaluation of shoulder disability questionnaires: a systematic review of the literature. Bot SDM, Terwee CB, van der windt DAWM *et al., Annals of Rheumatic Diseases*, Volume 63, Copyright 2004, with permission from BMJ Publishing Group, Ltd.

Exercises

1. Discuss the pros and cons of using nonexperimental research to evaluate treatment effectiveness.
2. Discuss the benefits and challenges of using secondary data to conduct outcomes research.
3. Define risk adjustment and the patient/client factors used in the adjustment process. Explain why risk adjustment is necessary when comparing outcomes.
4. Describe the circumstances necessary to make causal inferences in outcomes research.
5. Explain what it means if a self-report instrument does not demonstrate internal consistency.
6. Differentiate between floor and ceiling effects and discuss their implications for the use of a survey instrument.
7. Differentiate between the standardized effect size and the standardized response mean.
8. Describe how the meaning of self-report outcome scores is determined. Give an example of differing interpretations of a change in score provided by a physical therapist and his or her patient/client.

References

1. Helewa A, Walker JM. *Critical Evaluation of Research in Physical Rehabilitation: Towards Evidence-Based Practice*. Philadelphia, PA: W.B. Saunders Company; 2000.
2. Guyatt G, Rennie D. *Users' Guides to the Medical Literature: A Manual for Evidence-Based Clinical Practice*. Chicago, IL: AMA Press; 2002.
3. Domholdt E. *Rehabilitation Research: Principles and Applications. 3d ed.* St Louis, MO: Elsevier Saunders; 2005.
4. Portney LG, Watkins MP. *Foundations of Clinical Research: Applications to Practice*. 2d ed. Upper Saddle River, NJ: Prentice Hall Health; 2000.
5. Polit DF, Beck CT. *Nursing Research: Principles and Methods*. 7th ed. Philadelphia, PA: Lippincott Williams & Wilkins; 2003.
6. Straus SE, Richardson WS, Glaziou P, Haynes RB. *Evidence-Based Medicine: How to Practice and Teach EBM*. 3d ed. Edinburgh, Scotland: Elsevier Churchill Livingstone; 2005.
7. Batavia M. *Clinical Research for Health Professionals: A User-Friendly Guide*. Boston, MA: Butterworth-Heinemann; 2001.
8. Tabachnik BG, Fidell LS. *Using Multivariate Statistics*. 4th ed. Boston, MA: Allyn & Bacon; 2006.
9. Chan KBY, Man-Son-Hing M, Molnar FJ, Laupacis A. How well is the clinical importance of study results reported? An assessment of randomized controlled trials. *CMAJ*. 2001; 165(9):1197–1202.

10. American Physical Therapy Association. Guide to Physical Therapist Practice. 2d ed. *Phys Ther.* 2001; 81(1); 9–744.
11. Matchar DB, Rudd AG. Health policy and outcomes research 2004. *Stroke.* 2005; 36(2):225–227.
12. Knebel E. *Educating Health Professionals to Be Patient-Centered.* Institute of Medicine Web site. Available at: http://www.iom.edu/Object.File/Master/10/460/Patient.pdf. Accessed February 15, 2006.
13. Beaton DE, Bombardier C, Katz JN, Wright JG. A taxonomy of responsiveness. *J Clin Epidemiol.* 2001; 54(12):1204–1217.
14. Herbert R, Jamtvedt G, Mead J, Hagen KB. *Practical Evidence-Based Physical Therapy.* Edinburgh, Scotland: Elsevier Butterworth-Heinemann; 2005.
15. Britton A, McKee M, Black N, McPherson K, Sanderson C *et al.* Choosing between randomized and non-randomised studies: A systematic review. *Health Technol Assess.* 1998; 2(13):i–iv, 1–124.
16. MacLehose RR, Reeves BC, Harvey IM, Sheldon TA, Russell IT, *et al.* A systematic review of comparisons of effect sizes derived from randomised and non-randomised studies. *Health Technol Assess.* 2000; 4(34):1–154.
17. Outcomes Research Fact Sheet. Agency for Healthcare Research and Quality Web site. Available at: http://ahrq.gov/clinic/outfact.htm. Accessed March 15, 2006.
18. Iezzoni LI. Using administrative data to study persons with disabilities. *Millbank Q.* 2002; 80(2):347–379.
19. Focus on Therapeutic Outcomes, Incorporated. Available at: www.fotoinc.com. Accessed January 15, 2006.
20. Functional Independence Measure. Uniform Data System for Medical Rehabilitation Web site. Available at: http://www.udsmr.org/. Accessed April 1, 2006.
21. Freburger JK, Konrad TR. The use of federal and state databases to conduct health services research related to physical and occupational therapy. *Arch Phys Med Rehabil.* 2002; 83(6):837–845.
22. Grimes DA, Schulz KF. Bias and causal associations in observational research. *Lancet.* 2002; 359(9302):248–252.
23. Iezzoni LI. Risk adjusting rehabilitation outcomes. *Am J Phys Med Rehabil.* 2004; 83(4):316–326.
24. Iezzoni LI, ed. *Risk Adjustment for Measuring Health Outcomes.* 3d ed. Chicago, IL: Health Administration Press; 2003.
25. Retchin SM, Ballard DJ. Commentary: Establishing standards for the utility of administrative claims data. *HSR.* 1998; 32(6):861–866.
26. Concato J. Observational versus experimental studies: What's the evidence for a hierarchy? *NeuroRx.* 2004; 1(3):341–347.
27. Scientific Advisory Committee of the Medical Outcomes Trust. Assessing health status and quality-of-life instruments: Attributes and review criteria. *Qual Life Res.* 2002; 11(3):193–205.
28. Short Form-36. Medical Outcomes Study. Available at: http://www.rand.org/health/surveys_tools/mos/mos_core_36item.html. Accessed March 1, 2006.
29. Beaton DE, Boers M, Wells GA. Many faces of the minimal clinically important difference (MCID): A literature review and directions for future research. *Curr Opin Rheumatol.* 2002; 14(2):109–114.

30. Simm J, Wright CC. The kappa statistic in reliability studies: Use, interpretation and sample size requirements. *Phys Ther*. 2005; 85(3):257–268.
31. Bot SDM, Terwee CB, van der Windt DAWM, Bouter LM, Dekker J *et al.* Clinimetric evaluation of shoulder disability questionnaires: A systematic review of the literature. *Ann Rheum Dis*. 2004; 63(4):335–341.

Chapter 14

Appraising Systematic Reviews and Practice Guidelines

Traffic signals in New York are just rough guidelines.

—David Letterman

Objectives

Upon completion of this chapter the student/practitioner will be able to:

1. Discuss the purposes and potential benefits of systematic reviews and clinical practice guidelines.
2. Critically evaluate systematic reviews and clinical practice guidelines including the:
   a. Important questions to ask related to validity;
   b. The relevance of these products to physical therapy practice.
3. Apply the following concepts during the evaluation of systematic reviews:
   a. Effect size;
   b. Heterogeneity;
   c. Homogeneity;
   d. Meta-analysis;
   e. Publication bias;
   f. Relative risk;
   g. Selection bias;
   h. Subgroup analysis;
   i. Vote counting.
4. Interpret relative risks for beneficial and adverse outcomes.

5. Interpret forest plots and evaluate confidence intervals to determine the potential importance of reported findings in systematic reviews.
6. Discuss the potential benefits of using individual subject versus aggregate data in meta-analyses.
7. Discuss the challenges of creating evidence-based clinical practice guidelines.
8. Discuss considerations related to the application of systematic reviews and clinical practice guidelines to individual patients/clients.

Terms in This Chapter

Bias: Results or inferences that systematically deviate from the truth "or the processes leading to such deviation."[1(p. 251)]

Confidence Interval: A range of scores within which the true score for a variable is estimated to lie within a specified probability (e.g., 90%, 95%, 99%).[2]

Effect Size: The magnitude of the difference (or the relationship) between two mean values.[3]

Fixed Effects Model: A statistical method that assumes that all studies in a meta-analysis are measuring the same effect.[4]

Heterogeneity: In systematic reviews, differences in the results of individual studies that are more than a chance occurrence.

Homogeneity: The consistency of results of individual studies included in systematic reviews.

Likelihood Ratio: The likelihood that a rest result will be obtained in a patient/client with the condition of interest as compared to a patient/client without the condition of interest.[4]

Meta-Analysis: A statistical method used to pool data from individual studies included in a systematic review.[5]

Number Needed to Treat (NNT): The number of subjects treated with an experimental intervention over the course of a study required to achieve one good outcome or prevent one bad outcome.[6]

Odds Ratio: The odds that an individual with a prognostic (risk) factor had an outcome of interest, as compared to the odds for an individual without the prognostic (risk) factor.[7,8]

Power: The probability that a statistical test will detect, if it is present, a relationship between two or more variables or a difference between two or more groups.[2,9]

Practice Guideline: "Systematically developed statements to assist practitioner and patient decisions about appropriate health care for specific circumstances."[10(p. 2)]

Publication Bias: The tendency of health sciences and health policy journal editors to publish studies based on the direction and statistical significance of the outcomes.[7]

p-Value: The probability that a statistical finding occurred due to chance.

Random Effects Model: A statistical method that assumes that studies in a meta-analysis are measuring different effects.[4]

Relative Risk: In clinical trials, a ratio of the risk of the outcome in the experimental (intervention) group relative to the risk of the outcome in the control group.[7]

Research Validity: "The degree to which a study appropriately answers the question being asked."[7(p. 225)]

Selection Bias: Error that occurs as a result of systematic differences between individual studies included in, and those excluded from, a systematic review.[1]

Systematic Review: A method by which a collection of research is gathered and critically appraised in an effort to reach an unbiased conclusion about the cumulative weight of the evidence on a particular topic.[5]

Vote Counting: A method for generating a summary statement about the weight of evidence in a systematic review; for reviews about interventions, effectiveness is determined by the number of trials with positive results.[5]

INTRODUCTION

The previous four chapters have dealt with evidence for different topics—namely, diagnoses, prognoses, interventions, and outcomes. A variety of research designs typically used to address each of these patient/client management elements also were discussed. This chapter switches gears by focusing on evidence that is preappraised and summarized in one of two formats: systematic reviews and evidence-based practice guidelines. Although distinctly different in terms of purpose and content, both provide physical therapists with a broader view of the evidence than any single study may accomplish. However, just like individual studies, systematic reviews and evidence-based practice guidelines may be flawed in terms of their design and execution. Results from these lower quality products may be less trustworthy as a result. The purpose of this chapter is to discuss the nature and potential benefits of systematic reviews and evidence-based practice guidelines and to provide methods by which both may be appraised for their quality, meaningfulness, and usefulness.

SYSTEMATIC REVIEWS

A *systematic review* is a secondary analysis of original individual studies. Most commonly these analyses are performed using research about interventions, although systematic reviews of evidence about diagnostic tests or prognostic indicators relevant to physical therapy have been published.[11–14] The goal of conducting a review is to draw a conclusion based upon the cumulative weight of the evidence about an intervention (diagnostic test, prognostic indicator) of interest. As discussed in Chapter 5, systematic reviews are studies in their own right with specifically outlined 1) methods for identifying and selecting individual studies for evaluation, 2) review criteria to determine individual study quality, and 3) processes for drawing conclusions from the body of evidence. A formal results section also is included that may provide qualitative or statistical conclusions about whether the intervention works based on the studies included in the review. Qualitative judgments may be determined through *vote counting*, a process in which each individual trial included in the review receives one vote. A summary conclusion about evidence for an intervention's effectiveness may be made based on the number of votes that represent a positive treatment effect.[5] Alternatively, reviewers may qualify their judgments about the usefulness of a treatment (diagnostic test, prognostic indicator) by indicating the level of evidence, as determined by a specified hierarchy, used to support their statements. This approach commonly is used in the generation of clinical practice guidelines and will be discussed later in this chapter.

Qualitative judgments derived from vote counting are limited, in part, because they reduce the question of effectiveness down to a "yes/no" answer. There is no ability to assess the magnitude of the cumulative effect generated by gathering numerous studies. A levels-of-evidence approach is challenged by the inconsistencies among evidence hierarchies discussed in Chapter 2. The extent to which a judgment is supported may vary depending upon which hierarchy is applied. When possible, a quantitative analysis is preferred. Systematic reviews that use a quantitative method for drawing conclusions are referred to as meta-analyses. *Meta-analyses* pool data from individual studies, thereby creating larger sample sizes. For treatment studies, larger sample sizes have greater *power* to detect differences in outcome, if they exist, between the group that received the experimental intervention and the group that did not. In addition, the larger sample improves the estimate of the *effect size* as indicated by narrower *confidence intervals*. The same benefits may be achieved for reviews of prognostic indicators in the sense that larger sample sizes increase the power to detect relationships if they exist. Similarly, reviews of diagnostic tests have larger samples with which to examine the test's ability to correctly classify individuals with and without a condition of interest. Regardless of the focus of the review, meta-analytic techniques require that the interventions and outcomes of interest in individual studies be the same. Meta-analyses may be performed using aggregate data or using individual subject data from the studies reviewed.[8] The latter is preferable to obtain the most information from the data.

The most prolific source of systematic reviews is the Cochrane Collaboration.[15] This international organization has assembled multiple review groups (50 as of this publication) whose mission is to conduct systematic reviews of interventions relevant to their category (Table 14–1). As the titles suggest, evidence-based physical therapists will be interested in the products from many of these groups. Additional groups exist for the purpose of establishing methods for conducting systematic reviews. Of note are groups dedicated to the development of methods related to reviews of individual studies about diagnostic tests and measures, nonrandomized trials, qualitative studies, and patient-reported outcomes.[16] These studies potentially have more opportunities for *bias*; therefore, different approaches to

Table 14–1 Cochrane Review Groups.

Acute Respiratory Infections Group	Infectious Diseases Group
Airways Group	Inflammatory Bowel Disease and Functional Bowel Disorders Group
Anaesthesia Group	Injuries Group
Back Group	Lung Cancer Group
Bone, Joint and Muscle Trauma Group (formerly the Musculoskeletal Injuries Group)	Menstrual Disorders and Subfertility Group
Breast Cancer Group	Metabolic and Endocrine Disorders Group
Colorectal Cancer Group	Methodology Review Group
Consumers and Communication Group	Movement Disorders Group
Cystic Fibrosis and Genetic Disorders Group	Multiple Sclerosis Group
Dementia and Cognitive Improvement Group	Musculoskeletal Group
Depression, Anxiety and Neurosis Group	Neonatal Group
Developmental, Psychosocial and Learning Problems Group	Neuromuscular Disease Group
Drugs and Alcohol Group	Oral Health Group
Ear, Nose and Throat Disorders Group	Pain, Palliative and Supportive Care Group
Effective Practice and Organisation of Care Group	Peripheral Vascular Diseases Group
Epilepsy Group	Pregnancy and Childbirth Group
Eyes and Vision Group	Prostatic and Urologic Cancers Group
Fertility Regulation Group	Renal Group
Gynaecological Cancer Group	Schizophrenia Group
HIV/AIDS Group	Sexually Transmitted Diseases Group
Haematological Malignancies Group	Skin Group
Heart Group	Stroke Group
Hepato-Biliary Group	Tobacco Addiction Group
Hypertension Group	Upper Gastrointestinal and Pancreatic Diseases Group
Incontinence Group	Wounds Group

synthesizing and drawing conclusions from their data are warranted. The Cochrane Library houses the completed systematic reviews, which may be accessed online for a subscription fee. Updates are scheduled and performed regularly in order to incorporate new evidence as appropriate.

Systematic reviews also are conducted independently from the Cochrane Collaboration and published in numerous health sciences and health policy journals. Format and required content are established by each journal, a situation that poses a challenge to readers when appraising the review. Important questions related to the quality of the review may not be answered simply because of reporting differences in the various publications. In an effort to remedy this situation, Moher *et al.* developed a checklist and flow diagram, referred to collectively as the "Quality of Reporting of Meta-Analyses" (QUOROM) statement, for reporting meta-analyses conducted using clinical randomized controlled trials.[17] These authors expressed particular concern regarding the inclusion of information pertaining to:

- The evidence appraisal critieria;
- The quality of studies included in the meta-analysis, as judged by the appraisal criteria;
- The assessment of publication bias;
- The inclusion of unpublished studies or abstracts;
- The use of language restrictions as criteria for identification and selection of individual studies; and,
- The relationship between the findings from the meta-analysis and other results reported from similar reviews.

In addition, the statement included recommendations for report formats in order to standardize the look, along with the content, for easier reading and appraisal. Stroup *et al.* produced a similar statement—the Meta-Analysis of Observational Studies in Epidemiology (MOOSE)—addressing reporting issues for meta-analyses of studies using nonexperimental research designs.[18] These are the studies used to evaluate the usefulness of diagnostic tests, prognostic indicators, and patient/client outcomes. The degree to which journal editors have adopted either or both the QUOROM and MOOSE statements is not clear. The bottom line for readers, however, is that appraisal of systematic reviews will be more accurate and thorough if more details about the review's methods and results are provided by their authors.

Hierarchies developed for evidence-based medicine and practice generally rank systematic reviews at the top because their conclusions are based on a synthesis of several (sometimes many) studies rather than a single trial. This ranking assumes that the review in question is high quality in its own right, a fact which must be determined by the reader rather than taken for granted.

The potential for low quality exists both due to the manner in which the review is conducted and how the raw materials (e.g., the individual studies) were synthesized. For example, Jadad *et al.* compared the quality of reviews produced by the Cochrane Collaboration with reviews published in health sciences journals.[19] These authors found that Cochrane reviews appeared to be more methodologically sound based on their descriptions of processes used to identify, select, and appraise individual studies. On the other hand, reviews published in other health sciences journals were noted to contain a higher number of individual studies and larger sample sizes. As noted previously, Cochrane reviews are updated regularly, a fact that was supported to some extent by Jadad *et al.*'s work. Fifty percent (50%) of the Cochrane reviews were updated compared to only 2.5 percent of the reviews published in other journals. Shea *et al.* conducted a similar study, but appraised the included meta-analyses using an established checklist and scale.[20] These authors reported that the quality of reviews from both sources was low as demonstrated by the lack of a statistically significant difference in quality scale scores for the two groups of reviews. Both Jadad *et al.* and Shea *et al.'s* findings reinforce the need for evidence-based physical therapists to perform their own appraisal of systematic reviews rather than accepting them at face value.

STUDY CREDIBILITY

Evidence pertaining to systematic reviews physical therapists use first should be evaluated with the questions itemized in Table 14–2. These questions are adapted from the critical appraisal worksheets developed by the Oxford Center for Evidence-Based Medicine.[21] Their purpose is to help physical therapists determine whether there are problems with a review's design and execution that may have biased the results.[8] As most systematic reviews are about interventions, the questions focus on research designs relevant to these studies.

Table 14–2 Questions to determine the validity of systematic reviews.

1. Did the investigators limit the review to randomized controlled trials?
2. Did the investigators provide details regarding their search and study selection methods?
3. Did the investigators describe the processes and tools used to assess the quality of individual studies?
4. Did the investigators provide details about the research validity (or quality) of studies included in the review?
5. Did the investigators address publication bias?
6. If this is a meta-analysis, did the investigators use individual patient data in the analysis?

1. **Did the investigators limit the review to randomized controlled trials?**

   This question reflects the preference for experimental research designs in evidence about interventions. The assumption is that randomized controlled trials (RCTs) are better than quasi-experimental and nonexperimental designs because of the methods available to minimize bias in these experimental designs. As noted in Chapter 12, however, there is considerable debate about the usefulness of studies that lack randomization. In addition, many of the interventions available to physical therapists have yet to be studied using RCTs or may not be eligible for an experimental design because of ethical considerations. If review authors include studies with different types of designs, then they should make that point clear in their report. They also should provide a rationale for that decision and should describe methods for handling information from each type of design included.
2. **Did the investigators provide details regarding their search and study selection methods?**

   Systematic reviews may be limited by selection of a nonrepresentative sample just like individual research projects; the difference is that the "subjects" in the review are studies while the subjects in an individual study are people. To reduce the chances of committing *selection bias*, review authors should describe a process whereby all relevant electronic and print databases and collections are searched. Commonly cited sources include Medline (PubMed),[22] EMBASE,[23] the Cochrane Controlled Trials Register,[15] and CINAHL.[24] Databases also are available for identifying dissertations and unpublished studies.[5] Citation lists in the articles initially located also may be searched, along with Web sites of professional associations whose meetings include presentation of scientific reports. Thorough searches require both electronic and manual efforts to be successful.

   A related issue is the inclusion of studies published in languages other than English. Concerns have been expressed about the contribution to selection bias that language restrictions might create. Moher *et al.* compared meta-analyses that included non-English language studies to those that excluded them and found no difference in effect size between these groups.[25] Juni *et al.* reported a similar result.[26] These authors also indicated that the non-English language studies included in the meta-analyses studied had smaller sample sizes and lower methodological quality. In addition, these trials were more likely to demonstrate statistically significant results. However, they noted that individual meta-analyses might be differentially affected by the exclusion of non-English language works. Both Moher *et al.* and Juni *et al.* acknowledged the improved precision of effect size estimates that occurred by virtue of including foreign language studies in meta-analyses.[25,26] Ideally, authors of meta-analyses will make clear in their reports whether a language restriction was implemented so that readers may determine whether, and to what extent, bias may have been introduced into the review.

In addition, review authors should indicate whether they included both published and unpublished materials. This point refers to the editorial tendency to publish studies with statistically significant positive results rather than studies that demonstrate no difference.[26] McAuley *et al.* investigated the impact of including unpublished material in 41 meta-analyses published between 1966 and 1995.[27] These authors found that, on average, reviews that excluded unpublished works produced a 15 percent larger estimate of effect, as compared to reviews that included them. One approach to counteracting *publication bias* is to include "grey literature," such as unpublished studies, dissertations, theses, proceedings from meetings, and abstracts, in systematic reviews. Unfortunately, unpublished works are more time-intensive to locate and retrieve, a situation that likely deters some authors from pursuing this type of material. In addition, Egger *et al.* found that many unpublished works were of lower quality and cautioned that the extra effort put into searching for this material may not be fruitful.[28] Once again, authors should make clear whether they included unpublished works and, if not, why they were omitted.

Potential candidates for review should be identified using predetermined inclusion and exclusion criteria that are consistent with the purpose of the review. Criteria may refer to the study design, the type of intervention(s) investigated, the characteristics of subjects included in the individual trials, and the types of outcomes and the methods for their measurement. Ideally, authors will itemize studies that were excluded, as well as those that were included, so that readers can make their own judgments about the appropriateness of article selection.

3. **Did the investigators describe the processes and tools used to assess the quality of individual studies?**

The quality of individual studies is an essential ingredient for a successful systematic review. The phrase "garbage in, garbage out" illustrates the point. Individual trials that have weak *research validity* will only produce more misleading results when synthesized for the purposes of a review. Juni *et al.* argue that four types of threats to research validity in clinical trials are particularly concerning:[29]

- Bias that occurs when subject allocation to groups is manipulated by the researcher(s);
- Bias that occurs when groups are managed differently apart from the experimental treatment;
- Bias that occurs when outcome measures are collected by unmasked investigators; and,
- Bias that occurs when the loss of subjects produces systematic imbalances in group characteristics and/or when methods used to deal with this loss are inappropriate.

These sources of bias contribute to the research validity threats referred to in Chapter 8 as "assignment," "compensatory equalization of treatment," "testing," and "attrition." Recall that threats to research validity may introduce competing explanations for a study's results. Juni *et al.*, along with several others, demonstrated that the inclusion of lower quality trials suffering from one or more types of bias produced over-estimates of beneficial treatment effects in meta-analyses.[29,30,31]

The challenge for review authors is to determine the method by which the quality of individual studies will be assessed. In 1995, Moher *et al.* published an annotated bibliography of tools available to assess the quality of clinical trials.[32] These instruments were categorized either as checklists that itemized what design elements should be included in a trial or scales that produced quality scores. Only one of the 25 scales identified at that time was thoroughly tested for its reliability and validity, while several others had information about components of reliability or validity. This lack of methodological appraisal means that different scales may produce different quality ratings of the same clinical trial. In fact, Colle *et al.* investigated the impact of choice of scale on quality scores for studies included in a systematic review of exercise for the treatment of low back pain.[33] These authors reported that the quality scale implemented influenced conclusions regarding the effectiveness of exercise therapy. In addition, correlation among the different scale scores and inter-rater reliability was low. In a subsequent study, Moher *et al.* reported that masked quality appraisal provided higher quality scores using a validated scale, as compared to unmasked appraisals.[30] Until a methodologically sound and useful scale is developed, Juni *et al.* suggested that review authors assess the quality of individual trials using a descriptive component method that identifies the presence or absence of important elements of the review, such as allocation concealment, masking of investigators collecting outcome measures, and so forth.[29]

The bottom line for evidence-based physical therapists is that authors of a systematic review should clearly describe the method and instruments used to perform a quality assessment of individual trials. Ideally, they will have selected a validated instrument to perform the appraisal and will have masked those conducting the quality assessments.

4. **Did the investigators provide details about the research validity (or quality) of studies included in the review?**

   Appraising the quality of individual trials is not sufficient by itself; something should be done with the information acquired from the assessment. At a minimum, authors should report the level of quality for each trial reviewed. If a threshold quality score was required for study inclusion, then it should be stated along with a rationale for its selection. Moher *et al.* suggested incorporating quality scores into the meta-analysis calculation to reduce the over-estimate of effect size.[30] On the other hand, Juni *et al.* discourage this practice due to the variability in scales. Instead, these authors recommend conducting sensitivity analyses by performing the meta-analysis both with, and without, the lower quality individual trials.[29] Either way, a systematic review is likely to be more useful if the quality of individual trials is reported and results are interpreted in light of these appraisals.

5. **Did the investigators address publication bias?**

   As noted above, publication bias reflects the tendency of health sciences and health policy journal editors to publish studies based on the direction and statistical significance of the outcomes.[7] Specifically, preference is given to studies that have found statistically significant beneficial treatment effects (i.e., subjects improved or subjects' risk was reduced). The QUOROM statement recommends that review authors address explicitly the potential for publication bias by stating whether they included grey literature and/or non-English language publications.[17] Sterne *et al.* state that publication bias also may be detected by graphing effect sizes used in the meta-analysis.[34] A nonbiased review will result in a plot that looks like an inverted funnel with a wide base and narrow top. Bias will be suggested if pieces of the funnel are missing—that is, if effect sizes from studies that do not show treatment effects are not included in the plot. However, these authors also note that publication bias may be only one of several reasons for this result. Ultimately, readers must make a qualitative judgment about the potential role publication bias may have played in a review's findings.

6. **If this is a meta-analysis, did the investigators use individual patient data in the analysis?**

   As noted above, meta-analyses may be conducted using aggregate data—that is, summary scores for effect size—or individual patient data. Which data are selected depends entirely upon their availability. Review authors will start with the information that is included in written study reports. When possible, they may also contact investigators from the individual studies to request access to any data that have been maintained over time. Individual subject data are preferred because they provide more detail than summary scores. Of particular interest is the potential to create subgroups of subjects based on different prognostic indicators or other baseline characteristics.[8] Analysis with subgroups allows investigators to examine whether an intervention(s) has differential effectiveness. For example, a technique used to facilitate ventilator weaning in patients with tetraplegia may perform differently if some of these individuals were smokers, while others were not. Subgroup analysis using individual patient data would permit exploration of this hypothesized difference. Unfortunately, logistical impediments may prevent review authors from obtaining this level of information. From a review validity standpoint this is not a fatal flaw, but rather a lost opportunity. Resulting limitations in the interpretation of findings from a meta-analysis should be ackowledged.

STUDY RESULTS

One of the motivations to conduct a systematic review is to try to resolve conflicting results from individual studies. In order for this resolution to be meaningful, studies must not be extraordinarily divergent in their findings. Extreme differences in results suggest that these contradictory findings are more likely than a chance occurrence, which makes drawing conclusions about effectiveness, or lack of it, problematic. Review authors and readers may get a sense of the *homogeneity* of individual study findings by examining a plot of the individual effect sizes and associated confidence intervals. Overlapping confidence intervals indicate a more homogeneous collection of results.[34] Review authors also may perform chi-squared tests to determine the consistency of findings. In this case, a *p-value* below a specified threshold (e.g., alpha (α) = 0.05) indicates that *heterogeneity* of results is present more than chance alone would explain. Under these circumstances, review authors should offer their insights as to possible reasons for the divergence of study findings. Differences in sample composition, intervention protocol, or outcomes measured, are some of the commonly identified sources of heterogeneity. Depending upon possible reasons for the differences in results, review authors may either make statistical adjustments or conduct separate meta-analyses for identified subgroups in order to deal with heterogeneity. In situations where these adjustments are inappropriate, meta-analyses will be skipped altogether.[4]

Qualitative judgments about the strength of the evidence may be all that review authors can provide when individual studies have different methods for addressing the research question or when results are sufficiently heterogeneous that pooling data is not feasible. Under these circumstances, the outcomes of each trial usually are reported along with details about the relative strength of their designs. When meta-analyses are possible, review authors must decide which statistical methods to use to pool the data. The details of these approaches are beyond the scope of this textbook. In general, investigators must first determine whether individual studies are measuring a similar treatment effect or different treatment effects. In the former case they will report conducting a meta-analysis using a *fixed effects model* (also known as a Mantel-Haenzel test). In the latter case authors will describe the use of a *random effects model.*[4] Next, authors will pool the data by weighting each study based on its sample size. The larger the sample, the greater the weight assigned. Once the analysis is conducted the final product reported may be:

- A mean difference in outcomes between the groups (the effect size);
- The standardized mean difference in outcomes (the standardized effect size);
- Odds ratios; or,
- Relative risks.

The first two options are used with continuous data, while the latter two are used with dichotomous data.[5]

Reporting Formats

Review authors may present information from individual trials in a variety of formats. Descriptive details and qualitative assessments usually are summarized in tables. Table 14–3 is an example of descriptive information about each study included in a systematic review of manual therapy for tension-type headaches.[35] These details provide readers with a quick way to identify the subjects included, the interventions used, and the outcomes achieved—all of which are necessary to determine the relevance of the trials to an individual patient in the therapist's clinical setting. Table 14–4 elaborates on the qualitative assessment of the individual studies using the rating scale developed by PEDro, the Australian physiotherapy evidence database.[36] Note that this scale looks for the presence of key design components necessary to

Table 14–3 Descriptive information about articles included in a systematic review.[35]

Study	Design	PEDro Score	Diagnosis	Sample Size	Treatments (n patients)
Bove et al[28]	RCT	8/10	Episodic TTH	75 (26 men/49 women)	A) Spinal manipulation + soft tissue therapy (n = 38) B) Soft tissue therapy + placebo laser (n = 37)
Donkin et al[33]	RCT (No placebo group)	7/10 (rated by the authors)	TTH (subtype was not specified)	30 (10 men/20 women)	A) Spinal manipulation (n = 15) B) Spinal manipulation + cervical manual traction (n = 15)
Demirturk et al[31]	RCT (No placebo group)	7/10 (rated by the authors)	Chronic TTH	30 women	A) Connective tissue manipulation (n = 15) B) Dr. James Cyriax vertebral manipulation (n = 15)
Hanten et al[29]	RCT	6/10 (rated by the authors)	TTH (subtype was not specified)	60 (17 men/43 women)	A) CV-4 craniosacral technique (n = 20) B) Protraction-retraction neck exercises (n = 20) C) No treatment (n = 20)
Boline et al[30]	RCT	5/10	TTH (subtype was not specified)	126 (gender was not specified)	A) Spinal manipulation (n = 70) B) Amitriptyline doses between 10 mg to 30 mg/per day (n = 56)
Akbayrak et al[32]	Open non-controlled study	2/10 (rated by the authors)	TTH (subtype was not specified)	20 women	Connective tissue manipulation

Study	Outcome Measures	Number of Sessions	Follow Up	Results
Bove et al[28]	Daily hours of headache, headache intensity (VAS), daily analgesic use	8 sessions in 4 weeks (two sessions per week)	14 weeks after the intervention	Both groups obtained a significant reduction in outcome measures. No differences between groups
Donkin et al[33]	Headache diary, McGill Pain Questionnaire, Neck Disability Index, Numerical Pain Rating Scale	9 sessions in 5 weeks (two sessions per week)	4 weeks after the intervention	Group A obtained a greater improvement than group B
Demirturk et al[31]	Headache index value, active CROM, PPT	20 sessions in 4 weeks (5 sessions per week)	4 weeks after the interven-tion—(Immedi-ate effects)	No significant differences between groups were found
Hanten et al[29]	Headache pain intensity (VAS), affective component of pain (VAS)	1		Group A obtained a greater improvement than group B and C ($P < 0.05$)
Boline et al[30]	Headache pain intensity (VAS), weekly headache frequency, over the counter medication usage, functional health status (SF-36)	Group A received 12 ses-sions in 6 weeks (two ses-sions per week). Group B took a daily dose of amitriptyl during 6 weeks	4 weeks after the intervention	No significant differences between groups at the end of treatment. At 4-weeks follow up group A showed a greater improvement than group B
Akbayrak et al[32]	Headache intensity, frequency and duration, analgesic use and associated symptoms	20 sessions in 4 weeks (5 sessions per week)	6 months after the intervention	Patients showed a significant improvement in all the outcome measures ($P < 0.05$)

RCT, randomized controlled trial; TTH, tension type headache; PPT, pressure pain threshold; CROM, cervical range of motion; amitriptyl, amitriptyline; VAS, visual analogue scale.

Source: Reprinted with permission. Fernandez-de-las-Peñas C, Alonso-Blanco C, Cuadrado ML, Miangolarra JC, Bariiga FJ *et al.* Are manual therapies effective in reducing pain from tension-type headache? *Clinical Journal of Pain*. Copyright (2006); 22(3):278–285. Study source numbers are from original article.

Table 14–4 Qualitative assessment of individual trials in a systematic review of manual therapy for tension-type headaches.[35]

Study	PEDro Score Rated Details of the Trials Included in This Review					
	Random Allocation	Concealed Allocation	Baseline Comparability	Blind Assessors	Blind Subjects	Blind Therapist
Bove et al[28]	Yes	Yes	Yes	Yes	No	No
Donkin et al[33]*	Yes	Yes	Yes	No	Yes	No
Demirturk et al[31]*	Yes	Yes	Yes	No	Yes	No
Hanten et al[29]*	Yes	Yes	Yes	No	Yes	No
Boline et al[30]	Yes	Yes	Yes	No	No	No
Akbayrak et al[32]*	No	No	No	No	No	No

Study	Follow Up	Intention-to-Treat Analysis	Between-Group Comparisons	Points Estimates and Variability	Total Score
Bove et al[28]	Yes	Yes	Yes	Yes	8/10
Donkin et al[33]*	Yes	No	Yes	Yes	7/10
Demirturk et al[31]*	Yes	No	Yes	Yes	7/10
Hanten et al[29]*	No	No	Yes	Yes	6/10
Boline et al[30]	No	No	Yes	Yes	5/10
Akbayrak et al[32]*	Yes	No	No	Yes	2/10

*PEDro score calculated by the authors of this review.

Source: Reprinted with permission. Fernandez-de-las-Peñas C, Alonso-Blanco C, Cuadrado ML, Miangolarra JC, Bariiga FJ *et al.* Are manual therapies effective in reducing pain from tension-type headache? *Clinical Journal of Pain*. Copyright (2006); 22(3):278–285. Study source numbers are from original article.

optimize the research validity of a clinical trial. Readers of this review must make their own determination about whether a minimum threshold score is needed before the individual trial will be considered trustworthy. Cochrane reviews generally have the most comprehensive collection of descriptive and qualitative tables; however, access to this information generally means there are many pages to print!

Quantitative results from individual studies may be presented in table or in graph format. Table 14–5 illustrates a tabular summary of trials included in a systematic review of interventions for idiopathic scoliosis in adolescents.[37] Where possible Lenssinck *et al.* calculated the relative risk for individual trials. The *relative risk* is a ratio of the risk of the outcome in the experimental (intervention) group relative to the risk of the outcome in the control group.[7] A ratio less than one indicates that the outcome is less likely to occur in the experimental group versus the control group. A ratio greater than one indicates that the outcome is more likely to occur in the experimental group versus the control group. A ratio equal to one indicates no difference between the experimental group and the control group. In Table 14–5 the outcomes measured primarily are adverse events—surgery or progression of the spinal curvature. If the interventions studied are effective, then the relative risk should be less than one. Note that calculations were conducted only for individual trials; data could not be pooled to perform a meta-analysis because of the variety of manual therapeutic approaches investigated.

Results from systematic reviews also may be presented graphically using forest plots. These visual displays usually are designed to indicate treatment effect size, along with associated confidence intervals, for individual studies reviewed. If a meta-analysis was performed, then the cumulative effect size will be presented as well.[38] These same displays can be used to summarize *likelihood ratios, odds ratios*, and relative risks. Figure 14–1 is a forest plot from a Cochrane review of continuous passive motion (CPM) following total knee arthroplasty.[39] The plot summarizes results from each trial for the comparison between CPM combined with physical therapy versus physical therapy alone. The outcome of interest is active knee flexion two weeks following surgery (black oval, upper left). The midline of the graph is zero degrees or "no change" in active knee flexion (gray arrow). The positive values to the right of the midline indicate increased knee flexion—the outcome hypothesized to occur if CPM plus physical therapy is effective. The negative values to the left of the mid-line indicate decreased knee flexion—the outcome that is hypothesized to occur if CPM plus physical therapy is "harmful" (black arrows). The effect size, calculated as a weighted mean difference between the groups (gray oval, upper right), is measured

Table 14–5 Quantitative results from individual trials in a systematic review of interventions for scoliosis.[37]

Study	Intervention	Results	RR as Calculated by the Reviewers
Athanasopoulos et al[27]	I: Boston brace + training, n=20 C: Boston brace, n=20	I: increased ability to perform aerobic work, 48.1% C: decreased ability to perform aerobic work, 9.2%	
el-Sayyad and Conine[33]	I: exercise + Milwaukee brace, n=8 C1: exercise, n=10 C2: exercise + electrical stimulation, n=8	I change: −4.05° C1 change: −2.93% C2 change: −3.76°	
den Boer et al[29]	I: side shift therapy, n=44 C: brace therapy, n=120	I change: +2.6°, failure=34.1% C change: −1.5°, failure=31.7%	Failure I versus C: RR=1.08 (0.66−1.75), meaning no differences in failure rate between I and C
Birbaumer et al[28]	I: behaviorally posture-oriented training, n=15 C: noncompliers, n=4	I change: −6.14° C change: +8.20°	
Carman et al[30]	I: Milwaukee brace + exercises, n=21 C: Milwaukee brace, n=16	I (n=12) change: −3.7° C (n=12) change: −3.4°	Surgery I versus C: RR=1.52 (0.45–5.18), meaning no difference in surgery rate between I and C
Gepstein et al[35]	I: Charleston bending brace, n=85 C: thoraco-lumbo-sacral orthosis, n=37	Success: I=80%, C=81% Surgery: I=12.3%, C=11.8% Failure: I=7.4%, C=5.4%	Surgery I versus C: RR=1.09 (0.36–3.25), meaning no difference in surgery rate between I and C Failure I versus C: RR=1.31 (0.28–6.17), meaning no difference in failure between I and C

Nachemson and Peterson[38]	I: underarm plastic brace, n=111 C1: night-time electrical surface stimulation, n=46 C2: no treatment, n=129	Failure: I=15%, C1=48%, C2=45%	Failure I versus C1: RR=0.3 (0.16–0.56), meaning failure rate in I significantly lower compared with C1 Failure I versus C2: RR=0.28 (0.16–0.48), meaning failure rate in I significantly lower compared with C2 Failure C1 versus C2: RR=0.93 (0.62–1.41), meaning no difference in failure rate between both control groups
Dickson and Leatherman[32]	I: traction, n=? C: exercises, n=?	I change: standing curve in cast +3°, curve on lateral bending +1° C change: standing curve in cast +1°, curve on lateral bending −4°	
von Deimling et al[31]	I: Chêneau corset, n=21 C: Milwaukee brace, n=26	I change: +1.2°, 19% success C change: +2.9°, 3.8% success	Success I versus C: RR=0.84 (0.67–1.05), meaning no difference in success rate between I and C
Fiore et al[34]	I: 3-valve orthosis, n=15 C: Boston brace, n=15	I angle change: −6° C angle change: −3°	
Mulcahy et al[37]	I: Milwaukee brace, throat mold design, n=7 C: conventional Milwaukee brace, n=30	I: 42.85% remain in brace, 14.3% surgery C: 36.7% remain in brace, 16.7% surgery	Surgery I versus C: RR=0.86 (0.12–6.23), meaning no difference in surgery rate between I and C
Schlenzka et al[39]	I: lateral electrical surface stimulation, n=20 C: Boston brace, n=20	I (n=6) change: posttreatment +5°, follow-up (2.3 y) +8° C change: posttreatment −6°, follow-up (2.7 y) −2°	

continues

Table 14–5 Quantitative results from individual trials in a systematic review of interventions for scoliosis[37] *(continued)*.

Study	Intervention	Results	RR as Calculated by the Reviewers
Minami[36]	I: Milwaukee brace C: thoraco-lumbo-sacral orthosis, Boston-Milwaukee brace	No information about results of different treatment groups; results in curve and age groups	

[a] Degrees with "−" sign indicate a decrease of the spinal curvature; degrees with " +" sign indicate an increase of the spinal curvature. Failure is > 5 degrees progression of spinal curvature. RR = relative risk (95% confidence interval); RR < 1 means effect in favor of first-mentioned comparison. I = intervention, C = control.

Source: Reprinted from Lenssinck MLB, Frijlink AC, Berger MY, Bierma-Zeinstra SMA, Verkerk K *et al.* Effect of bracing and other conservative interventions in the treatment of idiopathic scoliosis in adolesents: A systematic review of clinical trials. *Phys Ther.* 2005; 85(12):1329–1339 with permission of the American Physical Therapy Association. Study source numbers are from original article.

in degrees and is represented by points on the plot (black circle). The boxes around each point indicate the weight assigned to each trial and coincide with the values in the second column from the right (weight %). A bigger box indicates a higher weight. Finally, the large diamond at the bottom of the plot (gray circle) represents the pooled estimate of the effect size which, based on the values in the far right column, is an increase of 4.3 degrees. Note that information regarding the test for heterogeneity also is printed on the plot; in this case, the high p-value indicates homogeneity of the trials (gray oval, bottom left).

Readers should examine all details of a forest plot to ensure accurate interpretation. In particular, it is important to note what outcome is being reported. In Figure 14-1, the outcome of interest is patient improvement reflected by increased range of motion at the knee. Studies demonstrating beneficial effects of the experimental intervention will have point estimates to the right of the midline. A later analysis in this review evaluated the effect of CPM plus physical therapy on hospital length of stay (Figure 14-2). The preferred outcome in that instance is a reduction, rather than an increase, in the number of days in the hospital. Therefore, the left side of the graph represents a beneficial effect of the experimental intervention.

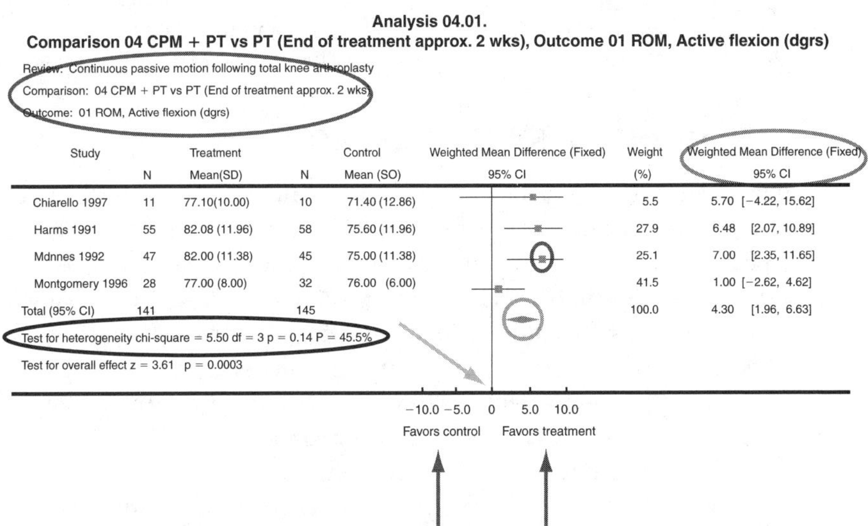

Study	Treatment N	Treatment Mean(SD)	Control N	Control Mean (SO)	Weight (%)	Weighted Mean Difference (Fixed) 95% CI
Chiarello 1997	11	77.10(10.00)	10	71.40 (12.86)	5.5	5.70 [−4.22, 15.62]
Harms 1991	55	82.08 (11.96)	58	75.60 (11.96)	27.9	6.48 [2.07, 10.89]
Mdnnes 1992	47	82.00 (11.38)	45	75.00 (11.38)	25.1	7.00 [2.35, 11.65]
Montgomery 1996	28	77.00 (8.00)	32	76.00 (6.00)	41.5	1.00 [−2.62, 4.62]
Total (95% CI)	141		145		100.0	4.30 [1.96, 6.63]

Figure 14-1 Forest plot of study results evaluating effect of experimental intervention on active knee flexion.

Source: Reprinted from Milne S, Brosseau L, Robinson V, Noel MJ, David J *et al.* Continuous passive motion following total knee arthroplasty. *The Cochrane Database of Systematic Reviews.* 2003; Issue 2. Article No.: CD004260. DOI: 10.1002/14651858. CD004260. Copyright 1999-2006, John Wiley & Sons, Inc. Reproduced with permission.

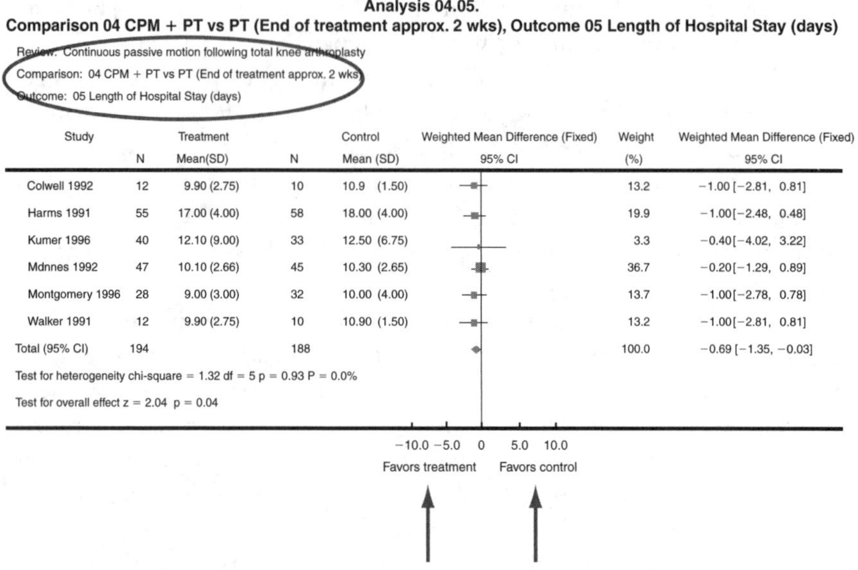

Analysis 04.05.
Comparison 04 CPM + PT vs PT (End of treatment approx. 2 wks), Outcome 05 Length of Hospital Stay (days)

Review: Continuous passive motion following total knee arthroplasty
Comparison: 04 CPM + PT vs PT (End of treatment approx. 2 wks)
Outcome: 05 Length of Hospital Stay (days)

Study	Treatment N	Treatment Mean(SD)	Control N	Control Mean (SD)	Weight (%)	Weighted Mean Difference (Fixed) 95% CI
Colwell 1992	12	9.90 (2.75)	10	10.9 (1.50)	13.2	−1.00 [−2.81, 0.81]
Harms 1991	55	17.00 (4.00)	58	18.00 (4.00)	19.9	−1.00[−2.48, 0.48]
Kumer 1996	40	12.10 (9.00)	33	12.50 (6.75)	3.3	−0.40[−4.02, 3.22]
Mdnnes 1992	47	10.10 (2.66)	45	10.30 (2.65)	36.7	−0.20[−1.29, 0.89]
Montgomery 1996	28	9.00 (3.00)	32	10.00 (4.00)	13.7	−1.00[−2.78, 0.78]
Walker 1991	12	9.90 (2.75)	10	10.90 (1.50)	13.2	−1.00[−2.81, 0.81]
Total (95% CI)	194		188		100.0	−0.69 [−1.35, −0.03]

Test for heterogeneity chi-square = 1.32 df = 5 p = 0.93 P = 0.0%
Test for overall effect z = 2.04 p = 0.04

Figure 14–2 Forest plot of study results evaluating effect of experimental intervention on length of hospital stay.

Source: Reprinted from Milne S, Brosseau L, Robinson V, Noel MJ, David J *et al.* Continuous passive motion following total knee arthroplasty. *The Cochrane Database of Systematic Reviews.* 2003; Issue 2. Article No.: CD004260. DOI: 10.1002/14651858. CD004260. Copyright 1999–2006, John Wiley & Sons, Inc. Reproduced with permission.

THE MEANING OF STUDY RESULTS

When meta-analyses cannot be performed, the "importance" of the findings are inferred from the extent to which individual studies report similar results. This determination is influenced by the quality of each trial, as well as by the statistical importance of their results as indicated by p-values, confidence intervals, or magnitude of the effect. Review authors will tell you what they think by creating summary statements about the weight of the evidence. A treatment effect will be considered likely if numerous studies all report beneficial outcomes from the intervention of interest.

Calculation of a cumulative effect size, odds ratio, relative risk, or likelihood ratio is the first step in making a decision about the weight of the evidence in a meta-analysis. These values are point estimates derived from the pooled sample; however, their statistical importance is determined based on the level of certainty that the treatment effect represents the "real effect," if it could be measured. The most useful way to demonstrate statistical importance in meta-analyses is to calculate *confidence intervals*. The confidence interval will provide a range within which the true effect is estimated to lie according to a specified probability.[2] Most often the probability selected is 95 percent. Interpretation of the confidence interval depends on the summary statistic used. For effect sizes, the confidence interval must *exclude* the value zero because that represents "no change." For odds ratios, relative risks and likelihood ratios the confidence interval must *exclude* the value one because that represents equal odds, risks, or likelihoods between the experimental and control groups.

Confidence intervals may be reported in text and/or graphic form. In forest plots, confidence intervals calculated for the individual trials are indicated by straight lines through the point estimates. In Figure 14–1, two of the studies have 95 percent confidence intervals that cross the midline of the plot indicating that the intervals include zero or "no change." The remaining two studies have confidence intervals that do not cross the midline of the plot, so a positive treatment effect is acknowledged. Note that all of the confidence intervals overlap, a situation that is consistent with the results of the heterogeneity test. The confidence interval for the cumulative effect size is represented by a diamond, a shape that reflects the increased precision of the estimate due to the increased sample size. Again in Figure 14–1, this confidence interval does not include zero. This result would be interpreted to mean that, based on the weight of the evidence included, CPM plus physical therapy is more effective than physical therapy alone for increasing active knee range of motion after total knee arthroplasty.

Another method by which to determine the importance of findings from a meta-analysis is to calculate the *number needed to treat* based on studies that use odds ratios. Fortunately, reference tables are available to make these conversions and are included on the systematic review worksheet in Appendix B.[8] What the therapist must determine is the rate with which their patients/clients will achieve the outcome of interest if provided with the experimental intervention. This value is a percentage expressed in decimal form and is referred to with the acronym "PEER" (patient's expected event rate). This step is comparable to determining a patient/client's pretest probability for a diagnostic test. Once the PEER has been identified on the y-axis of the table, then the odds ratio from the review can be identified on the x-axis. The number needed to treat is found at the intersection of the PEER row and the OR column. Not surprisingly, the lower the number needed to treat the more useful the experimental intervention may be.

Clinical Importance

As always, statistical importance should not be considered synonymous with clinical importance. This point is exemplified in Figures 14–1 and 14–2. Both figures indicate that a statistically significant benefit was achieved by CPM plus physical therapy because the confidence intervals do not include the value zero. However, the actual amount of change that occurred may be viewed by some as clinically unimportant because it is so small. Four additional degrees of active knee flexion two weeks after surgery likely would not translate into a detectable functional benefit for most individuals. Similarly, a reduction in length of stay of less than one full day may please the patient, but may or may not have an impact on the cost of the hospital stay. Once again, clinical judgment along with patient preferences and values, must be used to determine whether this evidence is convincing enough to support the additional cost, discomfort, and effort required to apply CPM.

EVIDENCE AND THE PATIENT/CLIENT

The same considerations outlined in Chapter 12 apply here with respect to using evidence from systematic reviews with a patient/client:

- The intervention (or diagnostic test, prognostic indicator, outcome) is appropriate and feasible in the physical therapist's practice setting;
- The subjects in the review resemble the patient/client to whom the evidence may be applied; and,
- The intervention (or diagnostic test, prognostic indicator, outcome) must be compatible with the patient/client's preferences and values.

Table 14-6 provides a checklist to guide the evaluation of systematic reviews for use in any practice setting. Answers to these questions should be considered in the context of the debate about the relative merits of experimental, quasi-experimental, and nonexperimental studies and their inclusion in systematic reviews.[20]

Table 14-6 Systematic reviews—Quality Appraisal Checklist.

Research Validity of the Study	
Did the investigators limit the review to randomized controlled trials?	___ Yes ___ No
Did the investigators provide details regarding their search and study selection methods?	___ Yes ___ No
Did the investigators describe the processes and tools used to assess the quality of individual studies?	___ Yes ___ No
Did the investigators provide details about the research validity (or quality) of studies included in the review?	___ Yes ___ No
Did the investigators address publication bias?	___ Yes ___ No

Research Validity of the Study

Do you have enough confidence in the research validity of this paper to consider using this evidence with your patient/client?	___ Yes ___ Undecided ___ No
If this is a meta-analysis, did the investigators use individual patient data in the analysis?	___ Yes ___ No
Were the results consistent from study to study (i.e., homogeneous)?	___ Yes ___ No

What results do the authors report related to your clinical question?

Effect Sizes ______________________________

Likelihood Ratios ______________________________

Odds Ratios ______________________________

Relative Risks ______________________________

Number Needed to Treat (Harm) ______________________________

Other ______________________________

How important are the results?

Obtained p-values for each statistic reported by the authors:

Obtained confidence intervals for each statistic reported by the authors:

If this paper is not a meta-analysis, is there a substantive conclusion that can be drawn about the cumulative weight of the evidence?	___ Yes ___ No
Do the subjects in the systematic review resemble your patient/client? If no, how are they different?	___ Yes ___ No
Can you perform this intervention(s) safely and appropriately in your clinical setting given your current knowledge and skill level and your current resources?	___ Yes ___ No
Does/(do) the intervention(s) fit within your patient/client's expressed values and preferences?	___ Yes ___ No
Do the potential benefits outweigh the potential risks of using the intervention(s) with your patient/client?	___ Yes ___ No
Will you use the intervention(s) for your patient/client?	___ Yes ___ No

Source: Based upon material developed by the Oxford Center for Evidence-Based Medicine (2006) (*www.cebm.net*), with permission.[20]

Readers should also consider the following questions pertaining to subgroup analysis in systematic reviews:[21]

1. "Do the qualitative differences in treatment effectiveness really make biologic and clinical sense?"
2. "Is the qualitative difference both clinically (beneficial for some, but useless or harmful for others) and statistically significant?"
3. "Was this difference hypothesized before the study began (rather than the product of dredging the data), and has it been confirmed in other independent studies?"
4. "Was this one of just a few subgroup analyses carried out in this study?"

These points challenge physical therapists to consider the extent to which meaningful subgroups are likely to exist among a population of patients/clients with a particular condition. Answers to these questions depend upon a physical therapist's knowledge and understanding of the condition of interest, as well as possible prognostic and risk factors with which it is associated. The potential for different responses to the experimental intervention must also be considered from a clinical and statistical perspective. Finally, differential effects that result from data dredging may be artifact and, therefore, clinically meaningless. Straus *et al.* argue that subgroup analysis should only be taken seriously if a reader can answer "yes" to all four questions.[8]

CLINICAL PRACTICE GUIDELINES

Clinical *practice guidelines* are defined as "systematically developed statements to assist practitioner and patient decisions about appropriate health care for specific circumstances."[10(p. 2)] Their intent is to improve the efficiency and effectiveness of health care through the use of summary recommendations about patient/client management. They may focus on the management of conditions or on specific aspects of care (Table 14–7).[40–46] If developed appropriately, practice guidelines reflect findings from current best evidence, as well as expert judgment and patient opinion or perspective. Often they are issued in two formats—one for health care professionals and one for the general public.

Practice guidelines are a phenomenon of contemporary health care. As of this publication, PubMed indexes 8278 English language practice guidelines about human subjects,[22] while PEDro lists 461 English and non-English language practice guidelines relevant to physical therapy.[36] Guidelines tend to be issued by government agencies or by professional societies; however, they may be developed by anyone with the motivation to organize the necessary resources to produce them. In the 1990s, the primary source of guide-

Table 14–7 Examples of clinical practice guidelines relevant to physical therapy.

Conditions

- Evidence-Based Guidelines for the Secondary Prevention of Falls in Older Adults [with systematic review].
- Increasing Physical Activity: A Report on Recommendations of the Task Force on Community Preventive Services [Quick Reference Guide for Clinicians].
- National Clinical Guidelines for Stroke. 2nd edition.
- Philadelphia Panel Evidence-Based Clinical Practice Guidelines on Selected Rehabilitation Interventions for Knee Pain [with systematic review].

Aspects of Patient/Client Management

- ACC/AHA 2002 Guideline Update For Exercise Testing. A Report of the American College of Cardiology/American Heart Association Task Force on Practice Guidelines (Committee on Exercise Testing).
- ATS Statement: Guidelines for the Six-Minute Walk Test.
- Ottawa Panel Evidence-Based Clinical Practice Guidelines for Electrotherapy and Thermotherapy Interventions in the Management of Rheumatoid Arthritis in Adults [with systematic review].

lines in the United States was the Agency for Health Care Policy and Research (AHCPR), now known as the Agency for Healthcare Research and Quality (AHRQ).[47] Physical therapists and their patients/clients can locate guidelines by using the usual electronic evidence databases or by online resources, such as professional societies and government agencies. An important resource is the National Guideline Clearinghouse (*http://www.guideline.gov/*), maintained by AHRQ, which offers a weekly electronic mail notification of changes in their catalog, as well as new guidelines under development.[48]

The proliferation of practice guidelines has prompted some concrete recommendations regarding their development. Evidence-based guidelines are preferred over expert-based products because the latter are likely to reflect practitioners' habits and preferences, as well as biases inherent in their professions.[49] Shekelle *et al.* have outlined the following steps specific to creating evidence-based practice guidelines:

- Identify and refine the topic and scope of the guideline;
- Identify and convene the appropriate stakeholders–such as clinicians, patients, caregivers, researchers, and technical support staff–to participate;
- Conduct or locate a systematic review of the evidence;
- Develop recommendations based on the systematic review, as interpreted by clinical expertise and patient experience, as well as on feasibility issues such as cost; and,
- Submit the guideline for external review.[50]

Central to this process is the quantity and quality of the evidence relating to the guideline topic. The number of studies addressing an aspect of patient/client management may be insufficient to create a true systematic review. In addition, the studies located may have varying degrees of bias associated with different research designs. As a result, authors of guidelines tend to rely on a "levels of evidence" approach to characterize the strength of their recommendations. As noted in Chapter 2, there is considerable variability in evidence hierarchy definitions, a situation that may create inconsistencies among guidelines addressing the same topic area (Table 14–8). In an effort to simplify mat-

Table 14–8 Examples of levels of evidence in clinical practice guidelines.

AHCPR (now AHRQ) Levels of Evidence	Alternative Classification Scheme
Recommendation is Supported by: A. Scientific evidence provided by well-designed, well-conducted, controlled trials (randomized and nonrandomized) with statistically significant results that consistently support the guideline recommendation. B. Scientific evidence provided by observational studies or by controlled trials with less consistent results to support the guideline recommendation. C. Expert opinion that supports the guideline recommendation because the available scientific evidence did not present consistent results, or controlled trials were lacking.	Category of Evidence 1a—Evidence from meta-analysis of randomized controlled trials. 1b—Evidence from at least one randomized controlled trial 2a—Evidence from at least one controlled study without randomization 2b—Evidence from at least one other type of quasi-experimental study 3—Evidence from nonexperimental descriptive studies, such as comparative studies, correlation studies, and case-control studies 4—Evidence from expert committee reports or opinions or clinical experience of respected authorities or both Strength of Recommendation A—Directly based on Category 1 evidence B—Directly based on Category 2 evidence or extrapolated recommendation from Category 1 evidence C—Directly based on Category 3 evidence or extrapolated recommendation from Category 1 or 2 evidence D—Directly based on Category 4 evidence or extrapolated recommendation from Category 1, 2, or 3 evidence

ters, the GRADE working group published the classification system in Table 14–9.[51] The apparent simplicity of this approach is somewhat deceptive as there are additional steps required to arrive at these grades. In order to develop a recommendation, guideline developers must integrate what is known about the quality and results of available evidence with the realities of the current practice environment, as well as patient/caregiver preferences and values. This process is characterized in Figure 14–3.

All guidelines are not created equal. Physical therapists using guidelines should assess them in the same way that they assess individual research studies. Unlike the critical appraisal of individual study types, the assessment process for guidelines is still a work in progress. The following questions and methods are provided to help organize one's thoughts as the guideline is considered.

IS THE GUIDELINE VALID?

Although guidelines are not research studies in their own right, they may still suffer from credibility issues. One of the first concerns is whether the guideline remains current. Guidelines may become outdated as a result of:

1. The introduction of new patient/client management techniques;
2. New evidence clarifying beneficial or harmful consequences of current patient/client management techniques;
3. Changes in which outcomes of care are considered important clinically and socially;
4. Full compliance with current guidelines, thus no longer necessitating their use;
5. Changes in health care resources.[52]

Shekelle *et al.* conducted a review of ACHPR guidelines and discovered that 75 percent were out of date at the time of their study. Survival analysis indicated that 10 percent of the guidelines reviewed were outdated at 3.6 years and 50 percent were lost at five years. These authors conservatively recommended that guidelines be reviewed every three years and updated as necessary.[53] Physical therapists using evidence-based practice guidelines should consider whether the age of the product makes its application unreasonable or inappropriate in the current practice environment. If not, then age alone should not be a reason to reject the guideline.

A second issue is the overall quality of the guideline. Hasenfeld and Shekelle compared AHCPR guidelines with subsequently developed products.[54] Using a 30-item checklist to determine the relative quality of the guidelines they located, these authors found that newer guidelines did not meet the majority

Table 14–9 Guideline rating systems from the GRADE working group.[51(p. 1493)]

	Quality of Evidence	Guideline Recommendation	
High	Further research is very unlikely to change our confidence in the estimate of effect.	*"Do It" or "Don't Do It"*	A judgment that most well-informed people would make.
Moderate	Further research is likely to have an important impact on our confidence in the estimate of effect and may change the estimate.	*"Probably Do It" or "Probably Don't Do It"*	A judgment the majority of well-informed people would make, but a substantial minority of people would not.
Low	Further research is very likely to have an important impact on our confidence in the estimate of effect and is likely to change the estimate.		
Very Low	Any estimate of effect is very uncertain.		

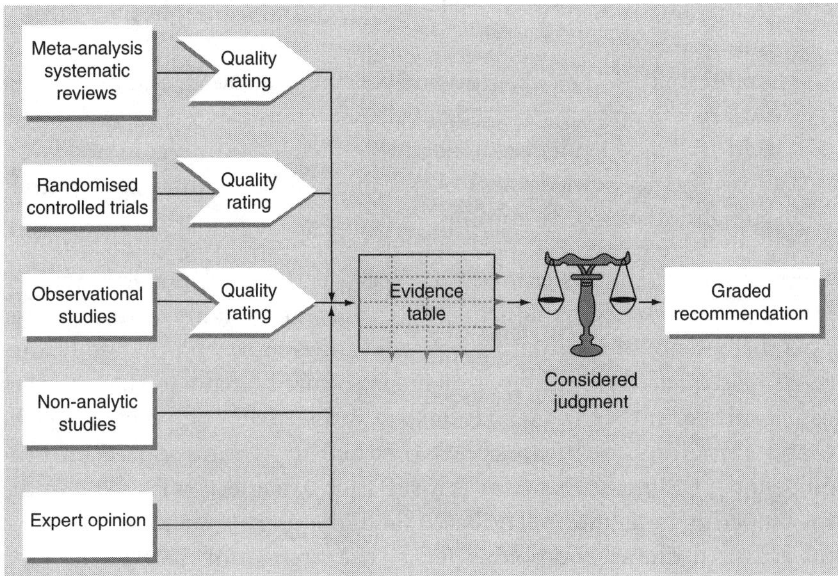

Figure 14–3 Overview of the process for developing and grading guideline recommendations.

Source: Reprinted from Robin Harbour and Juliet Miller. A new system for grading recommendations in evidence-based guidelines. *British Medical Journal*, Volume 323, Copyright 2001, with permission from BMJ Publishing Group, Ltd.

of the quality criteria. This apparent downward trend suggests that therapists must analyze guidelines carefully and use clinical judgment to determine their appropriateness for use with an individual patient/client.

Unfortunately, there is no consistently agreed upon method for analyzing the quality of guidelines. Most recently, an international working group was formed to address this issue. The Appraisal of Guidelines Research and Evaluation Collaboration (Agrec) created a 23-item instrument of which the reliability and validity was established prior to its release.[55] The instrument is comprised of the following six domains:

- Scope and purpose—"The overall aim of the guideline, the specific clinical questions, and the target patient population."
- Stakeholder involvement—"The extent to which the guideline represents the views of its intended users."
- Rigor of development—"The process used to gather and synthesise the evidence, the methods to formulate the recommendations and to update them."

- Clarity and presentation—"The language and format of the guideline."
- Applicability—"The likely organizational, behavioral, and cost implications of applying the guideline."
- Editorial independence—"The independence of the recommendations and acknowledgment of possible conflict of interest from the guideline development group."[56(p. 4)]

The extent to which this rating system has been adopted in North America is unclear. However, its demonstrated reliability and validity justifies its use.

In the absence of a formal tool, Straus *et al.* recommend that guidelines be evaluated based on the rigor of the literature search and the extent to which subsequent recommendations are supported by the evidence.[7] The first point addresses the possibility that bias will be introduced into the guideline if the literature review is insufficient. In effect, this is a reminder that superior guidelines will be based on high quality systematic reviews of the evidence. The second point refers to the strength of the evidence used to support each recommendation. Physical therapists must determine the system used to rate evidence and then consider whether to accept the recommendation in light of the evidence provided.

IS THE GUIDELINE APPLICABLE?

Once the credibility of a guideline has been determined, the question of its applicability should be explored. Whether implementation of the guideline is appropriate depends upon factors related to the condition of interest, the patient/client in question, other options available, and the practice environment in which the physical therapist is operating. First, the condition of interest covered by the guideline should have enough impact to make implementation worth the investment in time, resources, and energy. Impact may be determined by a high prevalence rate, as is the case with arthritis, or by the seriousness of the consequences it creates, such as falls in the elderly, or both. Evidence-based physical therapists determine the potential level of impact when they consider a patient/client's risk for the condition and its potential outcomes.

Second, the decision to implement the guideline is influenced by the congruence between its recommendations and the individual patient/client's preferences and values. Unlike research studies, practice guidelines often are produced in user-friendly formats that members of the general public will find easier to read and understand. As a result, it may be easier for physical therapists to provide information about guideline recommendations for patients/clients to consider during the decision-making process. Ideally, the guidelines will be explicit about what (and whose) preferences and values informed the development process. As will be discussed in Chapter 15, assessment of preferences and values is a process that may take many forms. An evaluation of the tradeoffs between the risks and benefits of various options for patient/client management is a common approach to this task. In effect, judgment in favor of, or opposed to, a particular option is determined based on its relative utility.[8] The challenge is to reconcile the utilities assumed in the guideline with those expressed by the individual patient/client.

Third, adoption of a guideline should be considered in terms of the outcomes achieved relative to the investment made. Comprehensive guidelines may require significant reorganization and reengineering in terms of the numbers and qualifications of health care staff, the type and amount of equipment and supplies, the methods and frequency with which care is delivered, and so forth. These changes may require considerable amounts of time, money, education, and training. If the anticipated outcomes are only incrementally better than current practice, then adoption of the guideline may not be worthwhile. Alternatively, even if the guideline is deemed beneficial, its adoption may be delayed or refused based on the nature and extent of local resource constraints.

Finally, successful implementation of a guideline is dependent upon the willingness of those involved to change their current behaviors and practice. The mere presence of a guideline will not ensure its use, no matter how well it is supported by high quality evidence. Potential barriers to change include provider preferences, habits, and concerns regarding loss of autonomy.[5] Guidelines also appear to contradict the mandate to individualize patient/client management. This last obstacle to implementation is perhaps the most legitimate—patient/client autonomy to make an informed decision to refuse a guideline recommendation should be respected. Strategies to overcome provider attitudes and behaviors are as complex as those used to encourage patients/clients to change their lifestyles. Whether or not to implement a guideline may depend on the extent of the effort required to facilitate this cultural shift, as well as the availability of resources to make it happen.

SUMMARY

Systematic reviews synthesize information from individual studies in order to arrive at a conclusion based on the cumulative weight of the evidence. Conclusions may be qualitative or quantitative in nature. Meta-analyses are a form of systematic review in which data are pooled to draw quantitative conclusions. These statistical assessments are possible when the types of subjects, procedures, and outcomes are consistent among the individual projects. Most systematic reviews relevant to physical therapy focus on therapeutic interventions; however, some reviews about diagnostic tests, measures, and prognostic indicators have been published. Systematic reviews are vulnerable to bias both due to the methods with which they are conducted, as well as the quality of the individual studies reviewed. Evidence-based physical therapists should evaluate systematic reviews carefully before accepting them at face value because of their high ranking on evidence hierarchies.

Clinical practice guidelines are statements developed to facilitate patient and provider decision making and to enhance quality of care. In their best form, these products combine a systematic review of the evidence with expert clinical judgment and patient/client preferences and values. There is some evidence to suggest that guideline quality may be declining; however, a widely accepted method for development and formatting is still evolving. Recently, an instrument was published to facilitate the evaluation of guideline quality. Other authors recommend focusing on the comprehensiveness of the literature review, the extent to which research validity is demonstrated by the evidence, and the applicability of the guideline to the local practice environment.

Exercises

1. Compare and contrast systematic reviews and clinical practice guidelines.
2. Discuss the potential sources of bias in systematic reviews and strategies to minimize their influence.
3. Describe the conditions under which a meta-analysis is appropriate to conduct.
4. Differentiate between the interpretation of relative risk for beneficial and adverse outcomes.
5. Forest plots may be used to illustrate effect sizes, odds ratios, relative risks, and likelihood ratios. Identify what the midline of the graph represents for each of these summary statistics.
6. Interpret the meaning of a confidence interval that crosses the midline of a forest plot for effect sizes, odds ratios, relative risks, and likelihood ratios.
7. Discuss the role of evidence in clinical practice guideline development and the challenges associated with linking evidence to recommendations.

8. Discuss potential barriers to clinical guideline implementation among your colleagues. Identify one strategy for each barrier you might implement in an effort to facilitate change.
9. Consider your own practice preferences and habits. What internal barriers can you identify regarding your willingness to adopt a clinical practice guideline? Will any of the strategies you identified in Question 8 help you to change?

REFERENCES

1. Helewa A, Walker JM. *Critical Evaluation of Research in Physical Rehabilitation: Towards Evidence-Based Practice.* Philadelphia, PA: W.B. Saunders Company; 2000.
2. Domholdt E. *Rehabilitation Research: Principles and Applications.* 3d ed. St Louis, MO: Elsevier Saunders; 2005.
3. Batavia M. *Clinical Research for Health Professionals: A User-Friendly Guide.* Boston, MA: Butterworth-Heinemann; 2001.
4. Diversity and Heterogeneity. The Cochrane Collaboration Open Learning Material. Available at: http://www.cochrane-net.org/openlearning/HTML/mod13-4.htm. Accessed April 25, 2006.
5. Herbert R, Jamtvedt G, Mead J, Hagen KB. *Practical Evidence-Based Physical Therapy.* Edinburgh, Scotland: Elsevier Butterworth-Heinemann; 2005.
6. Dalton GW, Keating JL. Number needed to treat: A statistic relevant to physical therapists. *Phys Ther.* 2000; 80(12):1214–1219.
7. Guyatt G, Rennie D. *Users' Guides to the Medical Literature: A Manual for Evidence-Based Clinical Practice.* Chicago, IL: AMA Press; 2002.
8. Straus SE, Richardson WS, Glaziou P, Haynes RB. *Evidence-Based Medicine: How to Practice and Teach EBM.* 3d ed. Edinburgh, Scotland: Elsevier Churchill Livingstone; 2005.
9. Portney LG, Watkins MP. *Foundations of Clinical Research: Applications to Practice.* 2d ed. Upper Saddle River, NJ: Prentice Hall Health; 2000.
10. Lohr KN, Field MJ. A provisional instrument for assessing clinical practice guidelines. In: Field MJ, Lohr KN, eds. *Guidelines for Clinical Practice: From Development to Use.* Washington, DC: National Academy Press; 1992.
11. Goodacre S, Sutton AJ, Sampson FC. Meta-analysis: The value of clinical assessment in the diagnosis of deep venous thrombosis. *Ann Intern Med.* 2005; 143(2):129–139.
12. MacDermid JC, Wessel J. Clinical diagnosis of carpal tunnel syndrome: A systematic review. *J. Hand Ther.* 2004; 17(2):309–319.
13. Pengel LH, Herbert RD, Maher CG, Refshauge KM. Acute low back pain: Systematic review of its prognosis. *BMJ.* 2003; 327(7410):323.
14. Yrjonen T. Long-term prognosis of Legg-Calve-Perthes disease: A meta-analysis. *J Pediatr Orthop B.* 1999; 8(3):169–172.
15. The Cochrane Collaboration Web site. Available at: http://www.cochrane.org/. Accessed April 23, 2006.

16. Methods Groups. Cochrane Collaboration Web site. Available at: http://www.cochrane.org/contact/entities.htm#MGLIST. Accessed April 23, 2006.
17. Moher D, Cook DJ, Eastwood S, Olkin I, Rennie D *et al.* Improving the quality of reports of meta-analyses of randomised controlled trials: The QUOROM statement. *Lancet.* 1999; 354(9193):1896–1900.
18. Stroup DS, Berlin JA, Morton SC, Olkin I, Williamson GD *et al.* Meta-analysis of observational studies in epidemiology. *JAMA.* 2000; 283(15): 2008–2012.
19. Jadad AR, Cook DJ, Jones A, Klassen TP, Tugwell P *et al.* Methodology and reports of systematic reviews and meta-analyses. *JAMA.* 1998; 280(3):278–280.
20. Shea B, Moher D, Graham I , Pham Ba', Tugwell P. A comparison of the quality of Cochrane reviews and systematic reviews published in paper-based journals. *Eval Health Prof.* 2002; 25(1):116–129.
21. Critically Appraising the Evidence. Worksheets for Systematic Reviews. Oxford Center for Evidence-Based Medicine Web site. Available at: www.cebm.net. Accessed July 15, 2005.
22. PubMed. National Library of Medicine Web site. Available at: http://www.ncbi.nlm.nih.gov/entrez/query.fcgi?DB=pubmed. Accessed February 20, 2006.
23. EMBASE. Elsevier. Available at: http://www.embase.com/. Accessed April 23, 2006.
24. Cumulative Index of Nursing and Allied Health Literature. Available via Ovid Web site at: http://www.ovid.com/site/catalog/DataBase/40.jsp?top=2&mid=3&bottom=7&subsection=10. Accessed February 20, 2006.
25. Moher D, Pham Ba', Klassen TP, Schulz KF, Berlin JA *et al.* What contributions do languages other than English make on the results of meta-analyses? *J Clin Epidemiol.* 2000; 53(9):964–972.
26. Juni P, Holenstien F, Stern J, Bartlett C, Egger M. Direction and impact of language bias in meta-analyses of controlled trials: Empirical study. *Int J Epidemiol.* 2002; 31(1):115–123.
27. McAuley L, Pham Ba', Tugwell P, Moher D. Does the inclusion of grey literature influence estimates of intervention effectiveness in meta-analyses? *Lancet.* 2000; 356(9237):1228–1231.
28. Egger M, Juni P, Bartlett C, Holenstein F, Sterne J. How important are comprehensive literature searches and the assessment of trial quality in systematic reviews? Empirical study. *Health Technol Assess.* 2003; 7(1):1–82.
29. Juni P, Altman DG, Egger M. Systematic reviews in health care: assessing the quality of controlled clinical trials. *BMJ.* 2001; 323(7303) 42–46.
30. Moher D, Pham Ba', Jones A, Cook DJ, Jadad AR *et al.* Does quality of reports of randomised trials affect estimates of intervention efficacy reported in meta-analyses? *Lancet.* 1998; 352(9128):609–613.
31. Moher D, Cook DJ, Jadad AR, Tugwell P, Moher M *et al.* Assessing the quality of reports of randomised trials: Implications for the conduct of meta-analyses. *Health Technol Assess.* 1999; 3(12):i–iv, 1–98.
32. Moher D, Jadad AR, Nichol G, Penman M, Tugwell P *et al.* Assessing the quality of randomized controlled trials: An annotated bibliography of scales and checklists. *Control Clin Trials.* 1995; 16(1):62–73.

33. Colle F, Rannou F, Revel M, Fermanian J, Poiraudeau S. Impact of quality scales on levels of evidence inferred from a systematic review of exercise therapy and low back pain. *Arch Phys Med Rehabil.* 2002; 83(12):1745–1752.
34. Sterne JAC, Egger M, Smith GD. Systematic reviews in health care: Investigating and dealing with publication and other biases in meta-analysis. *BMJ.* 2001; 323(7304):101–105.
35. Fernandez-de-las-Peñas C, Alonso-Blanco C, Cuadrado ML, Miangolarra JC, Barriga FJ *et al.* Are manual therapies effective in reducing pain from tension-type headache? A systematic review. *Clin J Pain.* 2006; 22(3):278–285.
36. Physiotherapy Evidence Database. Center for Evidence-Based Physiotherapy. Available at: http://www.pedro.fhs.usyd.edu.au/index.html. Accessed February 20, 2006.
37. Lenssinck MLB, Frijlink AC, Berger MY, Bierma-Zeinstra SMA, Verkerk K *et al.* Effect of bracing and other conservative interventions in the treatment of idiopathic scoliosis in adolescents: A systematic review of clinical trials. *Phys Ther.* 2005; 85(12):1329–1339.
38. Lewis S, Clarke M. Forest plots: Trying to see the wood and the trees. *BMJ.* 2001; 322(7300):1479–1480.
39. Milne S, Brosseau L, Robinson V, Noel MJ, Davis J *et al.* Continuous passive motion following total knee arthroplasty. *The Cochrane Database of Systematic Reviews.* 2003; Issue 2. Article No.: CD004260. DOI:10.1002/14651858.CD004260.
40. Moreland J, Richardson J, Chan DH, O'Neill J, Bellissimo A *et al.* Evidence-based guidelines for the secondary prevention of falls in older adults [with systematic review]. *Gerontology.* 2003; 49(2):93–116.
41. Kahn EB, Ramsey LT, Heath GW, Howze EH [Task Force on Community Preventive Services and the Centers for Disease Control and Prevention (CDC)]. Increasing physical activity: A report on recommendations of the Task Force on Community Preventive Services [quick reference guide for clinicians]. *MMWR.* 2001; 50(RR-18):i–18.
42. National Clinical Guidelines for Stroke. 2d ed. Royal College of Physicians Web site. Available at: http://www.rcplondon.ac.uk/pubs/books/stroke/ index.htm. Accessed April 26, 2006.
43. Brosseau L, Tugwell P, Wells GA, Robinson VA, Graham ID *et al.* Philadelphia Panel evidence-based clinical practice guidelines on selected rehabilitation interventions for knee pain [with systematic review]. *Phys Ther.* 2001; 81(10):1675–1700.
44. Gibbons RJ, Balady GJ, Bricker JT, Chaitman BR, Fletcher GF *et al.* ACC/AHA 2002 guideline update for exercise testing. A report of the American College of Cardiology/American Heart Association Task Force on Practice Guidelines (Committee on Exercise Testing). *Circulation.* 2002; 106(14):1883–1892.
45. Crapo RO, Casaburi R, Coates AL, Enright PL, MacIntyre NR *et al.* ATS statement: Guidelines for the six-minute walk test. *Am J Respir Crit Care Med.* 2002; 166(1):111–117.
46. Ottawa Panel. Ottawa Panel evidence-based clinical practice guidelines for electrotherapy and thermotherapy interventions in the management of rheumatoid arthritis in adults [with systematic review]. *Phys Ther.* 2004; 84(11):1016–1043.

47. Agency for Healthcare Research and Quality Web site. United States Department of Health and Human Services. Available at: http://ahrq.gov/. Accessed April 26, 2006.
48. National Guideline Clearing House Web site. Agency for Healthcare Research and Quality. Available at: http://www.guideline.gov/. Accessed April 26, 2006.
49. Scalzitti DA. Evidence-based guidelines: Application to clinical practice. *Phys Ther*. 2001; 81(10):1622–1628.
50. Shekelle PG, Woolf SH, Eccles M, Grimshaw J. Developing guidelines. *BMJ*. 1999; 318(7183):593–596.
51. GRADE Working Group. Grading quality of evidence and strength of recommendatios. *BMJ*. 2004; 328(7454):1490–1498.
52. Shekelle P, Eccles MP, Grimshaw JM, Woolf SH. When should guidelines be updated? *BMJ*. 2001; 323(7305):155–157.
53. Shekelle PG, Ortiz E, Rhodes S, Morton SC, Eccles MP *et al.* Validity of the Agency for Healthcare Research and Quality clinical practice guidelines. *JAMA*. 2001; 286(12):1461–1467.
54. Hasenfeld R, Shekelle PG. Is the methodological quality of guidelines declining in the US? Comparison of the quality of U.S. Agency for Health Care Policy and Research (AHCPR) guidelines with those published subsequently. *Qual Saf Health Care*. 2003; 12(6):428–434.
55. AGREE Collaboration. Development and validation of an international appraisal instrument for assessing the quality of clinical practice guidelines: The AGREE project. *Qual Saf Health Care*. 2003; 12(1):18–23.
56. The AGREE Collaboration Web site. Appraisal of Guidelines for Research & Evaluation. AGREE Instrument. Available at: www.agreecollaboration.org. Accessed April 26, 2006.

Part IV

EVIDENCE IN PRACTICE

Chapter 15

Patient/Client Preferences and Values

Everything depends on the value we give to things.

—Gustave Flaubert

Objectives

Upon completion of this chapter the student/practitioner will be able to:

1. Discuss the relationship among evidence, clinical judgment and expertise, and patient/client preferences and values.
2. Describe patient-centered care and its relationship to evidence-based physical therapy practice.
3. Discuss the ethical principles of autonomy, beneficence, and nonmaleficence and their relationship to evidence-based physical therapy practice.
4. Differentiate between shared decision making and the traditional biomedical model for determining a plan of care.
5. Discuss the incorporation of evidence into the shared decision-making process.
6. Differentiate among patient/client preferences, expectancies, and values.
7. Describe strategies for eliciting information about patient/client preferences, expectancies, and values.
8. Explain how subject preferences may undermine the research validity of a study.
9. Describe potential strategies investigators may implement to deal with subject preferences.

TERMS IN THIS CHAPTER

Autonomy: An individual's right to make decisions about his or her health care.

Beneficence: A commitment to helping others with minimal harm.

Cultural Competence: The knowledge, skills, and abilities needed to interact with individuals from different cultures in an appropriate, relevant, and sensitive manner.[1]

Expectancy: The belief that a process or outcome possesses certain attributes.[2]

Informed Consent: An individual's authorization of a procedure or technique following a conversation between the health care provider and patient/client about a proposed course of action, alternative courses of action, no action, and the risks and benefits of each of these options.[3]

Nonmaleficence: "First, do no harm."

Patient-Centered Care: Health care that "customizes treatment recommendations and decision making in response to patients' preferences and beliefs. . . . This partnership also is characterized by informed, shared decision making, development of patient knowledge, skills needed for self-management of illness, and preventive behaviors."[4(p. 3)]

Preference: The difference in the perceived desirability of two (or more) options related to health care.[2]

Shared Decision Making: An exchange of ideas between a health care provider and patient/client and collaboration in the decision itself.[3]

Values: Concepts or beliefs about desirable behaviors or states of being that are prioritized relative to one another.[5]

INTRODUCTION

Throughout this text readers have been reminded to integrate evidence with their clinical judgment and expertise, as well as with individual patient/client preferences and values. Evidence-based physical therapy practice (EBPT) is achieved only when these three information sources contribute to the final decision about how to address a patient/client's needs.[6] On one level, this integration process may sound counterintuitive given the emphasis on high quality evidence that has minimized bias. After all, both clinicians and patients/clients bring a level of subjectivity to their decision making that may result in choices that contradict valid and important findings from well-designed research. Nevertheless, health care is a human endeavor that, for many people, cannot and should not be reduced to complete dependence upon science in the absence of clinician or patient/client perspective and experience. In addition, the highest quality evidence usually provides information about groups rather than individuals, a fact that reinforces reluctance to accept the relevance of even the best evidence.[7]

The challenge for physical therapists, therefore, is to gather information from all three sources in the EBPT triad and to discuss all of it explicitly with the patient/client so that the relative merits of available options may be considered in a holistic fashion prior to establishing a plan of care. In order for physical therapists to be explicit about the nature and contribution of their expertise and judgment, they must routinely engage in self-reflection and appraisal. This process includes an acknowledgment of practice preferences and habits that have developed over the years, gaps in knowledge that would benefit from additional education or training, and enablers and barriers to change in their approach to patient/client management.[8] Patients and clients, on the other hand, require the opportunity to express their preferences and values in a decision-making process that traditionally has deemphasized their involvement. Physical therapists must provide this invitation early and often with each patient/client, as well as with family and/or caregivers, to facilitate this collaborative process. Meanwhile, evidence must be located and evaluated and its findings translated into meaningful information that all partners in the decision-making process can understand.

Needless to say, this integrated approach to patient/client management is probably easier to describe than to execute. There is no guarantee that patients/clients will respond to the available information in the same manner as their physical therapists. The stakes may be especially high when disagreement results between the provider and the patient/client over desired management approaches that are contrary to those supported by high level evidence. Potential conflict is not a reason to avoid the process, however. This chapter discusses the involvement of patients/clients in health care decision making and the contribution of their preferences and values to evidence-based physical therapy.

PATIENT-CENTERED CARE

Patient contribution to evidence-based physical therapy practice is an essential ingredient of *patient-centered care*. According to the Institute of Medicine, patient-centered care "is characterized by informed, shared decision-making, development of patient knowledge, skills needed for self-management of illness, and preventive behaviors."[4(p. 3)] This concept rejects the traditional biomedical model in which providers (e.g., physicians, physical therapists, etc.) make choices for patients based on superior knowledge and understanding of health-related issues and the options with which to address them.[9] Patients and their families (caregivers), no longer accept their role as passive recipients of biomedical expertise and skill; rather, they increasingly view themselves as partners in a health care system that should acknowledge and accept their unique culture and perspectives.[4,10]

Several factors are responsible for this shift of focus away from providers and onto patients and their families (caregivers). First, advances in biomedical technology and pharmaceuticals have transformed uniformly fatal diseases into chronic conditions with which individuals may live for decades.[4] Examples include heart failure, chronic obstructive pulmonary disease, diabetes, many forms of cancer, and acquired immune deficiency syndrome (AIDS), to name a few. The increased costs associated with the care of these long-term problems have resulted in disease management models focused on secondary prevention through patient and family education, self-management, and adherence to preventive treatment routines.[11] By definition, these approaches depend upon an informed partnership between the health care team and the patient and family (caregivers) rather than a unilateral decision-making structure.

Second, the Internet has increased the access of the general public to information about diseases and their management options. Numerous professional, patient advocacy, and government entities provide medical information in layman's terms through free Web sites. The National Library of Medicine,[12] the American Heart Association,[13] the American Diabetes Association,[14] the American Medical Association,[15] and the American Physical Therapy Association,[16] are just a few of the many groups offering this service. Many more sites from a variety of sources are available, the quality and accuracy of which are questionable. Nevertheless, patients and their families (caregivers) are arriving at health care appointments armed with information, including research findings that may reduce their reliance upon medical professionals for understanding about their situation.

Finally, the evidence itself indicates that increased availability of information and participation in health care decision making may enhance patient satisfaction, adherence to prescribed regimens, confidence in health care providers, adjustment to changes in health and, in some cases, psychological and physiological outcomes.[9] These findings are not conclusive because additional investigation is needed to determine patients' preferred level of participation in decision making, as well as the impact of that involvement across a wider range of diseases and disorders. In addition, the role of cultural and societal context in patient management and outcomes requires further study. Despite these knowledge gaps, patient-centered care is a concept that appears firmly embedded in contemporary health care. A similar focus may be applied to health promotion and primary prevention arenas if the phrase is changed to "client-centered care." Both terms reinforce the notion that evidence-based physical therapy practice is a collaborative and integrative process between the clinician and the patient/client.

Ethical Considerations

Beyond the epidemiological and societal changes promoting patient-centered care is a more fundamental obligation for physical therapists—patient/client management that is informed by a professional code of ethics (Table 15–1).[17] These statements are consistent with the concept of *autonomy*, which recognizes the right of patients/clients to make decisions about their health care. By definition, the patient/client is at the center of this ethical principle and physical therapists are duty-bound to honor this position. Describing and interpreting findings from the best available evidence can be argued to support autonomy by providing patients/clients with essential information to consider before making a final choice.[10] Similarly, therapists may view the use of evidence as consistent with two additional ethical principles: beneficence and nonmaleficence. *Beneficence* instructs physical therapists to make decisions with the patient/client's best interests in mind, while *nonmaleficence* states that harm should be avoided. Both of these dictates may be supported by well-designed research with compelling findings demonstrating a beneficial or harmful effect, respectively. On the other hand, therapists may find that these principles conflict with autonomy when high quality evidence recommends (or discounts) a management option that the patient/client is refusing (or requesting). Also at play in these situations is the therapist's clinical judgment and expertise and the patient/client's preferences and values, all of which influence perceptions about the meaning and relevance of the evidence beyond its stated results. Resolution of this potential dilemma is contingent upon a successful negotiation of a mutually agreeable plan of care.

Informed Consent and Shared Decision Making

Patient/client self-determination depends upon access to information. The opportunity to learn about the details relevant to a health care decision is the first step in the process referred to as informed consent. *Informed consent* requires formal conversations between physical therapists and patients/clients that result in unambiguous instructions regarding what services (e.g., procedures, techniques) will be accepted or refused.[3] During these

Table 15–1 Code of ethics for physical therapy practice.[8]

PREAMBLE
This Code of Ethics of the American Physical Therapy Association sets forth principles for the ethical practice of physical therapy. All physical therapists are responsible for maintaining and promoting ethical practice. To this end, the physical therapist shall act in the best interest of the patient/client. This Code of Ethics shall be binding on all physical therapists.

PRINCIPLE 1
A physical therapist shall respect the rights and dignity of all individuals and shall provide compassionate care.

PRINCIPLE 2
A phyical therapist shall act in a trustworthy manner towards patients/clients, and in all other aspects of physical therapy practice.

PRINCIPLE 3
A physical therapist shall comply with laws and regulations governing physical therapy and shall strive to effect changes that benefit patients/clients.

PRINCIPLE 4
A physical therapist shall exercise sound professional judgment.

PRINCIPLE 5
A physical therapist shall achieve and maintain professional competence.

PRINCIPLE 6
A physical therapist shall maintain and promote high standards for physical therapy practice, education and research.

PRINCIPLE 7
A physical therapist shall seek only such remuneration as is deserved and reasonable for physical therapy services.

PRINCIPLE 8
A physical therapist shall provide and make available accurate and relevant information to patients/clients about their care and to the public about physical therapy services.

PRINCIPLE 9
A physical therapist shall protect the public and the profession from unethical, incompetent, and illegal acts.

PRINCIPLE 10
A physical therapist shall endeavor to address the health needs of society.

PRINCIPLE 11
A physical therapist shall respect the rights, knowledge, and skills of colleagues and other health care professionals.

conversations, evidence-based physical therapists should supply details about the patient/client's diagnosis, prognosis, treatment options, and associated risks and benefits. In addition, therapists are responsible for translating available research findings into meaningful information that is applicable to the patient/client. In return, patients/clients hopefully will share their perceptions regarding their condition; understanding of, and preferences for different management options and their potential impact on daily life; as well as goals to be achieved at the conclusion of physical therapy. Respect for patient/client autonomy requires that this information exchange occur in an explicit manner.

The ability to exercise one's autonomy in health care implies an understanding of the potential consequences of the different choices outlined during the consent process. From a legal perspective, informed consent is particularly focused on the potential risk associated with elements of the plan of care. Risk in this sense reflects both the likelihood that harm will occur, as well as the severity of the adverse outcome itself, both of which may be defined by the provider's clinical experience and/or the available evidence.[3] Patients/clients may evaluate this risk within their sociocultural context and, in reference to available evidence or perceived knowledge about the situation. This potentially high-stakes evaluation process is most evident for surgical procedures. For example, the statement "arteriovenous (AV) malformation surgery is associated with an 8 percent risk of death"[18] suggests a low probability of a serious event occurring as a result of a proposed intervention. Whether 8 percent is low enough, however, is an individual decision that may be influenced by a patient's definition of acceptable risk,[9] as well as by cultural and social reactions to uncertainty about the future. Similarly, willingness to risk death in order to repair the AV defect may also be dependent on a patient's perspective about alternative outcomes without surgery—namely a 2–4 percent risk of stroke and associated loss of function.[18] Each of these factors may be influenced further by results from studies about prognostic factors associated with AV malformation rupture, or survival after repair, as well as by varying clinical judgments about the appropriateness of surgery, given a patient's clinical history and examination findings. The surgeon's job is to help the patient understand and consider all of this information thoroughly before making a decision. Physical therapists may find themselves in similar situations when proposed procedures are invasive (e.g., vaginal treatments for urinary incontinence) or potentially risky (e.g., cervical manipulation).

Once the information exchange has occurred, a clear, voluntary decision about the elements of patient/client management must be determined. How that decision is reached depends upon how the physical therapist and patient/client view the nature of their relationship. In the traditional biomedical model, the physical therapist is the expert who evaluates the risks and benefits of each management option on behalf of the patient and recommends (or makes) the decision within their frame of reference about what is in the best interests of the patient. Their evaluation may be derived from their clinical experience and judgment, and/or available evidence, depending upon the therapists' practice habits. The patient/client's sociocultural context and contribution to the decision is marginalized in this scenario. As stated above, this approach is the antithesis of patient-centered care. Shared decision making, on the other hand, is a process that supports an active partnership between therapists and patients/clients. *Shared decision making* is defined as "an exchange of ideas between a health care provider and patient and collaboration in the decision itself."[3(p. 55)] In other words, the therapist and the patient/client mutually accept responsibility for the decision and its consequences. In this model, all information relevant to the decision is incorporated, including culturally based patient/client preferences and values.[7] Moreover, in situations in which relatively equal management options exist, preferences and values may be the deciding factor in the selection process. When preferences and values are in conflict with the best available evidence, it is the physical therapist's responsibility to negotiate a suitable management option with the patient/client in a manner that is consistent with ethical codes and standards of conduct. In order to do that, therapists need to understand where preferences and values come from and how they may affect participation in, and outcomes of, care.

PREFERENCES, EXPECTANCIES, AND VALUES

For the purposes of this text, *preferences* are defined as the differences in the perceived desirability of two (or more) options related to health care.[2] These perceptions may be derived objectively from evidence, education, and observation, or they may be based on subjective interpretations and imprecise information about the potential benefits and risks of each choice. Unfortunately, the lack of quality control for the plethora of medical information on the Internet may contribute to patient/client misunderstandings of available evidence. Physical therapists often try to address detected inaccuracies in patient/client understanding through education, as well as through discussions about the best available evidence. Nevertheless, an individual's inner conviction about what is "right for me" may prevail, particularly when there is a high level of uncertainty about the outcomes of care. Bower *et al.* also point out that the strength of patient/client preferences may be more important than whether they are based on valid information.[2]

The desirability of one option over another may be stimulated in part by what patients/clients anticipate will happen when they participate in, or receive, health care.[19] This anticipation is reflected in the term *expectancy*, which is defined as the belief that a process or outcome possesses certain attributes.[2] Patients/clients reveal their "expectancies" in an explicit fashion when they define their goals for treatment. Physical therapists also may detect implicit expressions of "expectancies" when a patient guards an injured extremity during efforts to examine it or when clients perform more repetitions of an exercise than prescribed. In the first scenario, the patient likely anticipates (expects) pain when the extremity is moved, while in the second scenario the client likely believes that a higher volume of exercise will produce either a quicker result or a higher level of performance. In both situations, "expectancies" have helped to define the desirability (or lack thereof) of the examination technique or intervention.

Preferences about health care also may be shaped by the values patients/clients and their families (caregivers) use to guide their decisions and actions.[19] *Values* are defined as concepts or beliefs about desirable behaviors or states of being that are prioritized relative to one another.[5] Values may be global in perspective, as exemplified by beliefs in the importance of honesty, integrity, fairness, and so on. Values also may be defined more narrowly with reference to health care. Examples of patient/client values relevant to physical therapy may include, but are not limited to, the:

- Meaning of symptoms such as pain, shortness of breath, or fatigue;
- Importance of healthy lifestyles;
- Ability to minimize or avoid suffering;
- Preservation or restoration of self-image;
- Importance of work, school, and/or household responsibilities;
- Ability to care for and be involved with family and/or friends;
- Quality and consistency of the therapist-patient/client relationship; and the
- Importance and usefulness of research in health care decision-making;

and so on. By definition, all values are not equally important, although there is no uniformly accepted order for these beliefs. Patients/clients will prioritize them based on their own experiences and understanding of the world, as well as in response to sociocultural norms and expectations. The order also may shift depending upon the patient/client's health and/or psychological and emotional status at a given point in time.[5] Understandably, physical therapy management options are more likely to be desirable if they are consistent with a patient/client's values.

Assessment of Preferences and Values

The challenge for physical therapists, therefore, is to ascertain a patient/client's preferences, "expectancies," and values, so that this information may be integrated with clinical judgment and the best available evidence.

The process starts during the initial contact with the patient/client during which specific interview questions and/or spontaneous revelations might provide the necessary details. Family members and caregivers also may lend some insight into these issues; however, the inaccuracy of those speaking on behalf of the patient/client (e.g., the proxy) has been noted in several studies.[5] This disconnect may be attributable to a lack of knowledge about the patient/client's wishes or to the influence of the proxy's own preferences, "expectancies," and values. This substitution of one set of preferences, "expectancies," and values for another may be purposeful, as is the case in cultures in which family members are expected to make health care decisions for loved ones, or may be subliminal. In either case, physical therapists must determine whose preferences, "expectancies," and values are to be respected in regards to obtaining a final decision about how to proceed with care.

Assessment tools such as questionnaires, decision analyses, and rating scales also are available to facilitate the specification of preferences, "expectancies," and values. For example, Straus *et al.* include a 0–1 numerical rating scale in which 0 represents death and 1 represents complete health. Patients are asked to rate the relative value of the intended outcome of treatment on this scale in a fashion similar to that used with a visual analog scale for pain (Figure 15–1).[20] Inferences about preferences, "expectancies," and values also may be drawn from quality of life instruments, depending upon the phrasing of the survey items. However, when the information is gathered it must be discussed and interpreted with respect to the patient/client's sociocultural context as is consistent with *culturally competent* health care.

At the same time, physical therapists also must be aware of their own preferences, "expectancies," and values and evaluate how they influence clinical decision making. For example, therapists may indicate a preference for treatment techniques based in theoretical or biological plausibility, regardless of what the evidence indicates. Other clinicians may willingly use evidence about interventions, but only if it comes from randomized clini-

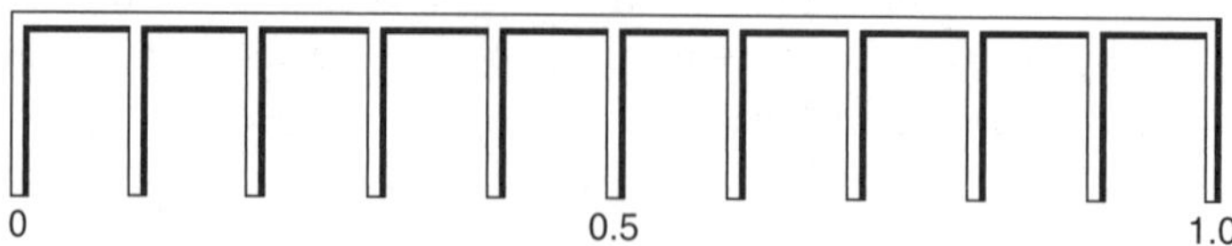

Figure 15–1 Rating scale for assessing values.[19]

Source: Reprinted from Straus SE, Richardson WS, Glaziou, P, Haynes RB. Evidence-Based Medicine. How to Practice and Teach EBM. 3d edition, p. 141. Copyright (2005), with permission from Elsevier.

cal trials. Experience also gives therapists an anecdotal perception about "what works," which can develop into an "expectancy" that is conveyed when describing a potential management option. Finally, physical therapists may value the achievement of a patient/client's full potential more than the individual with whom they are working. The issue is not the existence of these tendencies per se, but the potential lack of purposeful deliberation about their appropriateness for a specific patient/client. In the absence of such self-awareness and analysis, physical therapists may impose their own preferences and values relevant to the plan of care upon the patient/client rather than negotiate the outcome in an explicit fashion.

Incorporating evidence into this discussion requires physical therapists to clarify how the research findings are relevant to this specific individual. Of course, this task will be easier if the evidence includes subjects and circumstances that resemble the individual patient/client and his or her clinical situation. The manner in which the information is presented also matters. For therapists this means that explanations should be free from jargon and should be delivered in a way that accommodates individual patient/client learning needs and styles. Therapists must also be prepared to offer their objective opinion about the role the evidence plays in their decision making in general and in the specific situation. When evidence is inconclusive, or nonexistent, then decisions will be reached based on some combination of clinical judgment and patient/client preferences and values. Ultimately, the goal is to engage the patient/client in shared decision making in a culturally competent manner in an effort to minimize conflict between competing value systems and priorities and to reach a mutually agreeable approach to the plan of care.

Evidence about Preferences

As it turns out, preferences are both the focus of, and a potential concern for, health care research. Understanding preferences from a scientific point of view is consistent with evidence-based practice and has revealed some interesting findings. For example, Erkan *et al.* surveyed physicians to determine their preferences for rheumatoid arthritis medications and to evaluate whether cost influenced their choices.[21] The authors used three different patient scenarios to examine whether physicians were adopting more aggressive treatment strategies by using newly established drugs. The results indicated that 65 percent of the time physicians chose long-established medications for the mild case scenario, but preferred the newest medications, in combination with established regimens, for cases of increasing severity. However, this proportion dropped to 14 percent when cost was factored into the decision. A subsequent study by Fraenkel *et al.* evaluated patient preferences for rheumatoid arthritis treatment.[22] These authors used an interactive computer program to elicit subject preferences for four drugs based on tradeoffs between treatment side effects, effectiveness, and cost within different risk-benefit scenarios. Their results indicated that, on average, patients preferred drugs that reduced both rare and common side effects more than drugs with known benefits. Interestingly, the drug that was selected most often because of this characteristic was the same drug that physicians in the previous study reserved primarily for severe cases, and only when cost was not a factor. When considered together, these studies point to a potential disconnect between physicians and patients in the management of rheumatoid arthritis, although the physicians were not asked the same questions as the patients. At a minimum, studies of patient and provider preferences are warranted to better understand their nature and the factors that influence them in different disease states.

An additional concern about preferences is their potential influence on research outcomes. Specifically, preferences are assumed to be potential threats to research validity of intervention studies when subjects are aware of their group assignment.[2,19,23,24] Two mechanisms are proposed to explain the potential impact of preferences. First, subjects who receive their desired intervention may exhibit a response in excess of the actual treatment effect. This response is thought to share the same mechanism as the placebo effect and may be enhanced by higher-than-average compliance with the treatment protocol. Second, allocation to an undesired intervention may produce resentful demoralization thereby resulting in decreased adherence to the group protocol. This point is particularly salient when an experimental intervention is being compared to another treatment approach. King *et al.* outlined the proposed causal mechanisms that may produce exaggerated treatment effects (Figure 15–2).[19] Direct influences are attributed to purposeful changes in behavior (e.g., increased compliance), while indirect influences are attributed to the biopsychological effects of "expectancies" about preferred treatments.

Evidence about the extent of preference effects actually occurring in research is equivocal.[24] Several authors have suggested research designs that take subject preference into account. One option is to identify which subjects have strong preferences for the treatment options in the study and assign them to those groups, while randomizing everyone else who is preference-free. This approach requires larger sample sizes because of the increase in the number of groups and is likely to be logistically and financially prohibitive. An alternative approach is to identify subject preferences before randomization and then use this data as an adjustment factor in

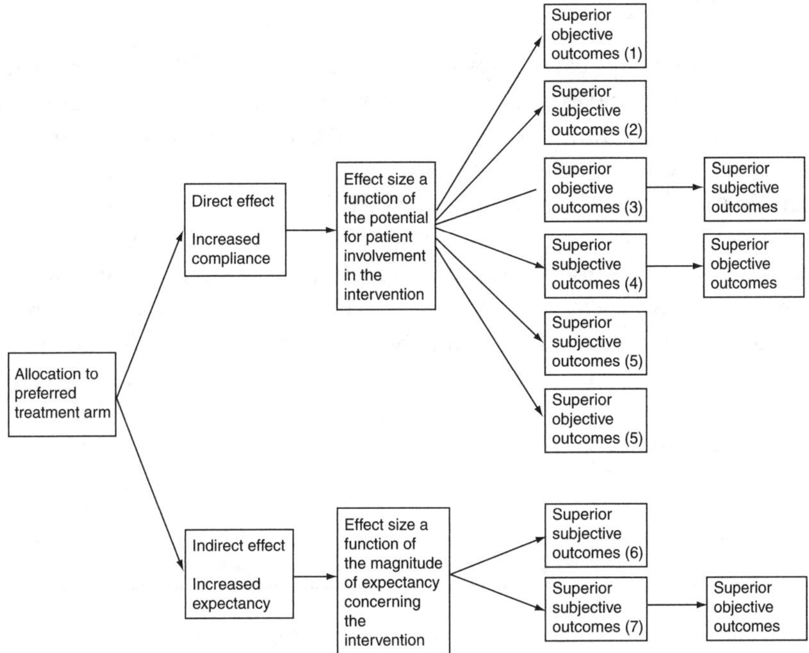

Figure 15–2 The proposed effects of subject preferences on research studies.[20]
Source: Reprinted from King M, Nazareth I, Lampe F, Bower P, Chandler F *et al.* Conceptual framework and systematic review of the effects of participants' and professionals' preferences in randomised controlled trials. *Health Technol Assess.* 2005; 9(35):1–191, with permission from the National Coordinating Center for Health Technology Assessment.

subsequent analyses. Two studies pertinent to physical therapy used the latter approach. Klaber Moffett *et al.* found that preference did not influence clinical outcomes following interventions for lower back pain,[25] but subsequently reported a potential (although nonsignificant) influence on outcomes following treatment of neck pain.[26]

The reality is that the majority of the research available does not address the potential influence of subject preferences on outcomes. Therefore, physical therapists should consider whether preferences may have played a role in individual studies. Designs in which subjects are randomly allocated and remain masked to group assignment are least vulnerable to this potential problem. Studies with unblinded assignment are at greater risk; however, until there is a better understanding of the extent of this effect, studies should not be rejected based on this issue alone.

SUMMARY

Evidence-based physical therapy integrates the best available evidence with clinical judgment and expertise, as well as with patient/client preferences and values. This definition is consistent with patient/client-centered care and supports the ethical principle of autonomy. Informed consent and shared decision making are the processes by which this integration occurs in practice. Determination of an evidence-based plan of care requires physical therapists to elicit and understand patient/client preferences and values within each individual's sociocultural context. Therapists also must be aware of their own preferences and values and how they shape clinical decision making. Finally, the nature of preferences in clinical practice and their influence on research validity requires further study to better understand their contribution to outcomes.

Exercises

1. Define patient-centered care in your own words. Explain how evidence-based physical therapy practice is consistent with this definition.
2. Discuss the ethical considerations related to evidence-based physical therapy practice.
3. Describe the elements of informed consent. Discuss the implications for presenting evidence to patients/clients during the consent process.
4. Differentiate shared decision making from the traditional biomedical model of determining a plan of care. Explain how this process relates to evidence-based physical therapy practice.
5. Define the concept of patient/client preferences and provide two examples to support your answer.
6. For each preference described in Question #5, identify two potential expectancies and two potential values that may influence the nature of the preference.
7. Identify one of your preferences, along with associated expectancies and values, related to patient/client management. Discuss how these issues may influence your approach to evidence-based physical therapy practice.
8. An elderly patient with a history of falls tells you she will not remove the area rugs in her home or change the shoes she wears despite numerous studies that indicate an increased fall risk due to these factors. During this exchange you learn that she values appearance and views these changes as concessions to old age and frailty. Discuss strategies you will use to help

the patient understand the evidence under these circumstances. Discuss what you will do if she continues to disagree with your recommendations.

9. Explain why individual preferences may be a threat to the research validity of a study. Describe one strategy with which investigators might address the challenge of subject preferences.

References

1. Purtilo RB, Jensen GM, Royeen CB. *Educating for Moral Action: A Sourcebook in Health and Rehabilitation Ethics*. Philadelphia, PA: F.A. Davis Company; 2005.
2. Bower P, King M, Nazareth I, Lampe F, Sibbald B. Patient preferences in randomised controlled trials: Conceptual framework and implications for research. *Soc Sci Med.* 2005; 61(3):685–695.
3. Whitney SN, McGuire AL, McCullough LB. A typology of shared decision making, informed consent, and simple consent. *Ann Intern Med.* 2003; 140(1):54–59.
4. Knebel E. *Educating Health Professionals to be Patient-Centered.* Institute of Medicine Web site. Available at: http://www.iom.edu/Object.File/Master/10/460/Patient.pdf. Accessed February 15, 2006.
5. Karel MJ. The assessment of values in medical decision making. *J Aging Studies.* 2000; 14(4):403–422.
6. Sackett DL, Rosenberg WMC, Gray JAM, Haynes RB, Richardson WS. Evidence-based medicine: What it is and what it isn't. *BMJ.* 1996; 312(7023):71–72.
7. Hasnain-Wynia R. Is evidence-based medicine patient-centered and is patient-centered care evidence-based? *Health Serv Res.* 2006; 41(1):1–8.
8. American Physical Therapists Association. Guide to Physical Therapist Practice. 2d ed. *Phys Ther.* 2001; 81(1):9–744.
9. Ford S, Schofield T, Hope T. What are the ingredients for a successful evidence-based patient choice consultation? A qualitative study. *Soc Sci Med.* 2003; 56(3):589–602.
10. Slowther A, Ford S, Schofield T. Ethics of evidence-based medicine in the primary care setting. *J Med Ethics.* 2004; 30(2):151–155.
11. Definition of Disease Management. Disease Management Association of America Web site. Available at: http://www.dmaa.org/definition.html. Accessed April 1, 2006.
12. MedlinePlus. The National Library of Medicine Web site. Available at: http://www.nlm.nih.gov/medlineplus/. Accessed April 1, 2006.
13. Diseases and Conditions. The American Heart Association Web site. Available at: http://www.americanheart.org/presenter.jhtml?identifier=1200002. Accessed April 1, 2006.
14. The American Diabetes Association Web site. Available at: http://www.diabetes.org/home.jsp. Accessed April 1, 2006.
15. Medem Web site. The American Medical Association Available at: http://www.medem.com/MedLB/medlib_entry.cfm?sid=103AF635-C640-11D4-8C0100508BF1C1F1&site_name=Medem. Accessed April 1, 2006.

16. Information for Consumers. American Physical Therapy Association Web site. Available at: http://www.apta.org/Content/NavigationMenu/Consumers/consumer1.htm. Accessed April 1, 2006.
17. Guide for Professional Conduct. American Physical Therapy Association Web site. Available at: http://www.apta.org/AM/Template.cfm?Section=Policies_and_Bylaws&Template=/CM/HTMLDisplay.cfm&ContentID=24781. Accessed April 1, 2006.
18. Arteriovenous Malformations and Other Vascular Lesions of the Central Nervous System Fact Sheet. National Institute of Neurological Disorders and Stroke. National Institutes of Health Web site. Available at: http://www.ninds.nih.gov/disorders/avms/detail_avms.htm. Accessed April 1, 2006.
19. King M, Nazareth I, Lampe F, Bower P, Chandler F *et al.* Conceptual framework and systematic review of the effects of participants' and professionals' preferences in randomised controlled trials. *Health Technol Assess.* 2005; 9(35):1–191.
20. Straus SE, Richardson WS, Glaziou P, Haynes RB. *Evidence-Based Medicine: How to Practice and Teach EBM.* 3d ed. Edinburgh, Scotland: Elsevier Churchill Livingstone; 2005.
21. Erkan D, Yazici Y, Harrison MJ, Paget SA. Physician treatment preferences in rheumatoid arthritis of differing disease severity and activity: The impact of cost on first-line therapy. *Arthritis Rheum.* 2002; 47(3):285–290.
22. Fraenkel L, Bogardus ST, Concato J, Felson DT, Wittink DR. Patient preferences for treatment of rheumatoid arthritis. *Ann Rheum Dis.* 2004; 63(11): 1372–1378.
23. Torgerson D, Sibbald B. Understanding controlled trials: What is a patient preference trial? *BMJ.* 1998; 316(7128):360.
24. McPherson K, Britton A. Preferences and understanding their effects on health. *Quality in Health Care.* 2001; 10(Suppl I):i61–i66.
25. Klaber Moffett J, Torgerson D, Bell-Syer S, Jackson D, Llewlyn-Phillips H *et al.* Randomised controlled trial of exercise for low back pain: Clinical outcomes, costs and preferences. *BMJ.* 1999; 319(7205):279–283.
26. Klaber Moffett JA, Jackson DA, Richmond S, Hahn S, Coulton S *et al.* Randomised trial of a brief physiotherapy intervention compared with usual physiotherapy for neck pain patients: Outcomes and patients' preference. *BMJ.* 2005; 330(7482)1–6.

Chapter 16

Putting It All Together

Understanding human needs is half the job of meeting them.

—Adlai E. Stevenson, Jr.

OBJECTIVES

Upon completion of this chapter the student/practitioner will be able to:

1. Use a hypothetical patient example to model the formulation of a clinical question, as well as the search for and evaluation of evidence pertaining to:
   a. A diagnostic test;
   b. Prognosis;
   c. An intervention;
   d. Outcomes.
2. Use a hypothetical patient example to model the use of physiologic studies to answer a clinical question pertaining to interventions.

INTRODUCTION

This chapter uses hypothetical patient cases to illustrate the process of evidence-based physical therapy practice described throughout this text. The first section contains four brief scenarios—one each for diagnosis, prognosis, interventions, and outcomes. Cases reflect patients across the lifespan in a variety of clinical settings. At the conclusion of each scenario, a clinical question is presented followed by a table that summarizes the search strategies used. For the sake of chapter length, only one article from each search is appraised using the relevant quality appraisal checklist. Worksheets adapted from the Oxford Center for Evidence-Based Medicine also are presented.

The second section illustrates the use of several physiologic studies as evidence during patient management. As noted in previous chapters, "physiologic studies" rank lower on the various evidence hierarchies because these projects focus on anatomy, physiology, and pathophysiology rather than on the "whole patient." The subjects of these studies are cells, tissues, or organ systems, and their properties and functions under healthy and diseased states. Observations and experimental manipulation usually are conducted in well-controlled laboratory conditions. As a result, it is often difficult to generalize findings from these studies directly to patients/clients in clinical settings. In spite of these potential drawbacks, physiologic studies may be the only form of evidence that is available to answer particular questions. Therefore, it is important for evidence-based physical therapists to understand how physiologic studies may inform their clinical decisions.

This chapter comes with an important caveat: These examples are not intended to serve as practice guidelines or standards of care for the conditions described.

SECTION ONE: CLINICAL CASE EXAMPLES USING EVIDENCE

Case #1: Diagnosis

This acute care patient is a 67-year-old African-American man who had elective double coronary artery bypass surgery using an internal mammary artery graft one day ago. His mediastinal chest tubes were removed early this morning. He is awake and anxious to get out of bed. He indicates that his previous limitations to activity over the last six months were pressure in his chest, as well as occasional fatigue and cramping in his legs. His goal is to return to his previous occupational and leisure activities as soon as possible. The physical therapist's initial clinical exam reveals the following:

- Observation: Moderately overweight man supine in bed with head elevated to 45 degrees. He is receiving three liters of oxygen via nasal cannula. His sternal incision is dressed and dry. There is an arterial line placed in the left radial artery. Bedside telemetry monitoring is in place. He has a Foley catheter that is draining clear yellow urine.
- Social History: He is widowed and lives in a two-story home. He operates the family farm raising soybeans and corn. He also maintains goats and chickens. His son, daughter-in-law, and two grandchildren live with him and help him with the farm duties. He enjoys bird hunting.
- Significant Medical History: Left anterior descending coronary artery disease treated with percutaneous transluminal angioplasty twice in

the last five years. He has a 25 pack per year smoking habit which was discontinued eight years ago and hyperlipidemia. He has been overweight for at least 15 years. He denies history of arthritis, previous trauma, or other documented neuro-musculoskeletal disorders related to his lower extremities.

- Medications: Oxycodone (pain), metoprolol (blood pressure and heart rate), and lovastatin (hyperlipidemia).
- Resting Vital Signs: Heart rate = 84 beats/minute with regular rhythm; Blood pressure = 112/74 millimeters of mercury; Respiratory rate = 16 breaths/minute; Oxygen saturation = 97%; Body mass index = 28.4 kilograms/meter^2.
- Mental Status: He is alert and oriented to person, place, and time. He follows multiple step commands and answers questions appropriately.
- Pain: 4/10 on a verbal pain rating scale for his chest incision.
- Auscultation: Heart sounds = normal S_1 and S_2; Lung sounds = clear in the upper and midzones, but crackles are present in both bases.
- Breathing Pattern: He demonstrates shallow inspirations with guarding due to incisional discomfort.
- Active Range of Motion: All joints in both upper and lower extremities are within normal limits except for shoulder elevation which is voluntarily restricted to 90 degrees of flexion due to incisional discomfort.
- Mobility: He is able to perform 75 percent of the effort to come to sitting at the edge of the bed and to execute a stand pivot transfer to a chair with assistance of one person.
- Vital Signs with Activity: Heart rate = 96 beats/minute; Blood pressure = 128/82 millimeters of mercury; Respiratory rate = 24 breaths/minute; Oxygen saturation = 94%.
- Pain with Activity: 7/10 on a verbal pain rating scale.
- Palpation: No edema is noted in his lower extremities while in the dependent position. His dorsal pedal pulse is absent on the right. Both posterior tibial pulses and his left dorsal pedal pulse are barely detectable.

The diminished lower extremity pulses and this patient's complaint of prior leg fatigue and cramping suggest that he is developing peripheral arterial disease; however, the physical therapist wonders how well palpation of peripheral pulses correctly identifies an individual with this problem. He decides to search the literature to answer the following clinical question:

> Is manual palpation of lower extremity pulses during a physical therapy examination sufficient to detect the presence of peripheral arterial disease in a 67-year-old man with coronary artery disease?

Table 16–1 details the results of a literature search using the National Library of Medicine's PubMed Clinical Queries function. Two articles were identified, both of which appear to address the clinical question based upon their titles and abstracts. The Collins *et al.* article[1] is selected for review because it compared pulse palpation to the ankle-brachial index (ABI), which is another clinical test performed by physical therapists. The second article compared pulse palpation with tests conducted in a vascular laboratory, as well as with the ABI.

Table 16–2 provides a critique of the Collins *et al.* article[1] using the quality appraisal checklist for evidence about diagnostic tests. Based upon the review findings, the physical therapist decides that the absence of a pulse on manual palpation is sufficient to rule in peripheral arterial disease (high specificity), but that the presence of a pulse is not useful for ruling out this condition (low sensitivity). Given that three out of four pulses are detectable, the therapist plans to measure this patient's ABI in both lower extremities. In light of the patient's desire to return to an active lifestyle, as well as his excellent rehabilitation potential, the therapist will report his findings to the attending physician with a recommendation for additional lower extremity vascular competency tests should the ABI results suggest the presence of peripheral arterial disease.

Table 16–1 Search results for a clinical question related to a diagnostic test for a patient with diminished lower extremity pulses.

Search Term	Study Category	Limits
"pedal pulse palpation"	Diagnosis with a narrow, specific search	• English language • Human subjects • Title/Abstract fields
Total Number of Citations Retrieved = 2		
Relevant Titles		
Collins TC, Suarez-Almazor M, Petersen NJ. An absent pulse is not sensitive for the early detection of peripheral arterial disease. *Fam Med.* 2006; 38(1):38–42.		
Kazmers A, Koski ME, Groehn H, Oust G, Meeker C *et al.* Assessment of non-invasive arterial testing versus pulse exam. *Am Surg.* 1996; 62(4):315–319.		

Table 16–2 Quality appraisal checklist for a diagnostic test for a patient with diminished lower extremity pulses.

Collins TC, Suarez-Almazor M, Petersen NJ. An absent pulse is not sensitive for the early detection of peripheral arterial disease. *Fam Med.* 2006; 38(1):38–42.

Research Validity of the Study	
Did the investigators compare results from the test of interest to results from a gold (or reference) standard test? Pedal pulses were compared to a bedside ankle-brachial index (ABI), not a vascular laboratory assessment.	___ Yes X No
Were the individuals performing and interpreting each test's results unaware (e.g., masked, or blinded) of the other test's results?	___ Yes X No
Did the investigators include subjects with all levels or stages of the condition being evaluated by the diagnostic test of interest? N = 403 (37.3% = No symptoms; 55.2% = "Atypical symptoms"; 7.5% = "Classic intermittent claudication")	X Yes ___ No
Did all subjects undergo the gold standard diagnostic test? All subjects underwent the ABI.	X Yes ___ No
Did the investigators repeat the study with a new set of subjects?	___ Yes X No
Do you have enough confidence in the research validity of this paper to consider using this evidence with your patient/client? Limitations include lack of a true "gold standard" comparison test, the potential for tester bias, and lack of validation in a second set of subjects.	___ Yes X Undecided ___ No

What results do the authors report related to your clinical question?

Sensitivity of Pulse Palpation = 18% (left leg) and 32% (right leg)

Specificity of Pulse Palpation = 99% (left leg) and 98% (right leg)

Positive Predictive Value(s) of pulse palpation = 67% (left leg) and 63% (right leg)

Negative Predictive Value(s) of pulse palpation = 89% (left leg) and 93% (right leg)

+ Likelihood Ratio(s) of nonpalpable pulse in patient with PAD = 18 (left leg) and 16 (right leg)

Likelihood Ratio(s) of palpable pulse in patient without PAD = 0.83 (left leg) and 0.69 (right leg)

How important are the results?

Obtained p-values for each statistic reported by the authors:

- Not reported for the measures listed above

Obtained confidence intervals for each statistic reported by the authors:

- Not reported for the measures listed above

continues

Table 16–2 Quality appraisal checklist for a diagnostic test for a patient with diminished lower extremity pulses *(continued).*

Is this test reliable and valid? If yes, continue below. The ABI is more reliable and valid than manual palpation of pulses.	___ Yes _X_ No
What is the pretest probability that your patient/client has the condition of interest?	~10%
What is the posttest probability that your patient/client has the condition of interest if you apply this test?	65–70% if pulse is absent; 6–7% if pulse is present
Do the subjects in the study resemble your patient/client? Mean age = 63.8 (SD 0.36); sample included African-American males and individuals with a history of smoking and hyperlipidemia.	_X_ Yes ___ No
Can you perform this test safely and appropriately in your clinical setting given your current knowledge, skill level and your current resources? Both manual palpation of pulses and the ABI are performed easily at the bedside by physical therapists.	_X_ Yes ___ No
Does the test fit within the patient/client's expressed values and preferences? The ABI is preferred over manual palpation of pulses as a screening test. The patient wants to resume an active lifestyle so he would benefit from more accurate tests to help determine the underlying cause of his leg cramping.	___ Yes _X_ No
Will you use this diagnostic test for this patient/client? The PT will use the ABI instead of relying on manual pulses.	___ Yes _X_ No

YOUR CALCULATIONS

Left LE		Peripheral Arterial Disease (PAD) Present (ABI < 0.90)	Peripheral Arterial Disease (PAD) Absent (ABI ≥ 0.90)	Totals
Palpation of Pedal Pulses	Positive (Absent Pulse)	**a** 8	**b** 4	**a+b** 12
	Negative (Present Pulse)	**c** 37	**d** 304	**c+d** 341
Totals		**a+c** 45	**b+d** 308	**a+b+c+d** 353

Sensitivity = a/(a+c) = 8/45 = 18%

Specificity = d/(b+d) = 304/308 = 99%

Likelihood Ratio for a Positive Test Result = LR+ = Sens/(1−Spec) = 0.18/1−0.99 = 18

Likelihood Ratio for a Negative Test Result = LR− = (1−Sens)/Spec = 1−0.18/0.99 = 0.83

Positive Predictive Value = a/(a+b) = 8/12 = 67%

Negative Predictive Value = d/(c+d) = 304/341 = 89%
Pretest Probability (Prevalence) = (a+c)/(a+b+c+d) = 45/353= 13%
Pretest Odds = Prevalence/(1−Prevalence) = 0.13/0.87 = 0.15
Posttest Odds = Pretest Odds × LR+ = 0.15 × 18 = 2.7
Posttest Probability = Posttest Odds/(Posttest Odds +1) = 2.7/3.7 = 73%
Posttest Odds = Pretest Odds × LR− = 0.15 × 0.83 = 0.12
Posttest Probability = Posttest Odds/(Posttest Odds +1) = 0.12/1.12 = 11%

		PAD		
		Present	Absent	
Right LE		(ABI < 0.90)	(ABI ≥ 0.90)	**Totals**
Palpation of Pedal Pulses	Positive (Absent Pulse)	**a** 12	**b** 7	**a+b** 19
	Negative (Present Pulse)	**c** 25	**d** 314	**c+d** 339
Totals		**a+c** 37	**b+d** 321	**a+b+c+d** 358

Sensitivity = a/(a+c) = 12/37 = 32%
Specificity = d/(b+d) = 314/321 = 98%
Likelihood Ratio for a Positive Test Result = LR+ = Sens/(1−Spec) = 0.32/1−0.98 = 16
Likelihood Ratio for a Negative Test Result = LR− = (1−Sens)/Spec = 1−0.32/0.98 = 0.69
Positive Predictive Value = a/(a+b) = 12/19 = 63%
Negative Predictive Value = d/(c+d) = 314/339 = 93%
Pretest Probability (Prevalence) = (a+c)/(a+b+c+d) = 37/358 = 10%
Pretest Odds = Prevalence/(1−Prevalence) = 0.10/0.90 = 0.11
Posttest Odds = Pretest Odds × LR+ = 0.11 × 16 = 1.8
Posttest Probability = Posttest Odds/(Posttest Odds +1) = 1.8/2.8 = 64%
Posttest Odds = Pretest Odds × LR− = 0.11 × 0.69 = 0.08
Posttest Probability = Posttest Odds/(Posttest Odds +1) = 0.08/1.08 = 7.4%

Case #2: Prognosis

This home health patient is a 78-year-old Caucasian woman diagnosed with Parkinson's disease seven years ago. Her modified Hoehn and Yahr stage score reported at her last neurologist's visit was 3.0. She fell for the first time turning from the counter to the kitchen table one week ago, resulting in a contusion and an extensive hematoma on her left hip. She denies any dizziness or other precipitating symptoms. Her primary complaint is increased difficulty coming to standing and walking because of pain with movement of her left lower extremity. Her family has expressed concern about her safety because of increasing loss of balance and near falls leading up to this recent event. However, they are committed to keeping her at home for as long as possible. The patient is worried that her declining function is a burden to her husband and wants to know what options are available to help them at home. The physical therapist's initial clinical exam reveals the following:

- Observation: Frail, elderly woman accompanied by her 80-year-old husband.
- Social History: Her home is a split-level ranch style with five steps to the bedroom and bathroom. Handrails are located on both sides of the stairs. Tight pile wall-to-wall carpets are in all rooms except the kitchen and bathroom. The entrance to the home is at ground level.
- Significant Medical History: Hypertension and depression.
- Medications: Levodopa-carbidopa (Parkinson's), hydrochlorothiazide (hypertension), and citalopram (depression).
- Resting Vital Signs: Heart rate = 76 beats/minute with regular rhythm; Blood pressure = 124/66 millimeters of mercury; Respiratory rate = 16 breaths/minute; Oxygen saturation = 98% on room air.
- Mental Status: She is alert and oriented to person, place, and time. She follows two-step commands with delayed motor response.
- Mobility: She is able to perform 50 percent of the effort to come to standing with assistance of one person. She stands using a rolling walker with a forward flexed posture and contact guard of one person. She ambulates with a festinating gait pattern, with decreased stance time on the left lower extremity due to pain, for a total distance of 50 feet. She is able to perform 75 percent of this task with assistance of one person to change directions and recover balance when turning.
- Vital Signs with Activity: Heart rate = 92 beats/minute with regular rhythm; Blood pressure = 140/60 millimeters of mercury; Respiratory rate = 28 breaths/minute; Oxygen saturation = 97%.

As the physical therapist considers this case, she recognizes that the patient has several characteristics that have been identified as risk factors for falls in the elderly. However, the therapist is not sure which of these factors is specifically relevant to individuals with Parkinson's disease. She decides to search for evidence to address the following clinical question:

> Which risk factors predict future fall risk for a 78-year-old woman with Parkinson's disease who has suffered a recent fall?

Table 16–3 details the results of a literature search using the National Library of Medicine's PubMed Medical Subject Headings (MeSH) search function. Nineteen citations were returned, eight of which look relevant to the question posed based upon their titles and abstracts. The Bloem *et al.* article[2] was

Table 16–3 Search results for a clinical question related to prognosis for a patient with Parkinson's disease.

Search Term	MeSH Term	Limits
Falls	"Accidental Falls"	• English language
Risk	"Risk Factors"	• Human subjects
Parkinson's	"Parkinson Disease"	• Title/Abstract fields
Final Search String: "Accidental Falls" AND "Risk Factors" AND "Parkinson Disease"		
Total Number of Citations Retrieved = 19		
Relevant Titles		
Robinson K, Dennison A, Roalf D *et al.* Falling risk factors in Parkinson's disease. *NeuroRehabilitation.* 2005; 20(3):169–182.		
Balash Y, Peretz C, Leibovich G, Herman T, Hausdorff JM, Giladi N. Falls in outpatients with Parkinson's disease: Frequency, impact and identifying factors. *J Neurol.* 2005; 252(11):1310–1315.		
Wood BH, Bilclough JA, Bowron A, Walker RW. Incidence and prediction of falls in Parkinson's disease: A prospective multidisciplinary study. *J Neurol Neurosurg Psychiatry.* 2002; 72(6):721–725.		
Bloem BR, Grimbergen YA, Cramer M, Willemsen M, Zwinderman AH. Prospective assessment of falls in Parkinson's disease. *J Neurol.* 2001; 248(11):950–958.		
Ashburn A, Stack E, Pickering RM, Ward CD. Predicting fallers in a community-based sample of people with Parkinson's disease. *Gerontology.* 2001; 47(5):277–281.		
Ashburn A, Stack E, Pickering RM, Ward CD. A community-dwelling sample of people with Parkinson's disease: Characteristics of fallers and non-fallers. *Age Ageing.* 2001; 30(1):47–52.		
Playfer JR. Falls and Parkinson's disease. *Age Ageing.* 2001; 30(1):3–4.		
Gray P, Hildebrand K. Fall risk factors in Parkinson's disease. *J Neurosci Nurs.* 2000; 32(4):222–228.		
Koller WC, Glatt S, Vetere-Overfield B, Hassanein R. Falls and Parkinson's disease. *Clin Neuropharmacol.* 1989; 12(2):98–105.		

selected for review because it was a prospective study examining fall risk in community-dwelling patients with Parkinson's disease, as compared to age-matched controls without Parkinson's disease. In addition, the authors specifically analyzed predictive factors related to recurrent falls.

Table 16–4 provides a critique of the Bloem *et al.* article[2] using the quality appraisal checklist appropriate for prognosis papers. Based upon the review findings, the physical therapist decides to inform the patient and her family about her increased risk for future "center of mass" falls like the one suffered last week. The therapist also decides to instruct the family on movement and guarding techniques in an effort to reduce that risk. Finally, she will explore the possibility of a personal care attendant, given the husband's age and everyone's desire for the patient to remain at home for as long as possible.

Table 16–4 Prognosis quality appraisal checklist for a patient with Parkinson's disease.

Bloem BR, Grimbergen YAM, Cramer M, Willemsen M, Zwinderman AH. Prospective assessment of falls in Parkinson's disease. *J Neurol.* 2001; 248(11):950–958.	
Research Validity of the Study	
Did the investigators provide sufficient information to describe the sample in their study? N = 59 (mean age = 60.8 ± 9.7 years; 36% female; mean modified Hoehn & Yahr stage score = 2.3 + 0.7 [2 = bilateral involvement without impairment of balance; 5 = Wheelchair-bound or bedridden] with 30 subjects scoring 2.5 or higher; mean Unified Parkinson's Disease Rating Scale score = 48.3 ± 15.2 (0 = no disability).	X Yes ___ No
Are the subjects representative of the population from which they were drawn?	X Yes ___ No
Did all subjects enter the study at the same (preferably early) stage of their condition? Mean duration of Parkinson's disease in the sample = 7.1 + 4.8 years	___ Yes X No
Was the study time frame long enough to capture the outcome(s) of interest? 6 months	X Yes ___ No
Did the investigators collect outcome data from all of the subjects enrolled in the study? 61 subjects with Parkinson's disease were enrolled originally. Two were lost to follow-up—one died and one could not be contacted. The authors reported the attrition, but did not replace the subjects or include their baseline data in the analyses. Characteristics of lost subjects also were not reported. However, the number of subjects lost was small and unlikely to have affected the outcome of the study.	___ Yes X No
Were outcome criteria operationally defined? Specific definitions of a "fall" were provided to subjects.	X Yes ___ No
Were the individuals collecting the outcome measures masked (or blinded) to the status of prognostic factors in each subject? Falls were measured by self-report of the subjects.	___ Yes X No
Does the sample include subgroups of patients for whom prognostic estimates will differ?	X Yes ___ No
If so, did the investigators conduct separate subgroup analyses or statistically adjust for these different prognostic factors? Predictive factors for recurrent fallers are analyzed separately. They did not adjust for differences in severity of Parkinson's disease.	X Yes ___ No
Did investigators repeat the study with a new set of subjects?	___ Yes X No

Do you have enough confidence in the research validity of this paper to consider using this evidence with your patient/client?

X Yes
___ Undecided
___ No

Limitations include differences in the stage of the disease among subjects, the potential for inaccurate reporting of falls, and the lack of validation in a second set of subjects.

What results do the authors report related to your clinical question?

Correlation Coefficient(s) ______

Coefficients of Determination ______

Odds Ratios ______

Relative Risk (RR) for Recurrent Falls:

Hoehn & Yahr Stage Score = 1–2.5	RR = 13.4
Hoehn & Yahr Stage Score ≥ 3.0	RR > 100
Fall in previous six months	RR = 5.0
Use of benzodiazapines	RR = 5.0

Other Important Findings for Subjects with Parkinson's Disease:

82% fell indoors
70% had intrinsic falls (not related to environmental factors)
72% had center of mass falls (turning around, standing up, and bending forward)
62% had injurious falls (mostly soft-tissue)
42% developed a fear of falling

How important are the results?

Obtained p-values for each statistic reported by the authors: N/A

Obtained confidence intervals for each statistic reported by the authors:

Hoehn & Yahr Stage Score = 1–2.5	CI 0.4–27
Hoehn & Yahr Stage Score > 3.0	CI 3.1–585
Fall in previous six months	CI 1.2–20.9
Use of benzodiazapines	CI 1.6–15.5

The CI for the "Hoehn & Yahr Stage Score = 1–2.5" includes the value 1 which indicates that the relative risk may be no better than chance. The CI for the "Hoehn & Yahr Stage Score ≥ 3.0" is very wide; however, the magnitude of the RR makes this predictive factor important to consider. The CIs for "fall in the previous six months" and "use of benzodiazapines" indicate reasonably precise estimates of risk.

How likely are the outcomes over time (based on your experience or on the proportion of subjects in the study who achieved the outcome)?

35% of subjects reported recurrent falls

Do the subjects in the study resemble your patient/client? If no, how are they different?

X Yes
___ No

Will sharing information from this study about prognostic indicators or risk factors help your patient/client given their expressed values and preferences?

X Yes
___ No

How will you use this information with your patient/client?

The patient and her family would benefit from understanding the nature of fall risk with Parkinson's disease. Specifically, the patient can be instructed regarding movement techniques to avoid center of mass falls, while the family can be instructed in guarding techniques during at risk movements. The possibility of a personal care attendant also should be explored given patient's husband's age.

Case # 3: Intervention

This outpatient is a 43-year-old right-handed woman of Asian descent who presents with progressive pain and stiffness that prevents her from lifting her right arm above her head to wash and dry her hair and to reach up into cabinets for dishes. She also complains of sudden sharp pain when she reaches to her right side at her desk or tries to reach into the back seat of her car. She denies previous trauma or similar problems but does recall an incident three months earlier in which her Labrador retriever nearly "pulled my arm out of its socket" trying to chase a cat during a morning walk. The physical therapist's initial clinical exam reveals the following:

- Observation: Fit-looking woman who maneuvers independently from the waiting room to the exam room guarding her right upper extremity.
- Social History: She is married with two children ages 11 and 14. She works as a grant reviewer for a charitable foundation where she spends an average of five hours a day on her computer. She attends the gym 4–5 days a week for strength and aerobic training, but has discontinued upper extremity activities.
- Significant Medical History: Type I diabetes diagnosed at age 12 and hyperlipidemia.
- Medications: Insulin (diabetes) and simvastatin (hyperlipidemia). Prescription strength ibuprofen "just takes the edge off" her shoulder pain.
- Resting Vital Signs: Heart rate = 60 beats/minute with regular rhythm; Blood pressure = 110/58 millimeters of mercury; Respiratory rate = 10 breaths/minute; Oxygen saturation = 99% on room air.
- Mental Status: Alert and oriented to person, place and time.
- Palpation: She complains of general tenderness over the right rotator cuff tendons with point tenderness at the subacromial space.
- Cervical Spine: No restrictions noted in active or passive motion or in segmental vertebral mobility. The therapist is unable to reproduce her upper extremity symptoms during this portion of the examination.
- Active Range of Motion: Her left glenohumeral joint is normal in all planes. Her right glenohumeral joint demonstrates 90 degrees of flexion, 70 degrees of abduction, 30 degrees of external rotation with her arm at her side, and 35 degrees of extension. When she tries to reach behind her back, she can only get to her pants pocket. All limitations are in response to increased pain provoked at the end of the achieved ranges.

- Passive Range of Motion: Her left glenohumeral joint is normal in all planes. Her right glenohumeral joint demonstrates 100 degrees of flexion, 82 degrees of abduction, 35 degrees of external rotation with her arm at her side, 40 degrees of extension with all limitations due to pain, producing an empty end feel.
- Motor Control: She initiates right shoulder elevation through activation of her upper trapezius in a hiking maneuver.
- Accessory Joint Motion: The left glenohumeral joint has normal accessory motion. Restriction to movement is noted with posterior and inferior glides of the right humeral head. Pain is reproduced when the humeral head is mobilized into the restriction.
- Pain (Verbal Pain Rating Scale): worst: 9/10; average: 5/10; today: 5/10
- Disability of Arm, Shoulder and Hand Scale (DASH) Score: 79 out of 100 possible points (higher score represents greater disability).

The physical therapist concludes that his examination findings are consistent with adhesive capsulitis of the right shoulder. The patient tells him that her physician recommended a corticosteroid injection for her shoulder, but she declined that option as she already has to inject herself with insulin daily. She also found information on the Internet that indicates that corticosteroids are "not good" for people with diabetes. She wants to know what the physical therapist can do to speed up her recovery. After considering the list of interventions that have potential to address this patient's problem, the therapist decides to review the evidence to answer the following clinical question:

> Which combination of interventions will produce the quickest improvement in pain and function for a 43-year-old woman with diabetes and adhesive capsulitis of the shoulder 1) joint mobilization and exercise or 2) joint mobilization, exercise and physical agents?

Table 16–5 details the results of a literature search using the Cochrane Library online database. Five citations were identified, the first of which appears most relevant to his clinical question. The Green *et al.* article[3] is a systematic review and meta-analysis of evidence regarding physical therapy interventions for shoulder pain; however, only one of the articles reviewed addresses patients with adhesive capsulitis. The majority of evidence includes patients with other disorders of the shoulder, such as rotator cuff tendonitis and subacromial bursitis. As a result, the therapist decides to retrieve the original article by van der Windt *et al.*[4] and review it to answer his question. The article compares physical therapy (exercise and joint mobilization, as well as electrical stimulation, hot or cold packs as needed for pain) to corticosteroid injections.

Table 16–5 Search results for a clinical question related to interventions for a patient with adhesive capsulitis of the shoulder.

Search Term	MeSH Term	Limits
Adhesive Capsulitis	"Bursitis"	• Search all text
Frozen Shoulder	No MeSH term available	
Exercise	"Exercise"	
Joint Mobilization	No MeSH term available	
Joint Manipulation	"Musculoskeletal Manipulations"	
Physical Agents	No MeSH term available	
Modalities	"Physical Therapy Modalities"	
Final Search String: "Adhesive Capsulitis" AND "Physical Therapy Modalities"		
Total Number of Citations Retrieved = 5		
Relevant Titles		
Green S, Buchbinder R, Hetrick S. Physiotherapy interventions for shoulder pain. *The Cochrane Database of Systematic Reviews.* 2003; 2:CD004258.		
Buchbinder R, Green S, Youd JM. Corticosteroid injections for shoulder pain. *The Cochrane Database of Systematic Reviews.* 2003; (1):CD004016.		
Green S, Buchbinder R, Hetrick S. Acupuncture for shoulder pain. *The Cochrane Database of Systematic Reviews.* 2005; (2):CD005319.		
Green S, Buchbinder R, Glazier SE, Bell SN. Interventions for shoulder pain. *The Cochrane Database of Systematic Reviews.* 1999;(4):CD001156.		
Coghlan JA, Buchbinder R, Green SE, Bell SN. Surgery for rotator cuff disease. *The Cochrane Database of Systematic Reviews.* 2006; (1):CD005619.		

Table 16–6 provides a critique of the van der Windt *et al.* article[4] using the quality appraisal checklist appropriate for intervention papers. Based upon the review findings, the physical therapist decides to inform the patient that the available evidence is limited and does not include patients with diabetes. Diabetes is known to delay healing time in general and may adversely influence this patient's prognosis in ways that cannot be estimated because subjects like her were not studied. However, he will discuss the findings from van der Windt *et al.* including a) the use of exercise and joint mobilization techniques as the primary physical therapy intervention methods; b) the potential for a longer recovery time during the first 2–3 months, as compared to corticosteroid injections; and c) the potential that her eventual improvement may be comparable over the long term to that achieved with injections. Based on the evidence and his prior experience with patients similar to this one, he also will offer electrical stimulation combined with ice for pain management as needed during her treatment.

Table 16–6 Intervention quality appraisal checklist for a patient with adhesive capsulitis of the shoulder.

van der Windt DAWM, Koes BW, Deville W, Boeke AJP, de Jong BA *et al*. Effectiveness of corticosteroid injections versus physiotherapy for treatment of painful stiff shoulder in primary care: Randomized trial. *BMJ*. 1998; 317(7168):1292–1296.

Research Validity of the Study	
Did the investigators randomly assign (or allocate) subjects to groups? Authors used a random number generator.	X Yes __ No
Was each subject's group assignment concealed from the people enrolling individuals in the study?	X Yes __ No
Did the groups have similar sociodemographic, clinical, and prognostic characteristics at the start of the study? More subjects in the physical therapy group were female and had: • Concomitant neck pain • An acute onset of shoulder pain and stiffness • Involvement of their dominant upper extremity. In comparison, more subjects in the corticosteroid group had: • Previous episodes of shoulder pain and stiffness • A higher rating of severity of pain associated with their main complaint • A higher rating of severity of pain at night.	__ Yes X No
Were subjects, clinicians, and outcome assessors masked (or blinded) to the subjects' group assignment?	X Yes (outcome assessors) X No (subjects)
Did the investigators manage all of the groups in the same way except for the experimental intervention(s)? Medication use and additional treatments outside of the study were not controlled.	__ Yes X No
Did subject attrition (e.g., withdrawal, loss to follow-up) occur over the course of the study? Two patients withdrew from the physical therapy group and four patients withdrew from the injection group. The investigators did not perform an analysis of the characteristics of those who withdrew to determine whether sampling bias had resulted.	X Yes __ No
Were subjects analyzed in the groups to which they were assigned? The investigators did perform an intention-to-treat analysis. They also analyzed their data excluding 12 patients that were not treated according to protocol for the purposes of comparison.	X Yes __ No
Did the investigators collect follow-up data on all subjects over a time frame long enough for the outcomes of interest to occur? Measures were collected at 3, 7, 13, 26, and 52 weeks, respectively.	X Yes __ No

continues

Table 16-6 Intervention quality appraisal checklist for a patient with adhesive capsulitis of the shoulder *(continued)*.

Did investigators repeat the study with a new set of subjects?

___ Yes
_X_ No

Do you have enough confidence in the research validity of this paper to consider using this evidence with your patient/client?

___ Yes
___ Undecided
_X_ No

What results do the authors report related to your clinical question?

Tests of Differences ______

Effect Sizes *Subjects in the corticosteroid group achieved a statistically significant greater improvement, as compared to subjects in the PT group, for the following measures*:

- Pain during the day mean difference between groups = 12 mm on a visual analog scale
- Pain at night mean difference between groups = 14 mm on a visual analog scale
- Shoulder disability mean difference between groups = 25 points on a 100 point scale
- External rotation of affected shoulder mean difference between groups = 15 degrees
- Therapist rating of success mean difference between groups = 15 mm on visual analog scale

Subjects in the physical therapy group did not improve their range of motion during the 7 weeks of treatment (Mean change in external rotation = − 2degrees (SD = 14); Mean change in abduction = −1 degree (SD = 14)).

Subjects in the corticosteroid group improved their external rotation (Mean change = 13 degrees (SD = 16), but not their abduction (Mean change = 4 degrees (SD = 11)).

Absolute Benefit Increases ______

Relative Benefit Increases ______

Absolute Risk Reductions ______

Relative Risk Reductions ______

Number Needed to Treat (Harm) ______

Other ______

How important are the results?

Obtained p-values for each statistic reported by the authors:

Obtained confidence intervals (CI) for each statistic reported by the authors:

Corticosteroid group versus physical therapy group

- Pain during the day 95% CI: 15, 37 mm; $p < 0.001$
- Pain at night 95% CI: 3, 25 mm; $p = 0.015$
- Shoulder disability 95% CI: 14, 35 points; $p = 0.024$
- External rotation of affected shoulder 95% CI: 9, 20°; $p = 0.002$
- Therapist rating of success 95% CI: 7, 22 mm; $p < 0.001$

Do these findings exceed a minimal clinically important difference?

MCID = 25% improvement of treatment group over control group; success rate in the study = 31%

_X_ Yes
___ No

Do the subjects in the study resemble your patient/client? ___ Yes
_X_ No

Subjects were older and individuals with diabetes were excluded from the study.

Can you perform this intervention safely and appropriately in your clinical setting given your current knowledge and skill level and your current resources? _X_ Yes
___ No

The physical therapist already uses the interventions described in this study.

Does the intervention fit within the patient/client's expressed values and preferences? _X_ Yes
___ No

The patient wants physical therapy rather than a corticosteroid injection.

Do the potential benefits outweigh the potential risks of using this intervention with your patient/client? _X_ Yes
___ No

The primary adverse reaction noted in the study was pain lasting >2 days in both groups.

Will you use this intervention for this patient/client? _X_ Yes
___ No

Case #4: Outcomes

This outpatient is a 6-year-old Caucasian male with spastic diplegia who has been referred to pediatric physical therapy to continue the progress he achieved with standing balance and gait over the school year. He was a full-term infant who was delivered vaginally without complication to a healthy 28-year-old mother following a normal pregnancy. APGAR (activity, pulse, grimace, appearance and breathing) scores were 6 and 9 at one minute and five minutes, respectively. He was diagnosed with cerebral palsy at 16 months of age when his parents noticed that he "wasn't moving like other babies." He has not suffered any seizures and is age-appropriate in his cognitive and emotional function. His primary method of locomotion is a wheelchair, but he can walk short distances in the classroom and at home using a posterior walker and bilateral solid ankle-foot orthoses (AFOs). His primary limitation to activity is fatigue and weakness. His goal is to walk without a walker back and forth to the cafeteria with his classmates when he returns to the school in the fall. The physical therapist's initial clinical exam reveals the following:

- Observation: Slender boy seated in a custom wheelchair, accompanied by his parents. He is wearing glasses and bilateral solid AFOs.
- Social History: He has an older sister and one younger brother. He has just completed the 1st grade. He is an avid baseball fan.

- Significant Medical History: He is being considered for botulinum toxin injections to his gastrocnemius, hamstrings, and hip adductors bilaterally. He also is nearsighted.
- Medications: None.
- Resting Vital Signs: Heart rate = 84 beats/minute with regular rhythm; Blood pressure = 92/58 millimeters of mercury; Respiratory rate = 20 breaths/minute; Oxygen saturation = 98% on room air.
- Mental Status: He is alert and oriented to person, place, and time. His answers to questions are age-appropriate. He follows two-step commands with motor limitations as described below.
- Pain: None
- Muscle Tone: Spasticity is present in the gastrocnemius, hamstrings, and hip adductors, bilaterally. Mild increased resting muscle tone is noted in the quadriceps, biceps, and triceps, bilaterally.
- Range of Motion: He has hip flexion and plantar flexion contractures bilaterally. He is lacking eight degrees of knee extension on the left and five degrees of knee extension on the right. His ankles can be passively dorsiflexed to neutral with significant resistance.
- Mobility (Independent): He can perform the following tasks:
    - Pushing up to stand from his wheelchair
    - Standing with unilateral upper extremity support
    - Manipulating objects with his free hand while standing
    - Ambulating 65 feet with the posterior walker; he stops due to fatigue and frustration with having to use the assistive device.
- Mobility (Assisted): He can perform the following tasks with assistance of one person for 25–50% of the effort:
    - Standing without upper extremity support
    - Walking without an assistive device
- Gait Pattern: His legs cross in a scissoring pattern when walking. He also has a crouched appearance which is exaggerated further if he does not wear his AFOs. Step length is short for his age and his upper extremities provide significant assistance for balance while advancing the swing leg.
- Vital Signs with Activity: Heart rate = 100 beats/minute with regular rhythm; Blood pressure = 112/64 millimeters of mercury; Respiratory rate = 30 breaths/minute; Oxygen saturation = 98%.
- Gross Motor Function Classification System Score: Level III (age 4–6 years)

The physical therapist's clinic has just purchased a body weight suspension harness system to use for gait training over ground, as well as on a treadmill. To date, the system has been used with children with incomplete spinal cord injuries and brain injuries. The therapist decides to review the evidence to answer the following clinical question:

> Will partial body weight-supported gait training on a treadmill improve functional outcomes in a 6-year-old male with spastic diplegia whose ambulatory ability is limited by weakness and fatigue?

Table 16-7 details the results of a literature search using the Cumulative Index of Nursing and Allied Health Literature (CINAHL) online database. Fourteen citations were returned, five of which look relevant to the question posed based upon their titles and abstracts. The Schindt *et al.* article[5] was selected for review because it focused on functional outcomes rather than on physiologic adaptations resulting from treadmill training. In addition, the subjects included several individuals diagnosed with spastic diplegia who had limited ambulation skills at the start of the study.

Table 16–7 Search results for a clinical question related to outcomes for a patient with spastic diplegia.

Search Term	CINAHL Heading Term	Limits
Spastic Diplegia	No CINAHL heading available	• English language
Cerebral Palsy	"Cerebral Palsy"	• Child 6–12 years old
Treadmill	"Treadmills"	
Outcome	"Treatment Outcomes"	
	"Outcome Assessment"	
Final Search String: "Cerebral Palsy" AND "Treadmills"		
Total Number of Citations Retrieved = 14		
	Relevant Titles	
Unnithan VB. The effect of partial body weight support on the oxygen cost of walking in children and adolescents with spastic cerebral palsy. *Pediatr Exerc Sci.* 2006; 18(1):11–21.		
Maltais D. Responses of children with cerebral palsy to treadmill walking exercise in the heat. *Med Sci Sports Exerc.* 2005; 84(1):36–49.		
Maltais D. Repeated treadmill walks affect physiologic responses in children with cerebral palsy. *Med Sci Sports Exerc.* 2003; 35(10):1653–1661.		
Schindl MR, Forstner C, Kern H, Hess S. Treadmill training with partial body weight support in nonambulatory patients with cerebral palsy. *Arch Phys Med Rehabil.* 2000; 81(3):301–306.		
Hoofwijk M. Maximal treadmill performance of children with cerebral palsy. *Pediatr Exerc Sci.* 1995; 7(3):305–313.		

Table 16–8 provides a critique of the Schindt *et al.* article[5] using the quality appraisal checklist appropriate for outcomes papers. Although the evidence is limited by the lack of randomly assigned groups that control for extraneous factors, the therapist decides to recommend body weight-supported treadmill training as an element of this patient's treatment plan because 1) the subjects with spastic diplegia demonstrated improvement in standing and walking ability, and 2) the outcomes documented in the article were achieved without any adverse treatment effects noted. Both the treadmill and the harness will allow the therapist to carefully titrate the patient's exertion levels to deal with his low level of aerobic conditioning, while simultaneously allowing interventions to improve his gait pattern. The patient is extremely enthusiastic about this option since he can "work out" like they do at his parents' fitness center and will not have to use his walker.

SECTION TWO: USING PHYSIOLOGIC STUDIES AS EVIDENCE

This outpatient is a 15-year-old male soccer player who reported gradual onset of pain in the region of his right knee over the course of his participation in a weekend soccer tournament approximately one week ago. He denies any previous injury to his knee. His mother reports that radiographs taken at the pediatrician's office were negative. Presently, the patient complains of intermittent pain with walking and ascending and descending steps. He has not attempted a return to soccer practice or gym class. The physical therapist's initial clinical exam reveals the following:

- Observation: Pleasant young male who ambulates independently to the examination room with a mildly antalgic gait pattern. He is accompanied by his mother.
- Social History: He is in the 10th grade and works for a local grocery store several nights a week. He is a starting halfback on the high school soccer team, as well as on a town league. College scouts have been evaluating his performance to determine his recruitment potential.
- Medications: 440 mg of naproxen sodium twice daily.
- Significant Medical History: None.
- Resting Vital Signs: Heart rate = 66 beats/minute with regular rhythm; Blood pressure = 104/50 millimeters of mercury; Respiratory rate = 12 breaths/minute; Oxygen saturation = 99% on room air.

Table 16–8 Outcomes quality appraisal checklist for a patient with spastic diplegia.

Schindl MR, Forstner C, Kern H, Hess S. Treadmill training with partial body weight support in nonambulatory patients with cerebral palsy. *Arch Phys Med Rehabil.* 2000; 81(3):301–306.

Research Validity of the Study	
Was this a study with more than one group? Two groups of children—ambulatory and nonambulatory. Both groups participated in the same treadmill training protocol. The study did not include a comparison group with a different form of gait training.	X Yes ___ No
Were the groups comparable at the start of the study? Group A consisted of 6 nonambulatory children with spastic tetraplegia. Group B consisted of 4 ambulatory children, 3 of whom had spastic diplegia, and 1 of whom had spastic tetraplegia. The mean age of both groups was 11 years old.	___ Yes X No
If groups were not equal at the start of the study was risk adjustment performed?	___ Yes X No
Were variables operationally defined and adequately measured by the data used for the study?	X Yes ___ No
Was a standardized outcomes instrument used? The Functional Ambulation Categories and the standing and walking section of the Gross Motor Function Measurement. Both have previously established reliability and validity in studies examining the effects of treadmill training.	X Yes ___ No
Were standardized data collection methods implemented? One physiatrist and one physical therapist performed the outcomes data collection 4 times during the study: 6 and 3 weeks before the study and at the start and conclusion of the treadmill training. Both were blinded to the stage at which the patient was being measured. Inter-rater reliability was 0.90 for the Functional Ambulation Categories and 0.81 and 0.83 for the two components of the Gross Motor Function Measurement.	X Yes ___ No
Did the intervention precede the outcome?	X Yes ___ No
Were other potentially confounding variables accounted for in the analysis?	___ Yes X No
Were missing data dealt with in an appropriate manner? The authors do not report any missing data.	X Yes ___ No
Did investigators respeat the study with a new set of subjects?	___ Yes X No
Do you have enough confidence in the research validity of this paper to consider using this evidence with your patient/client? Primary limitation is the lack of adjustment for confounding factors.	___ Yes X Undecided ___ No

continues

Table 16–8 Outcomes quality appraisal checklist for a patient with spastic diplegia *(continued).*

What results do the authors report related to your clinical question?

Tests of Differences ____________

Effect Sizes

- The mean increase in Functional Ambulation Categories = 0.8 points.
- The mean increase in the standing portion of the General Motor Function Measurement = 5.0 points.
- The mean increase in the walking portion of the Gross Motor Function Measurement = 4.3 points.

Absolute Benefit Increases ____________

Relative Benefit Increases ____________

Absolute Risk Reductions ____________

Relative Risk Reductions ____________

Number Needed to Treat (Harm) ____________

Other

Subjects and their caregivers also reported subjective assessments of improvement in standing balance and walking ability in 8 of 10 cases.

How important are the results?

Obtained p-values for each statistic reported by the authors:

- The mean increase in Functional Ambulation Categories = p = 0.02
- The mean increase in the standing portion of the General Motor Function Measurement = p = 0.018
- The mean increase in the walking portion of the Gross Motor Function Measurement = p = 0. 007

Obtained confidence intervals for each statistic reported by the authors: Not reported

Do these findings exceed a minimal clinically important difference?

___ Yes
_X_ No

The authors do not indicate an MCID threshold. Qualitatively, subjects in this study increased their postural control, ability to transfer without upper extremity push off, and walking ability. Gains in these areas are consistent with this patient's goals.

Do the subjects in the study resemble your patient/client?

_X_ Yes
___ No

Can you perform this intervention safely and appropriately in your clinical setting, given your current knowledge, skill level, and your current resources?

_X_ Yes
___ No

Does the intervention fit within your patient/client's expressed values and preferences?

_X_ Yes
___ No

Do the outcomes fit within your patient/client's expressed values and preferences?

_X_ Yes
___ No

Do the potential benefits outweigh the potential risks of using this intervention with your patient/client?

_X_ Yes
___ No

There were no adverse effects reported for any of the subjects during the study. In addition, 8 of 10 subjects and their caregivers recommended the technique because of the improvements they noted as a result.

Will you use this intervention for this patient/client?

_X_ Yes
___ No

- Mental Status: He is alert and oriented to person, place, and time and answers questions appropriately.
- Pain (Verbal Pain Rating Scale): worst: 8/10 average: 5/10 today: 4/10
- Palpation: There is tenderness over the anterior aspect of the medial tibial condyle with mild, localized swelling in the same region. The tibiofemoral and patellofemoral joint lines are nontender. No crepitus with active or passive knee flexion and extension is noted.
- Strength: Manual muscle testing of hamstrings, hip adductors, and sartorius on the right reproduces pain in the region of the medial condyle. Strength is at least full range of motion against gravity, but his effort is limited by pain. His left lower extremity strength is normal.
- Flexibility: Indirect assessment of hamstring length in supine (passive knee extension with hip at 90°) reveals a popliteal angle of approximately 30° bilaterally with reproduction of pain symptoms on the right at end range.
- Gait: He ambulates independently with decreased stance time and decreased knee flexion during the swing phase on his right.
- Special Tests: No laxity noted with stress tests of the medical collateral, lateral collateral, anterior cruciate, and posterior cruciate ligaments.

The physical therapist concludes that her findings are consistent with acute inflammation of the pes anserinus bursa and associated tendinous attachments secondary to overuse. Limitation in hamstring extensibility may be implicated as well. The prognosis for recovery is excellent and the patient's goal of unrestricted return to competitive soccer without pain is realistic. As part of the overall treatment plan for this patient, low intensity therapeutic ultrasound is considered to facilitate resolution of the acute inflammatory process. The intended treatment area, however, is in the region of the proximal tibial epiphysis and since the patient is a 15-year-old male, the therapist assumes that this growth plate is open. Prior to proceeding with ultrasound treatment, she decides to review the evidence to answer the following clinical question:

> Is therapeutic ultrasound contraindicated in the region of an open epiphyseal plate in a 15-year-old male?

Table 16–9 details the results of a literature search using the National Library of Medicine's PubMed online database. Unfortunately, none of the articles were from human studies so the physical therapist looked for the animal studies that most closely mimicked application of therapeutic ultrasound as used clinically by physical therapists on human patients. A review of the abstracts for the articles listed in the table indicated that the first study did not describe the intensity of the ultrasound used, while the second study discussed

Table 16-9 Search results for a clinical question related to use of ultrasound over an open epiphyseal plate.

Search String	Results
"Ultrasound" AND "epiphyseal plates"	32 citations are returned, most of which address diagnostic ultrasound; 3 citations are noted for possible review.
"Ultrasound" AND "epiphyseal plates" NOT "diagnostic"	8 citations are returned, one of which is in Russian. 2 of the 3 articles identified in the first search appear again in this search.
"Therapeutic ultrasound" AND "epiphyseal plates"	3 citations are returned, 1 of which appeared in the results of the first search. One of the new citations also is noted for possible review.
"Therapeutic ultrasound" AND "bone growth"	31 citations are returned, most of which address bone healing after fracture, rather than the growth of immature bone. One additional citation is added to the list of articles for potential review.

Relevant Titles
El-Bialy T, El-Shamy I, Graber TM. Growth modification of the rabbit mandible using therapeutic ultrasound: Is it possible to enhance functional appliance results? *Angle Orthod*. 2003; 73(6):631–639.
Lyon R, Liu XC, Meier J. The effects of therapeutic vs. high-intensity ultrasound on the rabbit growth plate. *J Orthop Res*. 2003; 21(5):865–871.
Ogurtan Z, Celik I, Izci C, Boydak M, Alkan F, Yilmaz K. Effect of experimental therapeutic ultrasound on the distal antebrachial growth plates in one-month-old rabbits. *Vet J*. 2002; 164(3):280–287.
Zhang ZJ, Huckle J, Francomano CA, Spencer RG. The influence of pulsed low-intensity ultrasound on matrix production of chondrocytes at different stages of differentiation: An explant study. *Ultrasound Med Biol*. 2002; 28(11–12):1547–1553. Erratum in: *Ultrasound Med Biol*. 2003; 29(8):1223.
Cadossi R, Cane V. Pathways of transmission of ultrasound energy through the distal metaphysis of the second phalanx of pigs: An in vitro study. *Osteoporos Int*. 1996; 6(3):196–206.

the acoustic properties of ultrasound energy in bone rather than the tissue-level effects of the ultrasound energy. As a result, these articles were not reviewed further. Critiques of the remaining three articles are provided here.

Article #1

Lyon *et al.*[6] examined the effects of ultrasound treatment on the epiphyseal plates and metaphyseal regions of the knee in growing rabbits. The investigators used a contralateral control design and compared two different treatment intensities in separate groups of rabbits. The two treatment intensities (0.5 and 2.2. W/cm^2) and the frequency (1 Mhz) were representative of those commonly used by physical therapists. However, the authors did not report the duty cycle used, making it impossible to calculate the total dose of ultrasound energy delivered. Following six weeks of treatment, the authors observed significant histological changes in the epiphyseal plates of knees in the higher treatment intensity group relative to both the low intensity group and controls. Plate height was greater and chondrocytes were less organized. Radiographically, growth plate lines were less distinct and metaphyseal wedging deformities were noted in the high dose group. During the course of treatment, skin burns developed in the treatment region on all the high dose knees. No significant changes were noted relative to controls in any of the dependent variables for the lower dose group.

The therapist concluded that the 1 Mhz at 0.5 W/cm^2 used in the study was consistent with the dose she considered using with her patient. Nonetheless, she noted the following major differences between the study's parameters and those under consideration a) 20 minute daily treatments for six weeks versus 7–10 minute treatments three times a week for a few weeks at most; b) stationary sound head versus moving sound head; and, c) pulsed mode versus continuous mode. Initially, the therapist was encouraged by the results of this study because she was considering a "low dose" for her patient, but she realized that she really could not determine a safe dosage range from reading this paper. Since the investigators used an unspecified pulsed ultrasound duty cycle, all she could conclude was that at some finite net intensity between 50 mW/cm^2 and 0.25 W/cm^2 (assuming an available duty cycle range of 10–50 percent) no deleterious changes occurred.

Article #2

Like the previous article, Ogurtan *et al.*[7] examined the effects of ultrasound treatment on the epiphyseal plates and bone growth rates in growing rabbits. Rather than the knee, Orgurtan *et al.* examined the distal radius and ulna. They too used a contralateral control design and compared two different treatment intensities in separate groups of rabbits. Groups were subdivided into those treated for 10, 15, or 20 days. The two treatment intensities (0.2 and 0.5 W/cm^2) and the frequency (1 Mhz) were representative of those commonly used by physical therapists. Treatments were delivered in pulsed mode, using a 20 percent duty cycle for five minutes. The authors reported treatment dose as spatial average temporal average ("SATA"), meaning that the temporal peak intensity (what would have been displayed on the intensity meter of the unit) during treatment was either 1.0 W/cm^2 for the 0.2 W/cm^2 SATA group or 2.5 W/cm^2 for the 0.5 W/cm^2 SATA group. The 0.5 W/cm2 SATA dose would be the same net energy output as a five minute treatment in continuous mode at 0.5 W/cm^2, a dose comparable to what the therapist was considering for her patient.

In comparison to controls, the authors found no difference in height of the growth plates, bone growth rates, or bone morphology in the radius and ulna of rabbits treated with either intensity ultrasound at any time period. However, the physical therapist realized that the treatment doses reported were not consistent with the maximum output intensity available for the ultrasound unit in the study. She concluded that the authors were reporting temporal peak intensities which would result in SATAs that were 20 percent of those reported. This difference would mean that the authors examined the effects of ultrasound at either 40 mW/cm^2 or 0.1 W/cm^2, both much lower doses than the therapist was considering for use with her patient.

Article #3

Zhang *et al.*[8] examined the effects of very low intensity ultrasound delivered using a commercially available unit with fixed parameters designed specifically for fracture healing. The target tissue was chick embryo sternum in culture. The proximal portion of the chick embryo sternum undergoes endochondral ossification, analogous to the bone growth that occurs at epiphyseal plates in immature humans. The ultrasound frequency used in this study was 1.5 MHz provided during 20 minute daily treatments. The authors reported an anabolic effect on chondrocytes and increased matrix production relative to control specimens that were not sonicated, despite a dose/intensity that was lower than the lowest dose that can be delivered by ultrasound units typically used in physical therapy clinics (0.2 W/cm^2 at 20 percent duty cycle, equivalent to 40 mW/cm^2). The tissue type studied and the treatment parameters used were considerably different than the scenario with which the physical therapist was dealing. However, she was concerned about the possibility that such a low dose of ultrasound may in fact be capable of facilitating bone growth.

Therapist's Decision

In her search, the therapist found one study in which she was unable to discern the actual ultrasound dosages used, but that nonetheless demonstrated the potential for deleterious effects on the epiphyseal plate. A second study did not find any deleterious effects, but appears to have examined two ultrasound dosages below that which she was considering for her patient. The final study, using an *in vitro* model and intensity lower than that achievable on any of the units available to her, showed a potential anabolic effect on bone growth.

In the absence of controlled studies describing human clinical trials, she would have been able to make a reasonable judgment based on animal studies had they used (or completely described the use of) similar ultrasound treatment parameters. The evidence she located suggests that very low intensity ultrasound may enhance cellular activity at the epiphyseal plate which may, in turn, facilitate increased bone growth. At some higher, undefined threshold, ultrasound may damage the epiphyseal plate and hinder growth. There *may* be some point in between that is "safe," but she was not comfortable defining this dosage based on a single study in which the dosages appeared to be inconsistent with the ultrasound unit's performance. Accordingly, the therapist decides to exclude therapeutic ultrasound for her patient's treatment plan.

SUMMARY

The cases in this chapter are intended to serve as models upon which students and clinicians may develop their own evidence-based practice skills. Readers should note that the "best available" evidence did not always represent the highest levels of evidence indicated by various published evidence hierarchies. In spite of these challenges, conclusions were drawn based upon the therapist's clinical judgment in conjunction with the patient's preferences and values. Readers are reminded that these examples are not intended to serve as practice guidelines or standards of care for the conditions described.

REFERENCES

1. Collins TC, Suarez-Almazor M, Petersen NJ. An absent pulse is not sensitive for the early detection of peripheral arterial disease. *Fam Med.* 2006; 38(1):38–42.
2. Bloem BR, Grimbergen YA, Cramer M, Willemsen M, Zwinderman AH. Prospective assessment of falls in Parkinson's disease. *J Neurol.* 2001; 248(11): 950–958.
3. Green S, Buchbinder R, Hetrick S. Physiotherapy interventions for shoulder pain. *The Cochrane Database of Systematic Reviews.* 2003; (2):CD004258.
4. van der Windt DAWM, Koes BW, Deville W, Boeke AJP, de Jong BA *et al.* Effectiveness of corticosteroid injections versus physiotherapy for treatment of painful stiff shoulder in primary care: Randomized trial. *BMJ.* 1998; 317(7168):1292–1296.

5. Schindl MR, Forstner C, Kern H, Hess S. Treadmill training with partial body weight support in nonambulatory patients with cerebral palsy. *Arch Phys Med Rehabil.* 2000; 81(3):301–306.
6. Lyon R, Liu XC, Meier J. The effects of therapeutic vs. high-intensity ultrasound on the rabbit growth plate. *J Orthop Res.* 2003; 21(5):865–871.
7. Ogurtan Z, Celik I, Izci C, Boydak M, Alkan F, Yilmaz K. Effect of experimental therapeutic ultrasound on the distal antebrachial growth plates in one-month-old rabbits. *Vet J.* 2002; 164(3):280–287.
8. Zhang ZJ, Huckle J, Francomano CA, Spencer RG. The influence of pulsed low-intensity ultrasound on matrix production of chondrocytes at different stages of differentiation: An explant study. *Ultrasound Med Biol.* 2002; 28(11–12): 1547–1553. Erratum in: *Ultrasound Med Biol.* 2003; 29(8):1223.

Appendix A

Evidence Hierarchies

HIERARCHY OF EVIDENCE FOR ARTICLES ABOUT DIAGNOSTIC TESTS

Level	Diagnosis and Differential Diagnosis
1a	**Diagnosis** • Systematic Review of Level 1 diagnostic studies that *do not* have statistically significant variation in the direction or degrees of results • Clinical Decision Rule[a] with 1b studies from different clinical centers **Differential Diagnosis** • Systematic Review of prospective cohort studies[b] that *do not* have statistically significant variation in the direction or degrees of results
1b	**Diagnosis** • Validating* cohort study with reference standards that were independent of the test and were applied blindly and objectively; • Clinical Decision Rule tested within one clinical center **Differential Diagnosis** • Single prospective cohort study with follow-up of >80% of subjects over 16 months if acute and 1–5 years if chronic
1c	**Diagnosis** • Studies that determine that a diagnostic test is an absolute SpPin (specificity = 100%) or absolute SnNout (sensitivity=100%) **Differential Diagnosis** • Studies that are all or none[c] case series[d]
2a	**Diagnosis and Differential Diagnosis** • Systematic Review of level 2b or higher studies that *do not* have statistically significant variation in the direction or degrees of results
2b	**Diagnosis** • Exploratory** cohort study with reference standards that were independent of the test and were applied blindly and objectively; • Clinical Decision Rule after derivation, or validated only on split-sample or databases

Level	Diagnosis and Differential Diagnosis
	Differential Diagnosis • Retrospective cohort study • Prospective cohort study with follow-up of < 80% subjects and/or insufficient follow-up time frames
3a	**Diagnosis and Differential Diagnosis** • Systematic Review of 3b and better studies that *do not* have statistically significant variation in the direction or degrees of results
3b	**Diagnosis** • Nonconsecutive study; or without consistently applied reference standards **Differential Diagnosis** • Nonconsecutive cohort study • Very limited population
4	**Diagnosis** • Case-control study,[e] poor or nonindependent reference standard **Differential Diagnosis** • Case series • Studies in which reference standards were overruled
5	**Diagnosis and Differential Diagnosis** • Expert opinion without explicit critical appraisal, or based on physiology, bench research, or "first principles"[f]

[a]*Clinical Decision Rule*: An empirically derived algorithm used to make decisions about diagnostic tests, prognostic indicators, or interventions.

[b]*Cohort Study:* In intervention papers, a prospective research design used to evaluate the relationship between a treatment and an outcome; two groups of subjects—one of which receives the intervention and one of which does not—are monitored over time to determine who develops the outcome and who does not. This label could be applied to quasi-experimental and nonexperimental research designs in which two nonrandomized groups of subjects are evaluated.

[c]*All or None:* A study in which some or all patients died before treatment became available, now none die.

[d]*Case Series:* A description of the management of several patients/clients for the same purposes as a case report; the use of multiple individuals increases the potential importance of the observations as the basis for future research.

[e]*Case-Control Study:* A retrospective epidemiological research design used to evaluate the relationship between a potential risk factor and a disease or disorder; two groups of subjects—one of which has the disease/disorder (the *case*) and one which does not (the *control*)—are compared to determine which group has a greater proportion of individuals with the risk factor.

[f]*First Principles:* Biologically plausible rationales for management of pathophysiology.

*Validating Study—Examines quality of diagnostic test based on prior research

**Exploratory Study—Initial examination of quality of diagnostic test

Source: Adapted with permission from Oxford Center for Evidence-Based Medicine (www.cebm.net).

HIERARCHY OF EVIDENCE FOR ARTICLES ABOUT PROGNOSIS

Level	Prognosis
1a	• Systematic Review of inception cohort[a] studies that *do not* have statistically significant variation in the direction or degrees of results; • Clinical Decision Rule[b] validated in different populations
1b	• Individual inception cohort study with >80% subject follow-up; • Clinical Decision Rule validated in a single population
1c	• All or none[c] case-series study[d]
2a	• Systematic Review of either retrospective cohort studies[e] or untreated control groups in randomized clinical trials that *do not* have statistically significant variation in the direction or degrees of results
2b	• Retrospective cohort study or follow-up of untreated control patients in an randomized clinical trial; • Derivation of Clinical Decision Rule or validated on split-sample only
2c	• "Outcomes" Research[f]
3	• N/A
4	• Case-series study • Prognostic cohort study in which: ◦ sampling was biased in favor of target outcome; or, ◦ measurement was accomplished in <80% of subjects; or, ◦ outcomes were measured in nonblinded or nonobjective method; or, ◦ no correction for confounding factors.
5	• Expert opinion without explicit critical appraisal, or based on physiology, bench research, or "first principles"[g]

[a]*Inception Cohort:* A group of subjects that are followed over time starting early in the course of their disease or disorder.

[b]*Clinical Decision Rule*: Algorithms or scoring systems that lead to a prognostic estimation or a diagnostic category.

[c]*All or None:* A study in which some or all patients died before treatment became available, now none die.

[d]*Case Series:* A description of the management of several patients/clients for the same purposes as a case report; the use of multiple individuals increases the potential importance of the observations as the basis for future research.

[e]*Cohort Study*: A prospective epidemiological research design used to evaluate the relationship between a potential risk factor and a disease or disorder; two groups of subjects—one of which has the risk factor and one of which does not—are monitored over time to determine who develops the disease/disorder and who does not. This label could be applied to quasi-experimental and nonexperimental research designs in which two nonrandomized groups of subjects are evaluated.

[f]*Outcomes Research:* Nonexperimental research that evaluates outcomes of care in "real world" clinical conditions.

[g]*First Principles:* Biologically plausible rationales for management of pathophysiology.

Source: Adapted with permission from Oxford Center for Evidence-Based Medicine. www.cebm.net.

HIERARCHY OF EVIDENCE FOR ARTICLES ABOUT THERAPY

Level	Therapy/Prevention, Etiology/Harm
1a	• Systematic Review of randomized clinical trials that *do not* have statistically significant variation in the direction or degrees of results
1b	• Individual randomized clinical trial with narrow confidence interval
1c	• All or none study[a]
2a	• Systematic Review of cohort studies[b] that *do not* have statistically significant variation in the direction or degrees of results
2b	• Individual cohort study (including low quality randomized clinical trial; e.g., <80% subject follow-up)
2c	• "Outcomes" Research[c]
3a	• Systematic Review of case-control studies[d] that *do not* have statistically significant variation in the direction or degrees of results
3b	• Individual Case-Control Study
4	• Case-series study[e] • Cohort or case-control study that did not: ◦ define comparison groups adequately; or, ◦ did not measure exposures and outcomes objectively or in a blinded fashion; or, ◦ control for confounders; or, ◦ have sufficient follow-up (cohort studies only).
5	• Expert opinion without explicit critical appraisal, or based on physiology, bench research, or "first principles"[f]

[a]*All or none:* A study in which some or all patients died before treatment became available, now none die.

[b]*Cohort Study*: In intervention papers, a prospective research design used to evaluate the relationship between a treatment and an outcome; two groups of subjects—one of which receives the intervention and one of which does not—are monitored over time to determine who develops the outcome and who does not. This label could be applied to quasi-experimental and nonexperimental research designs in which two nonrandomized groups of subjects are evaluated.

[c]*Outcomes Research:* Nonexperimental research that evaluates clinical and health outcomes of care in "real world" clinical conditions.

[d]*Case-Control Study:* A retrospective epidemiological research design used to evaluate the relationship between a potential risk factor and a disease or disorder; two groups of subjects—one of which has the disease/disorder (the *case*) and one which does not (the *control*)—are compared to determine which group has a greater proportion of individuals with the risk factor.

[e]*Case Series:* A description of the management of several patients/clients for the same purposes as a case report; the use of multiple individuals increases the potential importance of the observations as the basis for future research.

[f]*First Principles:* Biologically plausible rationales for management of pathophysiology.

Source: Adapted with permission from Oxford Center for Evidence-Based Medicine (www.cebm.net).

Appendix B

Additional Evidence Appraisal Worksheets†

DIAGNOSTIC TEST—EVIDENCE APPRAISAL WORKSHEET

Citation:

Are the results of this diagnostic study valid?

Appraisal Criterion	Comments
Was there an independent, masked comparison between the diagnostic test of interest and a "gold (reference) standard" diagnostic test? • If not, describe what was done, the limitations of this approach, and the potential consequences for the study's results.	
Was the diagnostic test evaluated in subjects with the range of presentation (i.e., different levels or stages) of the condition? • If not, briefly describe the sample and discuss the potential consequence that this limited sample has for the study results.	

†Adapted with permission from the Oxford Center for Evidence-Based Medicine (www.cebm.net).

Appraisal Criterion	Comments
Did the investigators perform the "gold standard" diagnostic test on every subject regardless of the result from the diagnostic test of interest? • If not, describe what was done, as well as the limitations of this approach.	
Was the test (or cluster of tests) evaluated in a second, independent group of subjects? • If no, describe the limitations resulting from the lack of a comparison group.	

Are the valid results of this diagnostic study important?

Appraisal Criterion	Comments
What were the statistical findings of this study? • When appropriate, use the calculation forms below to determine these values.	• Tests of Association? P-values? Confidence Intervals? • Sensitivity? • Specificity? • Positive Predictive Value? • Negative Predictive Value? • Positive Likelihood Ratios? Confidence Intervals? • Negative Likelihood Ratio? Confidence Intervals?
What is the meaning (application) of these statistical findings for your patient/client case?	

Can you apply this valid, important evidence about a diagnostic test in caring for your patient/client?

Appraisal Criterion	Comments
Does the test sound appropriate for use (available, affordable, reliable, and valid) in your clinical setting?	
Are the study patients/clients similar to your own? • If not, how are they different? • Can you use this test in spite of these differences?	
Can you generate a clinically sensible estimate of your patient's/client's pretest probability of the disorder (from personal experience, prevalence statistics, practice databases, or primary studies)? • Is it possible that the disease probabilities have changed since the data you are using were gathered? If so, how will you adjust your pretest probability?	
Would the test and its results, including the posttest probabilities, help your patient/client? • If so, how? • If not, could the test and its results cause harm to the patient/client?	
Does the test fit within your patient's/client's stated values or expectations? • If not, what will you do now?	

Additional notes:

SAMPLE CALCULATIONS

From Holtby and Razmjou[20]		**Target Disorder (Biceps Pathology & SLAP Lesion)**		**Totals**
		Present	**Absent**	**Totals**
Diagnostic Test Result (Yergason's)	Positive (Pain in Bicipital Groove or GH Joint)	**a** 9	**b** 6	**a+b** 15
	Negative (No Pain in Bicipital Groove or GH Joint)	**c** 12	**d** 22	**c+d** 34
Totals		**a+c** 21	**b+d** 28	**a+b+c+d** 49

Sensitivity = a/(a+c) = 9/21 = 43%

Specificity = d/(b+d) = 22/28 = 79%

Likelihood Ratio for a Positive Test Result = LR+ = Sens/(1−Spec) = 43%/21% = 2.05

Likelihood Ratio for a Negative Test Result = LR− = (1−Sens)/Spec = 57%/79% = 0.72

Positive Predictive Value = a/(a+b) = 9/15 = 60%

Negative Predictive Value = d/(c+d) = 22/34 = 65%

Pretest Probability (prevalence) = (a+c)/(a+b+c+d) = 21/49 = 43%

Pretest Odds = Prevalence/(1−Prevalence) = 43%/57% = 0.75

Posttest Odds = Pretest Odds × LR = 0.75 × 2.05 = 1.54

Posttest Probability = Posttest Odds/(Posttest Odds +1) = 1.54/2.54 = 61%

Holtby R, Razmjou H. Accuracy of the Speed's and Yergason's tests in detecting biceps pathology and SLAP lesions: Comparison with arthroscopic findings. *Arthroscopy*. 2004; 20(3): 231–236.

YOUR CALCULATIONS

		Target Disorder		
		Present	**Absent**	**Totals**
Diagnostic Test Result	Positive	**a**	**b**	**a+b**
	Negative	**c**	**d**	**c+d**
Totals		**a+c**	**b+d**	**a+b+c+d**

PROGNOSIS—EVIDENCE APPRAISAL WORKSHEET

Citation:

Are the results of this prognosis study valid?

Appraisal Criterion	Comments
Was a defined, representative sample of subjects included in the study? • If not, what are the sample's limitations and what are the potential consequences for this study's results?	
Were the subjects assembled at a common (usually early) point in the course of their disorder? • If not, what are the implications of multiple starting points for this study's results?	
Was the subject follow-up time sufficiently long to answer the question(s) posed by the research? • If not, what are the potential consequences of the follow-up time for the study's results?	
Did all subjects originally enrolled complete the study? • If not, how many subjects were lost? • What, if anything, did the authors do about this attrition? • What are the implications of the attrition and the way it was handled with respect to the study's findings?	
Were objective outcome criteria applied to the subjects in a masked ("blind") fashion? • If not, what are the potential consequences for the study's results?	

Appraisal Criterion	Comments
If subgroups with different prognoses are identified, was there adjustment for important prognostic (risk) factors? • If not, what should the investigators have included? • What are the potential consequences of the absence of adjustment for this study results?	
Was there validation in an independent group ("test set") of patients? • If not, what are the potential consequences for this study's results?	

Are the valid results of this prognosis study important?

Appraisal Criterion	Comments
How likely are the outcomes over time?	
What do the results for the predictors or risk factors indicate (e.g., odds ratios, relative risk)?	
How precise are the prognostic estimates?	**CI (%)** *Use the table at the end of this worksheet to calculate confidence intervals if not provided

Can you apply this valid, important evidence about prognosis in caring for your patient?

Appraisal Criterion	Comments
Were the study subjects similar to your patient/client? • If not, what are the differences and how do they affect your use of the study?	
Will this evidence make a clinically important impact on your conclusions about what to offer or tell your patient/client? • If yes, how so? • If not, why not?	

Additional notes:

*If you want to calculate a confidence interval around the event rate for one group:

Clinical Measure	Standard Error (SE)	Typical Calculation of CI
Proportion (i.e., the rate of some prognostic event, etc.) where: n = the number of patients p = the proportion of these patients who experience the event	$\sqrt{\{p \times (1 - p)/n\}}$	If p = 24/60 = 0.4 (or 40%) and n=60 SE = $\sqrt{\{0.4 \times (1 - 0.4)/60\}}$ = 0.063 (or 6.3%) 95% CI is 40% +/− 1.96 × 6.3% or 27.6%–52.4%
n from your evidence: ______ p from your evidence: ______	$\sqrt{\{p \times (1 - p)/n\}}$	Your calculation: SE: ________ 95% CI:

INTERVENTION—EVIDENCE APPRAISAL WORKSHEET

Citation:

Are the results of this therapeutic trial valid?

Appraisal Criterion	Comments
Did the investigators randomly assign subjects to treatment groups? • If no, describe what was done. • What are the potential consequences of this assignment process for the study's results?	
Did the investigators know who was being assigned to which group prior to the allocation? • If yes, what are the potential consequences of this knowledge for the study's results?	
Were the groups similar at the start of the trial? • If not, what differences existed? • How might the differences between groups affect the results of this study?	
Did subjects know to which treatment group they were assigned? • If yes, what are the potential consequences of the subjects' knowledge for this study's results?	
Did investigators know to which treatment group subjects were assigned? • If yes, what are the potential consequences of the investigators' knowledge for this study's results?	

Were the groups managed equally, apart from the experimental treatment? • If not, what are the potential consequences of this difference in management for the study's results?	
Was the subject follow-up time sufficiently long to answer the question(s) posed by the research? • If not, what are the potential consequences of the follow-up time for the study's results?	
Did all subjects originally enrolled complete the study? • If not, how many subjects were lost? • What, if anything, did the authors do about this attrition? • What are the implications of the attrition and the way it was handled with respect to the study's findings?	
Were all patients analyzed in the groups to which they were randomized (i.e., was there an intention-to-treat analysis)? • If not, what did the authors do with the data from these subjects? • If the data were excluded, what are the potential consequences for this study's results?	

Are the valid results of this randomized trial important?

Appraisal Criterion	Comments
What were the statistical findings of this study? • When appropriate, use the calculation forms below to determine these values.	• Tests of Differences? P-values? Confidence Intervals? • Effect Sizes? P-values? Confidence Intervals? • Absolute and Relative Benefit Increases? P-values? Confidence Intervals?

Appraisal Criterion	Comments
	• Absolute and Relative Risk Reductions? P-values? Confidence Intervals? • Number Needed to Treat (Harm)? Confidence Intervals? • Other?
What is the meaning (application) of these statistical findings for your patient/client's case?	
Do these findings exceed a minimal clinically important difference? • If not, will you still use this evidence?	

Can you apply this valid, important evidence about an intervention in caring for your patient/client?

Appraisal Criterion	Comments
Does the intervention sound appropriate for use (available, affordable) in your clinical setting?	
Are the study subjects similar to your patient/client? • If not, how different? Can you use this intervention in spite of these differences?	
Do the potential benefits outweigh the potential risks of using this intervention with your patient/client?	
Does the intervention fit within your patient/client's stated values or expectations? • If not, what will you do now?	

Additional notes:

SAMPLE CALCULATIONS—BENEFIT INCREASE

	+ Outcome	− Outcome
+ Intervention	A 72	B 55
− Intervention	C 40	D 78

CER = Control Group Event Rate = c / (c + d) = 0.25 = 34%

EER = Experimental Group Event Rate = a / (a + b) = 0.57 = 57%

		Relative Benefit Increase (RBI)	**Absolute Benefit Increase (ABI)**	**Number Needed to Treat (NNT)**
EER	CER	$\frac{\text{EER} - \text{CER}}{\text{CER}}$	EER−CER	1/ABI
57%	34%	56%	23%	4
		***95% CI**	10.9-35.1%	3-9

***95% Confidence Interval (CI) on an NNT = 1/(Limits on the CI of its ABI) =**

$$\pm 1.96 \sqrt{\left[\frac{\text{CER} \times (1 - \text{CER})}{\text{\# Control Pts}}\right] + \left[\frac{\text{EER} \times (1 - \text{EER})}{\text{\# Exper Pts}}\right]} =$$

$$\pm 1.96 \sqrt{\left[\frac{0.34 \times 0.66}{118}\right] + \left[\frac{0.57 \times 0.43}{127}\right]} = \pm 12.1\%$$

SAMPLE CALCULATIONS—RISK REDUCTION

	+ Outcome	− Outcome
+ Intervention	A 10	B 50
− Intervention	C 26	D 34

CER = Control Group Event Rate = c / (c + d) = 0.43 = 43%

EER = Experimental Group Event Rate = a / (a + b) = 0.17 = 17%

		Relative Risk Reduction (RRR)	Absolute Risk Reduction (ARR)	Number Needed to Treat (NNT)
CER	EER	$\frac{CER - EER}{CER}$	CER − EER	1/ARR
43%	17%	60%	26%	4
		***95% CI**	10.3–41.7%	2–10

***95% Confidence Interval (CI) on an NNT =**
1/(Limits on the CI of its ARR) =

$$\pm 1.96 \sqrt{\left[\frac{CER \times (1 - CER)}{\#\text{ Control Pts}}\right] + \left[\frac{EER \times (1 - EER)}{\#\text{ Exper Pts}}\right]} =$$

$$\pm 1.96 \sqrt{\left[\frac{0.17 \times 0.83}{60}\right] + \left[\frac{0.43 \times 0.57}{60}\right]} = \pm 15.7\%$$

YOUR CALCULATIONS

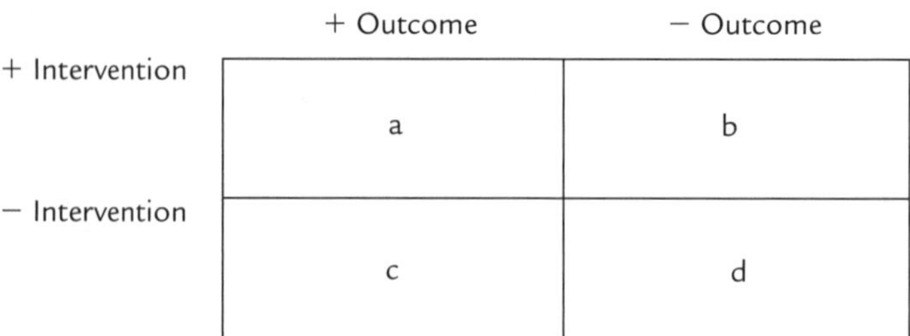

	+ Outcome	− Outcome
+ Intervention	a	b
− Intervention	c	d

CER = Control Group Event Rate = c / (c+d) =
EER = Experimental Group Event Rate = a / (a+b) =

		Relative Benefit Increase (RBI)	Absolute Benefit Increase (ABI)	Number Needed to Treat (NNT)
EER	CER	$\frac{EER - CER}{CER}$	EER−CER	1/ABI
		***95% CI**		

***95% Confidence Interval (CI) on an NNT =**
1/(Limits on the CI of its ABI) =

		Relative Risk Reduction (RRR)	Absolute Risk Reduction (ARR)	Number Needed to Treat (NNT)
CER	EER	$\frac{\text{CER} - \text{EER}}{\text{CER}}$	CER − EER	1/ARR
		*95% CI		

***95% Confidence Interval (CI) on an NNT =**
1/(Limits on the CI of its ABI) =

OUTCOMES—EVIDENCE APPRAISAL WORKSHEET

Citation:

Are the results of this outcomes measure study valid?

Appraisal Criterion	Comments
Was this a study with more than one group? • If not, describe the limitations resulting from the lack of a comparison group.	
Were the groups comparable at the start of the study? • If not, briefly describe the differences and discuss the potential consequences for this study's results.	
If groups were not equal at the start of the study, was risk adjustment performed? • If not, describe the potential consequences for this study's results.	
Were variables operationally defined and adequately measured by the data used for the study? • If not, describe what proxy measures were used and the implications of their use for this study's results.	
Was a standardized outcomes instrument used? • If not, describe how the outcomes were measured and the implications of this approach for the study's results.	

Appraisal Criterion	Comments
Were standardized data collection methods implemented? • If not, describe how data were collected and the implications of this approach for the study's results.	
Did the intervention precede the outcome? • If not, describe the potential consequences for this study's results.	
Were other potentially confounding variables accounted for in the analysis? • If not, describe the potential consequences for this study's results.	
Were missing data dealt with in an appropriate manner? • If not, describe the potential consequences for this study's results.	

Are the valid results of this outcomes study important?

Appraisal Criterion	Comments
What were the statistical findings of this study?	• Tests of Differences? P-values? Confidence Intervals? • Effect Sizes? P-values? Confidence Intervals? • Absolute and Relative Benefit Increases? P-values? Confidence Intervals? • Absolute and Relative Risk Reductions? P-values? Confidence Intervals? • Number Needed to Treat (Harm)? Confidence Intervals? • Other?

Appraisal Criterion	Comments
What is the meaning (application) of these statistical findings for your patient/client case?	

Can you apply this valid, important evidence about outcomes in caring for your patient/client?

Appraisal Criterion	Comments
Are the study subjects similar to your patient/client? • If not, how different? Can you use this intervention in spite of these differences?	
Do the potential benefits outweigh the potential risks of using this intervention to achieve the specified outcome with your patient/client?	
Do the interventions and related outcomes fit within your patient/client's stated values or expectations? • If not, what will you do now?	

Additional notes:

SYSTEMATIC REVIEW—EVIDENCE APPRAISAL WORKSHEET

Citation:

Are the results of this systematic review valid?

Appraisal Criterion	Comments
Is this a systematic review of randomized trials? • If not, what types of studies are included? • What are the potential consequences of including these studies for this review's results?	
Does the review include a methods section that describes identifying and selecting all relevant trials? • If not, what are the potential consequences for this review's results?	
Does the review include a methods section that describes the processes and tools used to assess the quality of individual studies? • If not, what are the potential consequences for this review's results?	
Was the quality of individual studies reported? • If not, what are the potential consequences for this review's results?	
Was publication bias addressed? • If not, what are the potential consequences for this review's results?	
If this is a meta-analysis, were the individual patient data used in the analysis (or aggregate data)? • If not, what are the implications of using aggregated data?	

Are the valid results of this systematic review important?

Appraisal Criterion	Comments
Were the results consistent from study to study (i.e., homogeneous)? • If not, what are the potential consequences for this review's results?	
If this paper is a meta-analysis, what are the statistical results (e.g., effect sizes, odds ratios, relative risks, likelihood ratios, numbers needed to treat) and associated confidence intervals?	
If this paper is not a meta-analysis, is there a substantive conclusion that can be drawn about the cumulative weight of the evidence (e.g., do the results all point in the same direction)?	

Can you apply this valid, important evidence from a systematic review in caring for your patient?

Appraisal Criterion	Comments
Is your patient different from those in the systematic review? • If yes, what are the important differences and what are their implications for your use of this study?	
Is the treatment feasible in your setting?	

Are your patient's values and preferences satisfied by the regimen and its consequences?

If subgroup analysis was performed, should you believe apparent qualitative differences in the effectiveness of the intervention in some subgroups of patients? Only if you can say 'yes' to all of the following:

Appraisal Criterion	Comments
Do the qualitative differences really make biologic and clinical sense? • If not, what are the potential consequences for this review's results?	
Is the qualitative difference both clinically (beneficial for some, but useless or harmful for others) and statistically significant? • If not, what are the potential consequences for this review's results?	
Was this difference hypothesized before the study began (rather than the product of dredging the data), and has it been confirmed in other independent studies? • If not, what are the potential consequences for this review's results?	
Was this one of just a few subgroup analyses carried out in this study? • If not, what are the potential consequences for this review's results?	

Additional notes:

Alternative ways to evaluate the importance of statistical results from meta-analyses or individual papers using odds ratios.

Translating odds ratios to numbers needed to treat (NNTs):

The numbers in the body of the tables are the NNTs for the corresponding odds ratio at that particular patient's expected event rate (PEER).

1. ***When the odds ratio (OR) < 1***
   This table applies when a bad outcome is prevented by therapy.

		OR < 1				
		0.9	**0.8**	**0.7**	**0.6**	**0.5**
Patient's Expected Event Rate (PEER)	**0.05**	2.09[a]	104	69	52	41[b]
	0.10	110	54	36	27	21
	0.20	61	30	20	14	11
	0.30	46	22	14	10	8
	0.40	40	19	12	9	7
	0.50	38	18	11	8	6
	0.70	44	20	13	9	6
	0.90	101[c]	46	27	18	12[d]

[a]The Relative Risk Reduction (RRR) here is 10%.

[b]The RRR here is 49%.

[c]The RRR here is 1%.

[d]The RRR here is 9%.

2. ***When the odds ratio (OR) > 1***
   This table applies both when a good outcome is increased by therapy and when a side effect is caused by therapy.

		OR > 1				
		1.1	**1.2**	**1.3**	**1.4**	**1.5**
Patient's Expected Event Rate (PEER)	**0.05**	212	106	71	54	43
	0.10	112	57	38	29	23
	0.20	64	33	22	17	14
	0.30	49	25	17	13	11
	0.40	43	23	16	12	10
	0.50	42	22	15	12	10
	0.70	51	27	19	15	13
	0.90	121	66	47	38	32

What are the potential benefits and harms to your patient from the therapy?

Method I: In the OR tables above, find the intersection of the closest odds ratio from the systematic review and your patient's expected event rate (PEER).	

What are the potential benefits and harms to your patient from the therapy?

Method II: To calculate the NNT from any RR or OR and any PEER:

For RR < 1:

$$NNT = 1/(1 - RR) \times PEER$$

For RR > 1:

$$NNT = 1/(RR - 1) \times PEER$$

For OR < 1:

$$NNT = \frac{1 - [PEER \times (1 - OR)]}{(1 - PEER) \times (PEER) \times (1 - OR)}$$

For OR > 1:

$$NNT = \frac{1 + [PEER \times (OR - 1)]}{(1 - PEER) \times (PEER) \times (OR - 1)}$$

Appendix C

Calculation of Confidence Intervals

Standard errors (SEs) and confidence intervals (CIs) for some clinical measures of interest

Clinical Measure	Standard Error (SE)	Typical Calculation of SE and CI[a]
I. THERAPEUTIC STUDIES		
(a) Outcome is an event—one group		
In general, r events are observed among n patients, so the observed proportion is $p = r/n$. In the illustrative example, $p = 24/60 = 0.4$ (or 40%).		
Proportion (event rate in one group)[b]	$SE = \sqrt{\frac{p \times (1 - p)}{n}}$ where p is proportion and n is number of patients	If $p = 24/60 = 0.4$ (or 40%): $SE = \sqrt{\frac{0.4 \times 0.6}{60}} = 0.063$ (or 6.3%) 95% CI is 40% ± 1.96 × 6.3% or 27.6 to 52.4%[b]
(b) Outcome is an event—comparison of two groups[c]		
In general, r_1 and r_2 events are observed among n_1 and n_2 patients in two groups, so the observed proportions are $p_1 = r_1/n_1$ and $p_2 = r_2/n_2$. In the illustrative example, $p_1 = 15/125$ (or 12%) and $p_2 = 30/120 = 0.25$ (or 25%).[d]		
Absolute risk reduction (ARR)	$SE = \sqrt{\frac{p_1(1 - p_1)}{n_1} + \frac{p_2(1 - p_2)}{n_2}}$	$ARR = p_2 - p_1 = 0.13$ (or 13%): $SE = \sqrt{\frac{0.12 \times 0.88}{125} + \frac{0.25 \times 0.75}{120}} = 0.049$ (or 4.9%) 95% CI is 13% ± 1.96 × 4.9%, i.e., 3.4% to 22.6%[b]
Number needed to treat (NNT)	Not calculated	NNT = 100/ARR = 100/13 = 7.7; CI is obtained as reciprocal of CI for ARR, so 95% CI is 100/22.6 to 100/3.4 or 4.4 to 29.4[e]

Relative risk (RR)	$RR = p_1/p_2$ $\text{SE of } \log_e RR = \sqrt{\frac{1}{r_1} + \frac{1}{r_2} - \frac{1}{n_1} - \frac{1}{n_2}}$	$RR = 0.12/0.25 = 0.48$ (48%); $\log(RR) = -0.734$; $\text{SE of } \log_e RR = \sqrt{\frac{1}{15} + \frac{1}{30} - \frac{1}{125} - \frac{1}{120}} = 0.289$; 95% CI for $\log_e RR$ is $-0.734 \pm 1.96 \times 0.289$, i.e., -1.301 to -0.167; 95% CI for RR is 0.272 to 0.846 or 27.2% to 84.6%
Relative risk reduction (RRR)	Not calculated	$RRR = 1 - RR = 1 - p_1/p_2 = 1 - 12/25 = 0.52$ (or 52%) 95% CI for RRR is obtained by subtracting CI for RR from 1 (or 100%), i.e., 0.154 to 0.728 or 15.4% to 72.8%
Odds ratio (OR)	$OR = \frac{r_1(n_2 - r_2)}{r_2(n_1 - r_1)}$ $\text{SE of } \log_e OR = \sqrt{\frac{1}{r_1} + \frac{1}{r_2} + \frac{1}{n_1 - r_1} + \frac{1}{n_2 - r_2}}$	$OR = \frac{15 \times 90}{30 \times 110} = 0.409$; $\log_e OR = -0.894$ $\text{SE of } \log_e OR = \sqrt{\frac{1}{15} + \frac{1}{30} + \frac{1}{90} + \frac{1}{110}} = 0.347$ 95% CI for $\log_e OR$ is $-0.894 \pm 1.96 \times 0.347$, or -1.573 to -0.214; 95% CI for OR is 0.207 to 0.807
(c) Outcome is a measurement		
Mean	If s is standard deviation (SD) of n observations, $SE = s/n$	95% CI is mean $\pm t \times SE$[f] If mean = 17.2, s = 6.4, n = 38, then SE = 6.4/38 = 1.038 and 95% CI is $17.2 \pm 2.026 \times 1.038$ or 15.1 to 19.3
Difference between two means	If s_1 and s_2 are SDs of n_1 and n_2 observations, SE(diff)=	95% CI is mean difference $\pm t \times$ SE(difference)[f] If $mean_1 = 17.2$, $s_1 = 6.4$, $n_1 = 38$, $mean_2 = 15.9$, $s_2 = 5.6$, $n_2 = 45$, then mean difference = d = 17.2 − 15.9 = 1.3, t = 1.99[f]

continues

Standard errors (SEs) and confidence intervals (CIs) for some clinical measures of interest *(continued)*

Clinical Measure	Standard Error (SE)	Typical Calculation of SE and CI[a]
	$\sqrt{\frac{(n_1-1)s_1^2+(n_2-1)s_2^2}{n_1+n_2-2} \times \left(\frac{1}{n_1}+\frac{1}{n_2}\right)}$	$SE(diff) = \sqrt{\frac{37 \times 6.4^2 + 44 \times 5.6^2}{38+45-2} \times \left(\frac{1}{38}+\frac{1}{45}\right)} = 1.317$ and 95% CI is $1.3 \pm 1.99 \times 1.317$ or -1.32 to 3.92
II. DIAGNOSTIC STUDIES		
(a) A single proportion		
In general, r diagnoses are observed among n patients, so the observed proportion is $p = r/n$. Using the notation of Chapter 3, the sensitivity is $a/(a + c)$, the specificity is $b/(b + d)$, the positive predictive value is $a/(a + b)$, and the negative predictive value is $d/(c + d)$.		
The illustrative example is from Table 3.3. The sensitivity is 731/809 = 90% or 0.90, and the specificity is 1500/1770 = 85% or 0.85, p = 73/82 = 0.89 (or 89%).		
Sensitivity, specificity, predictive values	$SE = \sqrt{\frac{p \times (1-p)}{n}}$ where p is proportion and n is number of patients	For the sensitivity, $p = 731/809 = 0.90$ (or 90%): $SE = \sqrt{\frac{0.90 \times 0.10}{809}} = 0.0105$ (or 1.05%) 95% CI is $90\% \pm 1.96 \times 1.05\%$ or 87.9% to 92.1%[b]
(b) Likelihood ratio		
In general, the likelihood ratios for positive or negative test results are, respectively, obtained as either LR+ = sensitivity/(1 − specificity) and LR− = (1 − sensitivity)/specificity.		
Likelihood ratio (LR)	$LR+ = [a/(a+c)]/[b/(b+d)]$ $LR- = [c/(a+c)]/[d/(b+d)]$ $SE\ of\ \log_e LR+ = \sqrt{\frac{1}{a}+\frac{1}{b}-\frac{1}{(a+c)}-\frac{1}{(b+d)}}$	$LR+ = (731/809)/(270/1770) = 0.9/(1-0.85) = 6.0$; $\log_e(LR+) = 1.792$; $SE\ of\ \log_e LR+ = \sqrt{\frac{1}{731}+\frac{1}{270}-\frac{1}{809}+\frac{1}{1770}} = 0.0572$;

$\text{SE of } \log_e \text{LR}- = \sqrt{\frac{1}{c} + \frac{1}{d} - \frac{1}{(a+c)} - \frac{1}{(b+d)}}$	95% CI for $\log_e$LR+ is 1.792 ± 1.96 × 0.0572, i.e., 1.680 to 1.904; 95% CI for LR+ is 5.37 to 6.71. A similar approach is used to derive a CI for LR−.

[a]In general a confidence interval is obtained by taking the estimate of interest and adding and subtracting a multiple of the SE. Except in the case of means or differences in means, the multiple is taken as a value from the standard normal distribution. For a 95% CI the multiplier is 1.96; for a 90% CI it is 1.645, and for a 99% CI it is 2.576. For proportions, this method is the traditional method referred to in footnote b. In some cases, such as for RR (and RRR) and OR, the CI is obtained for the logarithm of the quantity of interest and the values are antilogged (logs to base e are used in the table).
[b]The method illustrated is the traditional method. It works fine in most cases but is not recommended when sample sizes are small and/or proportions are near either 0% or 100% (in which case it is possible for the CI to include impossible values outside the range 0% to 100%). Newer methods are recommended both for general use and especially for the circumstances described. The methods are too complex to include here; they are described in reference 8 and incorporated into the software included with it.
[c]As used in this book, p_1 corresponds to the event rate in the experimental group (EER), and p_2 to the event rate in the control group (CER).
[d]The above calculations assume that comparisons are between two independent groups. For CIs derived from paired data (e.g., from crossover trials or matched case-control studies), and also CIs for some other statistics, see reference 8.
[e]When the ARR is not significantly different from zero, one limit of the 95% CI is negative. Taking reciprocals gives a CI for the NNT with one negative value, which corresponds to a harmful effect. We can write the CI in terms of both the NNT and NNH. For example, a 95% CI for the ARR of −5% to 25% gives the 95% CI for the NNT of 10 as −20 to 4, or from NNH = 20 to NNT = 4. However, the values included in this interval are NNH from 20 to ∞ (infinity) and NNT from 4 to ∞. We can write this as NNH = 20 to ∞ to NNT = 4 (see references 8 and 9).
[f]The calculation of a CI for a mean or the difference between means the multiplier for a 95% CI is not 1.96 but a value from the t distribution with $n - 1$ or $n_1 + n_2 - 2$ degrees of freedom (df), respectively. The appropriate value of t is found from statistical tables or software. As df increases, t approaches 1.96. For df larger than 40, t is close to 2.

Source: Reprinted from Straus SE, Richardson WS, Glaziou P, Haynes RB. Evidence-Based Medicine: How to Practice and Teach EBM. 3d edition, pages 267–272. Copyright (2005), with permission from Elsevier.

Index

Note: Italicized page locators indicate a figure; tables are noted with a *t*.

B

C

D

F

G

I

P

S

Y

Z